PHLEBOTOMY HANDBOOK

Seventh Edition

Blood Collection Essentials

Diana Garza, EdD, MT(ASCP)
Retired Professor—Health Sciences
Educational Consultant
Medical Writer/Editor
Houston, Texas

Kathleen Becan-McBride, EdD, MT(ASCP)
Director, Community and Educational Outreach
Coordinator, Texas-Mexico Border Health Services
Medical School Professor in the Department of Family & Community Medicine
The University of Texas Health Science Center at Houston
Texas Medical Center, Houston, Texas
Assistant Director for Academic Partnerships, Greater Houston AHEC

Contributing Author
Marilyn Wolfe-Kirk, RN, CIC
Infection Control/Employee Health Coordinator
Shriner's Hospital for Children
Texas Medical Center, Houston, Texas

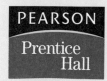

PEARSON

Prentice Hall

Upper Saddle River, New Jersey 07458

Library of Congress Cataloging-in-Publication Data

Garza, Diana.
  Phlebotomy handbook : blood collection essentials / Diana Garza, Kathleen Becan-McBride.—7th ed.
    p. ; cm.
  Includes bibliographical references and index.
  ISBN 0-13-113334-9
  1. Phlebotomy–Handbooks, manuals, etc.
  [DNLM: 1. Phlebotomy–Handbooks. QY 39 G245p 2005] I. Becan-McBride, Kathleen, (Date) II. Title.

  RB45.15.G37 2005
  616.07'561–dc22
                                    2004009835

Notice: The author[s] and the publisher of this volume have taken care that the information and technical recommendations contained herein are based on research and expert consultation, and are accurate and compatible with the standards generally accepted at the time of publication. Nevertheless, as new information becomes available, changes in clinical and technical practices become necessary. The reader is advised to carefully consult manufacturers' instructions and information material for all supplies and equipment before use, and to consult with a healthcare professional as necessary. This advice is especially important when using new supplies or equipment for clinical purposes. The author[s] and publisher disclaim all responsibility for any liability, loss, injury, or damage incurred as a consequence, directly or indirectly, of the use and application of any of the contents of this volume.

Publisher: Julie Levin Alexander
Publisher's Assistant: Regina Bruno
Senior Acquisitions Editor: Mark Cohen
Associate Editor: Melissa Kerian
Editorial Assistant: Jaquay Felix
Director of Production and Manufacturing: Bruce Johnson
Managing Editor for Production: Patrick Walsh
Production Liaison: Cathy O'Connell
Production Editor: Jessica Balch/Pine Tree Composition
Manufacturing Manager: Ilene Sanford
Manufacturing Buyer: Pat Brown
Creative Director: Cheryl Asherman

Senior Design Coordinator: Christopher Weigand
Cover Designer: Kevin Kall
Director of Marketing/Marketing Manager: Karen Allman
Channel Marketing Manager: Rachele Strober
Marketing Coordinator: Janet Ryerson
Media Editor: John Jordan
Media Production Manager: Amy Peltier
Media Project Manager: Stephen Hartner
Photographer: Rocky Kneten Photography
Photography Consultant: Michal Heron
Composition: Pine Tree Composition, Inc.
Printer/Binder: R.R. Donnelley & Sons, IN
Cover Printer: Phoenix Color Corp.

Pearson Education Ltd.
Pearson Education Australia Pty. Limited
Pearson Education Singapore, Pte. Ltd.
Pearson Education North Asia Ltd.
Pearson Education Canada, Ltd.

Pearson Educación de Mexico, S.A. de C.V.
Pearson Education—Japan
Pearson Education Malaysia, Pte. Ltd.
Pearson Education, Upper Saddle River, New Jersey

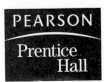

10 9 8 7 6 5 4 3
ISBN 0-13-113334-9

To my husband, Peter McLaughlin; my children, Lauren, Kaitlin, and Kevin; and my parents for their affection, patience, and constant support.

Diana Garza

To my husband, Mark; my sons, Patrick and Jonathan; my grandson, Finnaveir; my parents; my sister; and my parents-in-law for their support and devotion.

Kathleen Becan-McBride

BRIEF CONTENTS

CONTENTS

Chapter 16   **Forensic Toxicology, Workplace Testing, Sports Medicine, and Related Areas   431**

Preface

Phlebotomy Handbook: Blood Collection Essentials, seventh edition, is designed for health care students and practitioners who are responsible for blood and specimen collections (i.e., nurses, phlebotomists, clinical laboratory technicians and technologists, respiratory therapists, and others). The primary goal of the book is to link the phlebotomist (blood collector) to the latest information, techniques, skills, and equipment for the provision of safe and effective collection procedures, for the improvement of diagnostic and therapeutic laboratory testing, for enhancement of customer satisfaction, and ultimately, for the promotion of better health outcomes. This textbook is the most comprehensive compilation of information about phlebotomy available. It provides a wide range of competencies, including communication, clinical, technical, and safety skills that any health care worker will use in the practice of phlebotomy and other specimen collection procedures. In addition, the book provides a background of general knowledge and insights to support the technical skills.

The book highlights the professional role that phlebotomists play as essential members of the health care team. The role of the blood collector has expanded to encompass additional patient care duties and clinical responsibilities, a more patient-sensitive role, and improved interpersonal communication skills to deal effectively with patients, their families, and health care teams.

The order in which the material is presented generally follows the way in which a phlebotomist approaches the patient (i.e., beginning with important communication skills, knowledge of ethical behavior and legal implications, and a basic understanding of physiologic aspects, and moving to safety and infection control considerations in preparation for the phlebotomy procedure, preparation of supplies and equipment, actual venipuncture or skin puncture, and potential complications). Specialized specimen collection procedures, along with focused sections on pediatric care and considerations for the elderly are included. Problem-solving cases integrate the information into real-life situations. And the glossary and appendices provide useful procedures and important terms, phrases, and symbols.

The content is divided into four major parts:

PART I: Overview provides a knowledge base of the roles and functions of a phlebotomist in the health care industry and the basics of anatomy and physiology with an emphasis on the circulatory system.

PART II: Safety Procedures and Equipment provides information about safety and infection control in the workplace and the documentation and transportation procedures needed for safe handling of biohazardous specimens, and comprehensive coverage on the latest equipment and supplies available to phlebotomists.

PART III: Phlebotomy Procedures provides the most updated information and comprehensive description of the actual techniques used in phlebotomy, and reviews clinical and technical complications that may occur during the procedure.

PART IV: Special Procedures and Point-of-Care Testing provides information about pediatric phlebotomy procedures, arterial and IV collections, and special considerations for the elderly, homebound, and long-term care patients.

KEY FEATURES OF THE 7TH EDITION

- Colorful photographs show procedural steps and equipment.
- New case studies encourage problem solving and troubleshooting.
- Equipment chapter is the most comprehensive ever with emphasis on the most recent safety features of phlebotomy supplies and equipment.
- The glossary terms have been updated.
- Latest information about health-related infections and the standards related to the Needlestick Prevention Act and the Joint Commission on Accreditation of Healthcare Organization's 2004 National Patient Safety Goals.
- Expanded discussion addresses age-related competencies and transcultural communication.
- Self-assessment exercises have been added. Exercises for improving communication skills are included to "get the feel" of being a patient and being an effective part of a health care team.
- The "Clinical Alerts," a feature that our readers think highly of, have been expanded. Clinical alert symbols indicate procedures or concepts that have vitally important clinical consequences for the patient. The clinical alert indicates that "extra caution" should be taken by the health care worker to comply with the procedure, thereby avoiding adverse outcomes for the patient.
- Procedural information is presented in comprehensive descriptions, using an "on the job" perspective.
- Key terms, objectives, and study questions are provided for each chapter.
- A color chart of types of blood collection tubes relates appropriate color codings with additives.
- Appendices have been expanded and contain essential elements for finding a job, hand-hygiene recommendations, basic procedures for taking vital signs, Spanish phrases, units of measurement and symbols, laboratory tests and blood requirements, blood donations, military time, and formulas and calculations used in laboratories.

COMPANION CD-ROM

A companion CD was newly developed to integrate knowledge in a multisensory manner. It is organized to correlate with the textbook chapters and is a valuable tool for students and instructors. Features of this exciting new ancillary include interactive quizzes and games, animations, and videos.

ANCILLARY RESOURCES

Phlebotomy Handbook: Blood Collection Essentials, 7th edition, has companion resources that are cross-referenced to the text. The Instructor's Resource Guide contains a wealth of material to help faculty plan and manage their course. It includes a detailed lecture outline, a complete test bank, teaching tips and more for each chapter. Packaged with the Instructor's Resource Manual is the Instructor's Resource CD-ROM. The CD-ROM includes the complete test bank as well as PowerPoint lectures which contain discussion points with embedded color images from the book as well as animations and videos. In addition, Prentice Hall's *Q&A Review for Phlebotomy,* 5th edition, is an aid to students and health care workers preparing for a certification examination. It also has an accompanying CD-ROM with a simulated board examination consisting of 100 multiple-choice questions and referenced explanatory answers. Students can practice taking the simulated examination in print or via computer. A diagnostic report identifies those topics that need further review and study and provides the score for each content area.

In summary, the authors have created a book that health care professionals and students will use as a central authority on blood collection practices. Instructors can also use this as the central text for teaching specimen collection skills.

Acknowledgments

We are grateful to many generous people, product suppliers, manufacturing companies, professional organizations, and health care organizations for their assistance in preparing the previous editions of this text. The first edition was conceptualized in the early 1980s, when phlebotomy was learned in an apprentice-type situation and teaching materials were scarce. As licensing, credentialing, manufacturing of new products, procedures, competencies, hazards, and safety measures expanded, so did our text. Each version used previous versions as a framework for updating, redesigning, and improving the next. We thank many phlebotomists, medical technicians and technologists, artists, photographers, and educators who have given us countless editorial tips and practical advice over the years. We thank health care workers around our country and the world who have taken the time to read about new and better ways of improving the practice of phlebotomy.

We are particularly indebted to BD Vacutainer Systems, Greiner Bio-One, the American Society of Clinical Pathology, The University of Texas M.D. Anderson Cancer Center, Memorial Hermann Health Care System, The University of Texas Houston Health Science Center for their support throughout many stages of our previous and current editions. We thank Marilyn Wolfe, RN for her expertise in pediatrics, Barbara Davis, MT (ASCP), Carol Singer MT(ASCP), MBA for sharing procedural information, Estella Woodard, MT (ASCP), and Benjamin Lichtiger, MD, for their clinical expertise and in coordination of the on-site photography. We also thank J. Alexander Manos, Yvette M. Bobb, Tammie Brown, Kellan Caldwell, Jason Pigott, Troy Fields, and especially Willie Singleton (the Diva of Phlebotomy) and Peter McLaughlin, MD, for their positive encouragement and modeling for photography. Thanks go to Rocky Kneten, the photographer, and Michal Heron for her input on the photography.

We greatly appreciate our working relationships with editors and copy editors, past and present, who have encouraged us and improved our writing through seven editions. Special thanks go to Jane Licht, Cheryl Mehalik, Lin Marshall, Melissa Kerian, and Mark Cohen.

Last, and most important, we are thankful to our families who have proudly grown up with this text as part of their lives. They have continued to encourage us and supportively tolerated the thousands of hours over many years that we have spent writing the previous and current editions of this textbook. They will always hold a special place in our hearts.

Diana Garza
Kathleen Becan-McBride

Reviewers

Lana J. Anderson, RN, MA, Ed.
Assistant Professor
HHS Coordinator
Ivy Tech State College
Indianapolis, Indiana

Patricia DeiTos, RN, MSN
Program Developer
Continuing Education and Workforce Development
for Health Care Programs
Northern Virginia Community College
Annandale, Virginia

Evelyn Glass, MS, MT(ASCP)
Program Coordinator
Medical Laboratory Technology
Navarro College
Corsicana, Texas

Ernest Dale Hall, MAEd, MT(ASCP)
Clinical Coordinator
Medical Laboratory Technology/Phlebotomy
Southwestern Community College
Sylva, North Carolina

Lynnette Hobbs, MS, MT(ASCP)
Director/Chairperson
Phlebotomy Program
Tyler Junior College
Tyler, Texas

Jeanne R. Phelps, MEd., MT(ASCP), CLS(NCA), SM(ASCP)
Instructor
Medical Laboratory Technology and Phlebotomy
Wake Technical Community College
Raleigh, North Carolina

Harry Wandell, M.Ed, MT(ASCP)
Assistant Professor
Medical Laboratory Technician Department
Broome Community College
Binghamton, New York

PROCEDURES

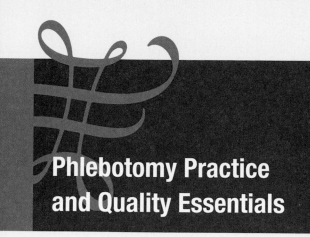

Phlebotomy Practice and Quality Essentials

CHAPTER OBJECTIVES

Upon completion of Chapter 1, the learner is responsible for the following:

1. Define phlebotomy and identify health professionals who perform phlebotomy procedures.
2. Identify the importance of phlebotomy procedures to the overall care of the patient.
3. List professional competencies for phlebotomists and key elements of an employer's performance assessment.
4. List skills for active listening and effective verbal communication.
5. List examples of positive and negative body language.
6. Describe health care settings where phlebotomy services are routinely performed.
7. Give examples of how a phlebotomist can participate in quality improvement activities.

 MediaLINK

Access the accompanying CD-ROM to explore a wide variety of review questions and interactive activities for this chapter, including multiple choice, true/false, and video exercises.

■■■■■ PHLEBOTOMY PRACTICE, DEFINITION, AND DUTIES

The development of modern diagnostic techniques, clinical laboratory automation, computer technology, and changes in the delivery of health care services have increased the variety and number of laboratory testing options available for clinical decisions. As a result, various health care workers (e.g., phlebotomists, laboratorians, nurses, respiratory therapists, medical assistants, and others) are taking greater roles in phlebotomy and other specimen collection processes. Regardless of specific job backgrounds, however, there are common elements about the practice of phlebotomy that should be known by all who perform or are responsible for blood collections. The term *phlebotomy* is derived from the Greek words, *phlebo,* which relates to veins, and *tomy,* which relates to cutting. Therefore the definition can be summarized as the incision of a vein for blood letting (i.e., blood collection). Synonomous words are venesection or venisection.

The **phlebotomist**, or blood collector, is the individual who performs phlebotomy. The term phlebotomist will be used throughout this book even though it is interchangeable with blood collector. Phlebotomists often assist in the collection and transportation of specimens other than venous blood (e.g., arterial blood, urine, tissues, sputum) and may perform clinical, technical, or clerical functions. However, the primary function of the phlebotomist is to assist the health care team in the accurate, safe, and reliable collection and transportation of specimens for clinical laboratory analyses.

Laboratory analyses of a variety of specimens are used for *three* important clinical purposes:

Diagnostic testing—to figure out what is wrong with the patient, e.g., tests that detect abnormalities.

Therapeutic assessments—to develop the appropriate therapy or treatment of the medical condition, e.g., tests that predict the most effective treatment or the drug of choice.

Monitoring—to make sure the therapy or treatment is working to alleviate the disease or illness, e.g., tests to confirm that the abnormality has returned to normal or that the drug is reaching its effective dosage.

Thus the requirement for a high quality specimen that is correctly identified, collected, and transported is vital to the overall care of a patient. Phlebotomists' duties vary in scope and range, depending on the setting. They may have duties related to all phases of laboratory analysis or may be assigned to only specimen collection duties in one area of a hospital. Technology has enabled laboratory testing to be performed closer to the point of care (e.g., at the patients' bedside, at ancillary or mobile sites, or even in the home). Phlebotomists' duties have become more coordinated with other health care processes. In some cases, health professionals, such as nurses, respiratory therapists, patient care technicians, and others, have been cross-trained to assume phlebotomy duties; in other cases, traditional laboratory-based phlebotomists have been cross-trained to assume expanded clerical or patient care duties such as electrocardiograms and low-risk laboratory procedures. Whatever the case, the workplace settings and roles and responsibilities of the phlebotomist will continue to evolve and change.

Box 1–1	Job Sites for Phlebotomists
HOSPITAL (INPATIENT) SETTINGS	**AMBULATORY (OUTPATIENT) SETTINGS**
Acute-care hospitals	Health department clinics
Specialty hospitals (cancer centers, psychiatric, long-term care, pediatric)	Community health centers (CHCs)
Urban or rural hospitals	Rural health clinics
Hospital-based clinics	Community-based mental health centers
Hospital-based emergency centers	School-based clinics
	Prison health clinics
	Dialysis centers
	Multiphasic screening centers
	Home health agencies
	Home hospice agencies
	Durable medical equipment suppliers
	Health maintenance organizations (HMOs)
	Insurance companies
	Physician group practices
	Individual or solo medical practices
	Specialty practices
	Rehabilitation centers
	Mobile vans for blood donations
	Mobile vans for primary care delivery
	Mobile mammography units
	Free-standing surgical centers

HEALTH CARE ORGANIZATIONS

Health care organizations in the United States vary widely but most fit into two categories: inpatient or hospital care, and outpatient or ambulatory care. Traditional hospitals are organized into departments according to medical/surgical specialties and/or around organs systems as shown in Table 1–1. Sometimes, departments are organized by therapy services or procedures offered to the patient. Phlebotomists should become knowledgeable about these areas of the hospital because patients spend time in them prior to, during, and/or after their phlebotomy procedures. There are factors that relate to these departments that may affect the outcome of the laboratory test.

PROFESSIONAL COMPETENCIES AND CERTIFICATIONS

A high school diploma or its equivalent is most often required to enter a phlebotomy training program in hospitals, community colleges, or technical schools. Typically, the length of training varies from a few weeks to months, depending on the location, size of the facility, and the complexity of patients being served. Employers often require phlebotomy certification, which is accomplished by passing a national certification examination. Certification

TABLE 1–1.   Medical, Surgical, and Ancillary Service Departments Found in Large Health Care Facilities

DEPARTMENT	BRIEF DESCRIPTION
Allergy	Diagnosis and treatment of persons who have allergies or "reactions" to irritating agents
Anesthesiology	Preparing the patient for specialized treatment and/or surgery
Cardiology	Medical diagnosis and treatment of conditions relating to the heart and circulatory medical conditions
Cardiovascular	Surgical diagnosis and treatment of heart and blood circulation disorders
Dermatology	Diagnosis and treatment of conditions relating to the skin
Diagnostic imaging/Radiology	Uses ionizing radiation for treating disease, fluoroscopic and radiographic x-ray instrumentation and imaging methods for diagnosis, and radioisotopes for both diagnosing and treating disease. Sometimes patients are injected with dye that might interfere with some laboratory tests. The phlebotomist should document the circumstances as appropriate. In addition, the phlebotomist should be aware of applicable safety requirements.
Electrocardiography	Uses the electrocardiograph (ECG or EKG) to record the electric currents produced by contractions of the heart. This assists in the diagnosis of heart disease.
Electroencephalography	Uses the electroencephalograph (EEG) to record brain wave patterns
Endocrinology	Diagnosis and treatment of disorders in the organs and tissues that produce hormones (e.g., estrogens, testosterone, cortisol)
Family medicine/General practice	Care of general medical problems of all family members
Gastroenterology	Diagnosis and treatment of conditions relating to esophagus, stomach, and intestines
Geriatrics	Diagnosis and treatment of the elderly population
Hematology	Diagnosis and treatment of conditions relating to the blood
Immunology	Diagnosis and treatment of conditions relating to the immune system
Internal medicine	General diagnosis and treatment of patients for problems of one or more internal organs
Laboratory medicine/Pathology	Uses sophisticated instrumentation to analyze blood, body fluids, and tissues for pathological conditions. Laboratory results are used in diagnosis, treatment, and monitoring of patients' health status.
Neonatal/Perinatal	Study, support, and treatment of newborn and prematurely born babies and their mothers
Nephrology	Kidneys
Neurology	Nervous system
Nuclear medicine	Uses radioactive isotopes or tracers in the diagnosis and treatment of patients and in the study of the disease process. The radioactive substance is injected into the patient and emits rays that can be detected by sophisticated instrumentation. Phlebotomists should be knowledgeable of special safety requirements for entering this area. Also, the radioisotopes may interfere with laboratory testing, so documentation of this therapy may be required.

TABLE 1–1.   Continued

DEPARTMENT	BRIEF DESCRIPTION
Nutrition and dietetics	Perform nutritional assessments, patient education, and design special diets for patients who have eating-related disorders (e.g., diabetes, obesity)
Pathology	See Laboratory medicine/Pathology above.
Pediatrics	General diagnosis and therapy for children
Psychiatry/Neurology	Diagnosis and treatment for people of all ages with mental, emotional, and nervous system problems, using primarily nonsurgical procedures
Radiology/Medical imaging	Diagnosis and treatment, primarily through the use of x-ray, ultrasonography, and other internal imaging procedures
Obstetrics/Gynecology	Diagnosis and treatment relating to the sexual reproductive system of females, using both surgical and nonsurgical procedures
Occupational therapy	Assists the patient in becoming functionally independent within the limitations of the patient's disability or condition. Occupational therapists (OTs) collaborate with the health care team to design therapeutic programs of rehabilitative activities for the patient. The therapy is designed to improve functional abilities or activities of daily living (ADLs).
Oncology	Diagnosis and treatment of malignant (life-threatening) tumors
Ophthalmology	Diagnosis and treatment of the eyes and vision related medical problems
Orthopedics	Care of medical concerns related to bones and joints
Otolaryngology	Diagnosis and treatment of medical problems related to ears, nose, and throat
Pharmacy	Dispenses medications ordered by physicians. Pharmacists also collaborate with the health care team on drug therapies. Phlebotomists may collect blood specimens at timed intervals to monitor the level of the drug in the patient's bloodstream.
Physical medicine	Diagnosis and treatment of disorders and disabilities of the neuromuscular system
Physical therapy	Assists in restoring physical abilities that have been impaired by illness or injury. Rehabilitation programs often use heat/cold, water therapy, ultrasound or electricity, and physical exercises designed to restore useful activity.
Plastic surgery	Cosmetic surgery or surgical correction of the deformity of tissues, including skin
Proctology	Diagnosis and treatment of diseases of the anus and rectum
Pulmonary	Diagnosis and treatment of conditions relating to the respiratory system
Radiotherapy	Uses high-energy x-rays, such as from cobalt treatment, in the treatment of disease, particularly cancer. Safety precautions are important to avoid unnecessary irradiation.
Rheumatology	Diagnosis and treatment of joint and tissue diseases, including arthritis
Surgery	Diagnosis and treatment in which the physician physically alters a part of the patient's body
Urology	Diagnosis and treatment of medical conditions related to sexual/reproductive system in men, and renal system for men and women

---

Box 1-2   Hospitals in the United States

There are approximately 6,000 hospitals in the U.S. They vary according to the following:

- Mission (patient care, education, research).
- Bed size.
- Ownership (public or nonprofit, governmental, for profit or proprietary).
- Length of stay (short-term [e.g., less than 30 days]; long-term [e.g., greater than 30 days]).
- Type of care provided (general acute care hospitals or specialty care hospitals, such as birthing centers, cancer centers, psychiatric hospitals, pediatric hospitals, and rehabilitation hospitals).
- Location (urban or rural).
- Relationship to other health facilities (integrated hospital systems, religious multihospital systems, independent hospitals).

---

provides career advantages through job opportunities, career advancement, and portability (i.e., recognized from state to state).

Professional organizations that recognize phlebotomists are listed in Table 1–2. Many of these organizations have developed competency statements to describe the entry-level skills, tasks, and roles performed by designated health care workers. In addition, some offer continuing educational opportunities via conferences, online coursework, or

---

Box 1-3   Typical Examples of Clinical, Technical, and Clerical Duties of Phlebotomists

What are the clinical duties for phlebotomists?

- Identify the patient correctly
- Assess the patient prior to blood collection
- Prepare the patient accordingly
- Perform the puncture
- Withdraw blood into the correct containers/tubes
- Assess the degree of bleeding and pain
- Assess the patient after the phlebotomy procedure

What kind of technical duties do phlebotomists have to perform?

- Manipulate small objects, tubes, needles
- Select and use appropriate equipment
- Perform quality control functions
- Transport the specimens correctly
- Prepare/process the sample(s) for testing/analysis
- Assist in laboratory testing procedures, washing glassware, cleaning equipment

What clerical duties are expected of phlebotomists?

- Print/collate/distribute laboratory requisitions and reports
- Answer the telephone
- Answer all queries as appropriate
- Demonstrate courtesy in all patient encounters
- Respect privacy and confidentiality

TABLE 1–2. Professional Organizations for Phlebotomists

The organizations listed below have an interest in promoting and improving the practice of phlebotomy. They differ slightly in their membership requirements, fees, member benefits, continuing education courses, and/or to the degree that they offer certification examinations specifically for phlebotomists. The eligibility requirements and documentation for each certification also differ among these groups. Before applying for one or more of the certification examinations, the phlebotomist should check to see which ones are more accepted in the local community or state. Sometimes health care organizations have preferences for specific certifications and will adjust salaries accordingly. Likewise, local community colleges and universities can also provide recommendations about which certification examination to take.

The American Society for Clinical Pathology (ASCP)
ASCP
Board of Registry
P.O. Box 12277
Chicago, IL 60612-0277
(312) 738-1336 or (800) 621-4142
www.ascp.org

ASCP allows clinical laboratory personnel to gain associate membership status in the organization. ASCP offers many levels of certification and educational programs for laboratory personnel. Through the ASCP Board of Registry, a Phlebotomy Technician Examination, PBT (ASCP), is offered quarterly. It covers the entry-level skills of a phlebotomist and uses taxonomy levels that assess recall (recognize facts), interpretive skills (use knowledge to interpret numeric data), and problem-solving skills (use applications of specific information to solve problems). Over 13,000 phlebotomists have been certified by ASCP since 1989, when the first phlebotomy examination was administered. ASCP is the oldest and one of the most widely recognized certifications in the field of laboratory medicine.

The National Phlebotomy Association (NPA)
NPA
1901 Brightseat Road
Landover, MD 20785
(301) 386-4200
(301) 386-4203 (fax)
www.scpt.com/NationalPhlebotomyAssociation.html

NPA was established in 1978 to recognize the phlebotomist as a distinctive and identifiable part of the health care team. NPA has established professional standards, a code of ethics, educational opportunities, and an annual certification examination resulting in a CPT (NPA). NPA has trained and certified approximately 15,000 phlebotomists in all 50 states and abroad and has accredited 75 teaching programs. Accredited programs must include the following topic areas: Historical Perspective, Medical Terminology, Anatomy and Physiology, Communication, Phlebotomy Practical, Cardio-Pulmonary Resusitation (CPR), Stress Management, Phlebotomy Techniques, Human Relations, Legal Aspects, Infection Control, and Drug Awareness.

The American Society for Clinical Laboratory Science (ASCLS)
and The National Credentialing Agency for Laboratory Personnel, Inc. (NCA)

NCA	ASCLS
P.O. Box 15945-289	7910 Woodmont Aven,ue Suite 530
Lenexa, KS 66285	Bethesda, MD 20814
(913) 438-5110	(301) 657-2768
www.nca-info.org	www.ascls.org

(continued)

TABLE 1–2. Continued

ASCLS has recognized clinical laboratory personnel for more than 50 years. Several types of memberships are available, depending on the education and experience of the individual. Phlebotomists may join ASCLS as associate members in the Phlebotomy Section and take a certification examination through the NCA. The certification is a CLP1b (NCA).

American Medical Technologists (AMT)
AMT
710 Higgins Road
Park Ridge, IL 60068-5765
(847) 823-5169 or (800) 275-1268
(847) 823-0458 (fax)
www.amt1.com

AMT offers a certification examination for Registered Phlebotomy Technician (RPT).

American Society of Phlebotomy Technicians (ASPT)
P.O. Box 1831
Hickory, NC 28603
(828) 294-0078
(828) 327-2969 (fax)
www.aspt.org

ASPT offers a certification examination that results in a CPT (ASPT) certification. They also offer certification examinations for Point-of-Care Technician, EKG Technician, Drug Collection Specialist, Paramedical Insurance Examiner, and Patient Care Technician.

National Accrediting Agency for Clinical Laboratory Sciences (NAACLS)
8410 West Bryn Mawr Avenue, Suite 670
Chicago, IL 60631
(773) 714-8880
(773) 714-8886 (fax)

NAACLS accredits educational programs in clinical laboratory sciences including phlebotomy. No certification examinations are provided.

National Healthcareer Association (NHA)
NHA-National Headquarters
134 Evergreen Place, 9th floor
East Orange, NJ 07018
(800) 499-9092
(973) 678-7305 (fax)
www.nha2000.com

Established in 1989, NHA was formed to create a network for health care professionals. NHA offers a certification examination for phlebotomists, CPT(NHA).

correspondence courses. Table 1–3 is an example of one organization's list of competencies for entry-level phlebotomy technicians. At minimum, these are the types of competencies that an employer might assess for the phlebotomist's performance evaluation.

Other more specific competencies that vary by employer but are nevertheless important might include those listed in Table 1–4. There are many ways for supervisors to assess competency: for example, direct observation, videotaping, reviewing worksheets or log books, reviewing quality control records, providing simulations similar to real-life situations, and providing written examinations. Performance evaluations are important to both the employee and the employer because they provide feedback, identify problems early, promote consistency in the evaluation process, encourage employees to stay abreast of policies and procedures, target improvement and high quality, and document that personnel are competent to perform tasks.[1]

PROFESSIONAL CHARACTER TRAITS

Within the health professions, organizations such as ASCP and NPA have developed standards of ethical conduct and behavior for members, and members are expected to adhere to those standards of performance. The major points common to most ethical standards are:

- Do no harm to anyone intentionally.
- Perform according to sound technical ability and good judgment.
- Respect patients' rights (which include confidentiality, privacy, the right to know about their treatment, and the right to refuse treatment).

For phlebotomists, ethical conduct involves responsibilities for accuracy and reliability of laboratory specimen integrity, respect for patient confidentiality and privacy, honesty, integrity, and regard for the dignity of all human beings. Many hospitals and health service organizations across the country have also established specific codes of ethics for their employees and/or statements of organizational values. For further discussion of ethical issues in phlebotomy, refer to Chapter 2.

Before entering the field of phlebotomy, one should reflect on the important character attributes for this career. Generally speaking they include the following:

- **Sincerity and compassion**—Phlebotomists should possess an intense desire to serve people and a sincere interest in learning about blood and specimen collection practices.
- **Emotional stability and maturity**—Phlebotomists must cope daily with seeing others in pain, handling blood and body fluids, facing injury and trauma, seeing disease sites, and the possibility of observing death. Responses of health care workers to harsh situations must be prompt, professional, and reassuring to the patient, their families, and the health care team.
- **Accountability for doing things right**—Personal integrity, veracity (telling the truth), or "doing what's right when no one is looking" (e.g., washing hands between patient collections, observing precautions to gown and scrub in isolation, reporting one's own mistakes, and collecting timed tests at the proper time), reflects a health care worker's personal responsibility for actions.
- **Dedication to high standards of performance and precision**—Phlebotomists must continually upgrade and maintain the quality of their skills. Phlebotomists must seek knowledge about new techniques and safety procedures, new supplies and equipment, and computer technology through continuing education. They

TABLE 1–3.   American Society for Clinical Pathology (ASCP) Board of Registry Competency Statements for the Phlebotomy Technician

Competency statements describe the entry-level skills and tasks performed by phlebotomy technicians and measured on the certification examination. In regard to Anatomy and Physiology, Specimen Collection, Specimen Processing and Handling, and Laboratory Operations related to Phlebotomy, and in accordance with established procedures, the Phlebotomy Technician, PBT(ASCP), at career entry should be able to accomplish the following:

Applies knowledge of	• Principles of basic and special procedures • Potential sources of error • Standard operating procedures • Fundamental biological characteristics
Selects appropriate	• Course of action • Equipment/methods/reagents
Prepares patient and equipment	
Evaluates	• Specimen and patient situation • Possible sources of error or inconsistencies • Quality control procedures • Common procedural/technical problems • Appropriate actions and methods • Corrective actions

(From the American Society for Clinical Pathology Board of Registry, www.ascp.org, 2004, with permission.)

should be willing to ask for assistance when dealing with a difficult patient or procedure and have the desire to follow rigid standards of performance. They should only collect the specimens ordered and only those that they have been trained to collect.

- **Respect for patients' dignity, privacy, confidentiality, and the right to know—** Phlebotomists have an obligation to respect all patients' rights regardless of their personal opinions and biases. All patients must be treated with dignity and respect regardless of race, culture, religion, gender, age, or disabling conditions. Phlebotomists should have a full understanding of patients' rights to privacy, confidentiality, and to knowing what procedures are being performed and by whom.

- **Propensity for cleanliness—**Phlebotomists must protect themselves and patients by accepting that sterile techniques, good personal hygiene, and cleanliness affect safety and the quality of health care. This is more important than saving time or cutting corners to save money.

- **Pride, satisfaction, and self-fulfillment in the job—**Phlebotomists should attain professional satisfaction from continually improving their professional skills and knowledge, from knowing that others are dependent on the quality of their work, and from knowing that their skills contribute to the betterment of patients. The most successful, highly regarded phlebotomists are those who are most gratified with their work.

TABLE 1–4.   Additional Measures of Phlebotomist's Performance

In addition to the competencies above, this list encompasses professional attributes, ability, and performance measures that employers might use for a phlebotomist's performance evaluation. Performance measures are observed through the phlebotomist's behavior, approach to the job, knowledge and skills.

ATTRIBUTES/ABILITY/PERFORMANCE/ KNOWLEDGE	EXAMPLES
Adherence to policies • Organizational policies • Safety • Infection control • Fire and safety	• Unexcused absences or tardiness • Dress code • Handwashing • Waste disposal • Gowning and gloving • Handling of fire extinguishers
Communication skills • Verbal • Nonverbal • Listening skills	• Management of angry patients • Interactions with peers and coworkers • Telephone etiquette • Satisfaction of the patients • Courtesy • Use of appropriate medical and/or laboratory terminology
Efficiency and quality • Productivity • Quality	• Waiting times • Complications during procedures • Number of uncomplicated blood draws in a specified time period • Blood culture contamination rate • Number of unacceptable laboratory specimens

- **Working with team members**—Phlebotomists are obliged to be flexible enough to work with a variety of health care professionals in a wide range of settings. Health care teams can improve skills (more talent, expertise, and technical competence), communication (more ideas, mutual respect, crossing departmental lines), participation (increased job satisfaction, combined efforts valued above individual efforts), effectiveness (solutions likely to be implemented; the team has ownership of the shared decisions).[2]
- **Take pleasure in communicating with patients**—The quality and ease of collecting blood specimens depends both on the technical skills of the health care worker and successful interactions with the patient. Phlebotomists should learn about transcultural communication strategies, communication barriers, and gender or age-related issues that affect communication.

The decision to become a phlebotomist requires a special person with multiple talents and internal drive. The choice of this career path should not be taken lightly.

Box 1–4	How Can I Be a Better Team Member? What Do I Need To Do To Maximize Team Effectiveness?

Every team member should:

1. Understand the mission of the organization
2. Know the basic skills for group process and team dynamics (e.g., active listening, setting norms)
3. Understand relevance and commitment to team goals
4. Show reliability and dependability in work assignments
5. Communicate own ideas and feelings
6. Actively participate in decision making
7. Learn how to be flexible in decision making
8. Constructively manage conflicts
9. Contribute to the cohesion of the team
10. Contribute to problem-solving strategies
11. Support and encourage other team members

Individuals should reflect on this list periodically as they go through this textbook and through their career. To make it a self-assessment, simply add the words "Do I . . ." to each phrase above. Professional growth and maturity occur if one can honestly answer these questions and strive for improvement if there are deficits.

ROLE OF THE CLINICAL LABORATORY IN SPECIMEN COLLECTION SERVICES

A typical hospital-based clinical laboratory has two components: clinical pathology and anatomic pathology. Laboratories can also be independently owned and operated outside the hospital setting.

Regardless of the type or size of the laboratory, it is important to understand that the phlebotomist plays a vital role early in the process of producing laboratory results/reports. Reliability and accuracy of *all* patient test results depend on the **preanalytic phase** of specimen collection, that is, the part of the process that occurs before the actual testing and analysis is performed. The preanalytic process is the fundamental and crucial domain of every phlebotomist. Figure 1–1 ■ depicts the functional phases of laboratory testing, the preanalytic, analytic, and postanalytic phases.

Smaller clinical laboratories can be located in remote locations or clinics, physicians' offices, and in mobile vans. Health care workers who perform the testing must maintain the same high standards of quality as are found in larger, high-volume laboratories.

The federal government regulates all clinical laboratories through the Clinical Laboratory Improvement Amendments of 1988 (CLIA 1988). Regulations apply to any site that tests human specimens, including small physician's office laboratories (POLs), and to screening tests done at a hospital bedside. The regulations include establishing qualifications for health care personnel who perform the tests, periodic inspections, proficiency assessments, and the investigation of complaints.

Other regulatory agencies also have oversight of clinical laboratories, depending on the type of testing they do and the reimbursement they receive for the procedures. Among

Box 1–5	Phlebotomy Career Self-Assessment

To consider a career in phlebotomy ask yourself the following questions. If there are doubts in your mind about your answers, think about whether you are willing to change or learn new ways of behaving.

1. Do I pay attention to details?
2. Do I like to work with small objects such as needles and test tubes?
3. Do I follow procedures exactly?
4. Does it bother me if I am closely watched or supervised?
5. Do I mind seeing blood, sick patients, body tissues or fluids, or smelling unpleasant odors?
6. What is my reaction to inflicting the pain of a needlestick on someone?
7. Am I willing to admit my own mistakes?
8. Do I like working with a team? Do I get along well with other people?
9. Am I willing to stand for long periods of time, walk extensively, reach, stoop, lift, or carry equipment?
10. Am I willing to work on holidays and weekends occasionally?

these are the Health Care Financing Administration (HCFA), the Food and Drug Administration (FDA), the American Association of Blood Banks (AABB), the American Society for Clinical Pathologists (ASCP), and the Joint Commission for the Accreditation of Healthcare Organizations (JCAHO).

■■■■■■ COMMUNICATION STRATEGIES FOR PHLEBOTOMISTS

Communication is essential for everyday success in all areas of the workplace. Effective verbal interactions can be depicted as a communication loop. The message must leave the sender and reach the receiver as depicted in Figure 1–2 ■. The receiver usually provides feedback to the sender. Without feedback, the sender has no way of knowing whether the message was accurately received or if the message was somehow blocked by extraneous factors. The factors can "filter out" meaning from a message. Filters can be damaging to effective communication. When there are cultural, behavioral, or language differences among health care workers and patients, there is an increased risk that patients will not understand care instructions. Phlebotomists need to be sure that the message they send is

Box 1–6	Clinical and Anatomical Pathology

In the *clinical pathology* area, blood and other types of body fluids and tissues are analyzed (e.g., urine, cerebrospinal fluid [CSF], sputum, gastric secretions, synovial fluid). In the *anatomic pathology* area, autopsies are performed, histologic and cytologic procedures are utilized for tissue and fluid specimens, and surgical biopsy tissues are analyzed.

Figure 1–1. Phases of Laboratory Testing: Preanalytic, Analytic, Postanalytic

 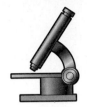

Pre-analytical	Analytical	Post-analytical
What happens before testing.	What happens during testing.	What happens after testing.

the same message received by the patient. In the following sections, communication is broken down into its three more detailed components:

1. Verbal communication
2. Nonverbal communication
3. Active listening

VERBAL COMMUNICATION

Keep in mind that talking with strangers about personal things such as your body is never easy and can be particularly difficult for young teenage patients or patients from cultural

---

Box 1–7   Clinical Laboratory Personnel

Aside from the actual phlebotomist, personnel who work on the *analytic* phase, or testing phase, of producing laboratory results may have different educational backgrounds:

- **Pathologists:** physicians who have extensive training in pathology, which is the study and diagnosis of disease through the use of laboratory test results.
- **Administrative staff:** usually individuals who have a graduate degree in health care administration or business. Often these individuals have extensive clinical experience as well.
- **Technical supervisors:** clinical laboratory scientists (also known as medical technologists) with additional experience and education in a laboratory specialty area, such as hematology, microbiology, or clinical chemistry.
- **Clinical Laboratory Scientists (CLS) or Medical Technologists (MT):** individuals with a bachelor's degree in a biological science. Educational requirements include 1 or more years of study in a CLS program. Licensing is required in some states. Roles and responsibilities include performing chemical, microscopic, microbiologic, or immunologic tests pertaining to patient care; recording and reporting test results; participating in research and development of new test methods; performing preventive maintenance, troubleshooting, and quality control of instruments and reagents; maintaining safety in the clinical laboratory; and teaching residents and fellows in pathology and laboratory sciences.
- **Medical Laboratory Technicians (MLT) or Clinical Laboratory Technicians (CLT):** these individuals have a two-year certificate or associate degree. The MLT may perform designated tests and procedures, prepare specimens for testing and transport, prepare reagents, perform quality control measures, and assist the CLS in numerous preanalytic and postanalytic processes.
- **Other laboratory personnel:** laboratory information systems (LIS) operators and programmers, clerical staff, quality management staff, infection control officers, and biomedical equipment specialists.

Box 1-8   Sections of a Clinical Laboratory

Large clinical laboratories cluster testing processes according to the following sections:

- Clinical chemistry
- Hematology and coagulation
- Microbiology and parasitology
- Immunohematology (blood banking) or transfusion medicine
- Immunology and serology
- Cytology
- Histology
- Cytogenetics
- Urinalysis

---

backgrounds that are different from the phlebotomist's. Encouraging patients to accept an unfamiliar phlebotomist or to talk about themselves usually involves the following:[2]

- Show empathy (for waking them up, disturbing them, or interrupting their meal)
- Show respect (for their privacy, for their condition, for their family members)
- Build trust (maintain confidentiality, explain procedures clearly, tell the truth)
- Establish rapport (common courtesy, show interest)
- Listen actively (face the patient, maintain nonauthoritative posture, lean toward the patient, establish eye contact, relax and listen intently)
- Provide specific feedback (about their behavior, about a procedure)

Language

Health care workers often explain procedures to patients using complex jargon or medical terminology that can be confusing to laypeople. In addition, the meaning of words varies with context and the age of the speaker. To promote understanding, phlebotomists should

---

Box 1-9   CLIA Approval for Laboratories

CLIA categorizes laboratory tests according to the level of complexity of the testing procedure and the risk involved for the patient if errors are made in performing or interpreting the test. The tests may also be reclassified from one category to another as technology advances.

Waived tests are those tests that are the easiest to perform, the least susceptible to error, and the least risky to patients. Examples include urinalysis, urine pregnancy tests, blood glucose screening tests, rheumatoid factor tests or mononucleosis tests using blood agglutination, occult blood detection from stool samples, spun microhematocrits, and erythrocyte sedimentation rates. These are tests that are commonly done in ambulatory settings, on hospital units near the bedside, and in other remote locations.

Moderate complexity tests are those tests that are simple to perform but may involve more risk to the patient if results are inaccurate. Examples include white and red blood cell counts, hemoglobin, hematocrit, blood chemistries, and urine cultures.

High complexity tests are those tests that are complex to perform and may allow for reasonable risk of harm to the patient if results are inaccurate. These include tests that require sophisticated instrumentation and oversight by a pathologist or Ph.D.-level scientist. Examples include molecular probe analyses, bone marrow evaluations, immunoassays, flow cytometry, cytogenetics analysis, and electrophoresis.

Figure 1–2. Patient–Phlebotomist Communication Loop

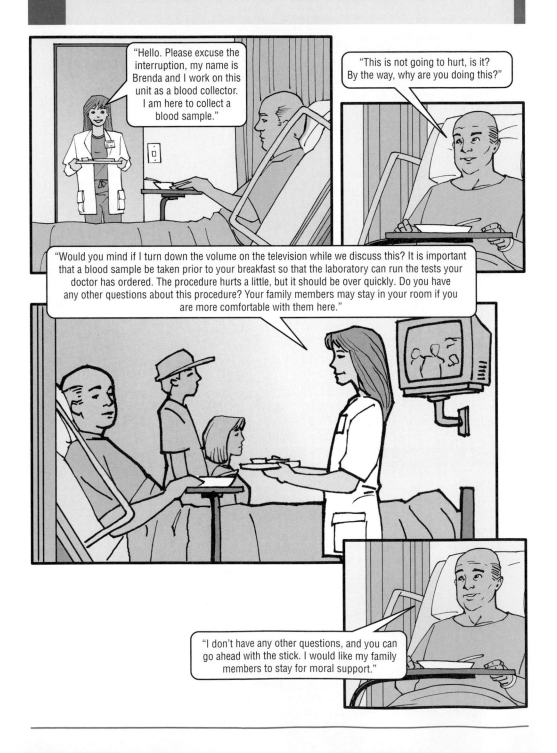

use simple vocabulary, particularly with children. Patients must *not* be told, "This won't hurt." Most blood collection procedures are indeed slightly painful; therefore, it is important that the patient be forewarned and prepared.

Hearing Impairments

Phlebotomists should be sensitive to patients who have impaired hearing. A question such as, "Is there a step you would like me to repeat before we begin?" yields better clues that the patient has heard and understood than saying, "Do you understand?" If it is obvious that the patient did not hear, all efforts should be made to write down instructions for the patient. It is recommended that writing tools be kept at the bedside of these patients and also be accessible in ambulatory settings.

Languages other than English

The diversity of languages spoken in this country is extensive. In large metropolitan areas of the United States (and the world), one sees signs in multiple languages. Patients who do not speak English can understand some basics from nonverbal cues, but the phlebotomist must know how to locate an interpreter when possible. In hospitals and larger clinics, there may be personnel available to perform language interpretations. In the absence of an interpreter, written instructions in other languages may facilitate the process. Printed cards in different languages can be used to transmit information about the venipuncture procedures.

United States census data from 2000 indicate large increases in the Spanish-speaking population, particularly in specific parts of the country. In these areas it is beneficial for phlebotomists to develop some skill in Spanish; however, it is recommended that the health care worker practice the phrases with someone who can speak the language before attempting to communicate with a patient, because mispronounced words may lead to more confusion. (Basic requests in Spanish/English are listed in Appendix 11.)

Regardless of the patient's language, the health care worker is responsible for communicating essential information. The phlebotomist should always speak respectfully, in a highly professional manner, and with phrases that are clearly articulated. If a health care worker feels

---

Box 1–10   Overcoming Barriers to Effective Communication

Distracting noises can interfere with hearing. A busy hallway, visitors, a television or radio in the room, or headphones can prevent the patient from hearing accurately. In these cases, the phlebotomist should take steps, in a polite and professional manner, to reduce the sound level so the patient can hear necessary instructions. Examples might include phrases such as the following:

To visitors: "Excuse me please, it is important for me to explain this procedure to Mr. Jones. Would you mind if we have a quiet moment together for a few minutes? Thank you for your cooperation."

For the television: "Mr. Jones, I am sorry to disrupt your television show, but would you mind if we lower the volume for a few minutes so we can go over the procedure for collecting your blood sample? Thank you, this should only take a few minutes."

For headphones: "Mr. Jones, it is important that we discuss this procedure before beginning. Would you mind taking off your headphones for a few minutes? I will be brief. Thank you for your cooperation."

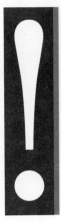

Clinical Alert

In some states, children are not permitted to serve as translators for their parents when health care issues are discussed. Phlebotomists should check with their supervisors about the applicable laws in their states.

frustrated by an inability to communicate with a patient, he or she should seek assistance from a supervisor, translator, family member, or physician. Each patient should be treated compassionately, fairly, and with the utmost of dignity, regardless of language abilities.

Age

The vocabulary of a teenager is different from that of an elderly person. Phlebotomists should be sensitive to word usage for each age. Communication issues for various age groups are discussed in later chapters.

Tone of Voice

The tone of one's voice and the inflection used can change a positive sentence into a negative-sounding statement. The tone of voice should match the words that are spoken. Sarcasm is usually communicated just by tone of voice. Health care workers can avoid sending mixed messages to patients by practicing a calm, soothing, and confident tone of voice. Box 1–11 is a practice exercise for health care professionals to use in observing their own facial expressions and voice tones.

Emergency Situations

Emergency, or "STAT," blood collections are common in emergency rooms and in some complicated surgical or medical cases. These phlebotomy procedures require extra speed and accuracy without jeopardizing the "personal touch." Patients in emergency rooms may not have identification information with them and/or may be unconscious. All facilities, however, should have documented procedures for the identification process with which phlebotomists should be familiar. Individual patients should be considered in terms of their privacy, dignity, and individual needs, not by nicknames such as "Mr. L down the hall" or "the broken leg in 3C." Each is entitled to professional, respectful care in all circumstances.

Bedside Manner

The climate established by a phlebotomist upon entering a patient's room will affect the entire patient encounter. The feeling of confidence that comes from the knowledge that the collection tray is clean and well stocked is the first step in a good bedside manner. A pleasant

Box 1–11	Improving Tone of Voice and Facial Expression

The following exercise is useful for improving verbal and nonverbal communication skills. Practice it in front of a mirror or with a coworker.

Step 1. Using a nice tone of voice (i.e., calm, compassionate, clear, professional tone), with a smile on your face, practice saying the following phrases:

- "Please . . ."
- "Good morning."
- "How was your breakfast?"
- "Have you had lunch?"
- "May I check your identification bracelet?"
- "Thank you."

Step 2. Now, using a degrading tone of voice (i.e., sarcastic, whiny, angry tone), with a frustrated, disdainful look on your face, repeat the phrases listed in step 1.

Step 3. List the specific features you liked about the first method with those features you disliked about the second method. Try to contrast details of facial features (wrinkled eyebrows or smiling face), how the voice lowers or raises at the end of the statements, and how you feel when speaking in the two manners.

Step 4. Keep a mental impression (or actually take a picture) of the way you look and sound during the first step. Remember: A simple smile can often force a positive change in voice tone.

facial expression, neat appearance, and professional manner set the stage for a positive interaction with the patient. The first 30 seconds after the phlebotomist enters the patient's room determines how that patient perceives the quality of patient care offered by that hospital. Most patients admit that the procedure they dread most is being "stuck" for blood collection, so phlebotomists should make every effort to minimize the negative effects of the situation.

When encountering the patient for the first time, either after knocking (not pounding) on the door to his or her room or after calling a patient from a clinic waiting room, the phlebotomist should introduce him- or herself and state that he or she is part of the hospital unit or laboratory staff, whichever is the case. The patient should be informed that the specimen is being collected for a test ordered by the physician. A statement indicating that this is routine hospital protocol often reassures the patient. A lengthy discussion of why a certain test was ordered or what tests were ordered is inappropriate. These questions should be referred to the patient's physician.

During all the steps of the venipuncture, the health care worker should remain calm, compassionate, and professional with conversations limited to essential information. Sometimes patients are comforted by letting them know about how the procedure is going (e.g., "this is going well," or "it is almost over"). Care should be taken not to be distracted from the phlebotomy procedure by excessive talk of unrelated issues. And before leaving the phlebotomist should thank the patient for cooperating.

COMMUNICATION FOR CONFIRMING PATIENT IDENTIFICATION

Health care organizations differ slightly in their guidelines for patient identification but all agree that proper identification is essential. If the patient is hospitalized, this should be accomplished by a match between the test requisition or labels and the armband, and by

Box 1-12   Greeting a Patient

The following scenario is a typical one that might occur at the opening greeting between a phlebotomist and a hospitalized patient. Imagine both the verbal and non-verbal factors involved. The *wrong responses* are suggested in italics. They can be used as a discussion tool of how the phlebotomist can have a negative impact.

Phlebotomist: Good morning, my name is Sally and I am here to collect a blood sample for your laboratory tests. Could you state your name please? *Wrong response: Hi, are you Mrs. Betty Smith?*

Patient (softly): My name is Betty Smith.

Phlebotomist: Could you repeat that please? *Wrong response: Huh? What did you say?*

Patient: My name is Betty Smith.

Phlebotomist: Thank you, I think I have it now but I also need to check your identification bracelet. I will be taking a blood sample from your arm so that the laboratory can perform tests that your doctor ordered. Have you had breakfast yet? *Wrong response: Okay, let's get on with it.*

Patient: No breakfast yet; I just woke up.

Phlebotomist: I need to look at your arms. Would you prefer your right side or left side?

Patient: Nobody ever gets blood on the left side so we'd better try the right side.

Phlebotomist: Thanks for that info; we can check the right side. Please hold out your arm so that I can feel for your veins. *Wrong response: Oh, don't worry about a thing. I'm pretty good at drawing from tough veins.*

Patient: Okay, but will it hurt?

Phlebotomist: It will hurt a little, but I'll do my best to have it done quickly. Do you have any other questions? *Wrong response: No, it doesn't hurt.*

Patient: Not really, just get it over with.

Phlebotomist: Thanks for your cooperation, Mrs. Smith. *Wrong response: Well, I'm just doing what I was told!*

Box 1-13   Communication in Ambulatory Settings or in the Home Usually Requires More Time for the Following Reasons:

- The phlebotomist must introduce him- or herself and clearly explain the purpose of the interaction.
- The patient should be directed to an appropriate place to sit or recline during the procedure. This may involve walking to a private area, blood collection booth, or special recliner.
- If the phlebotomy procedure is taking place in an unfamiliar setting, such as the patient's home, the phlebotomist must take extra time to find the nearest bathroom (for hand washing, blood spillage) and the nearest bed in case there are complications to the phlebotomy procedure (fainting).
- In a patient's home, the phlebotomist may need to find a phone or bring a mobile phone to clarify laboratory orders or inquire about patient information.
- Information about the procedure should be fully explained (especially if it is a first-time blood collection for the patient or if it has been a long time since the last blood collection).
- Identifying the patient should be done meticulously and cautiously, using various methods to identify the patient positively (e.g., driver's license or identification card, confirmation of birthday and home address, or social security number, if available).
- The puncture site must be appropriately cared for and it should be clear that the patient is physically fit to leave the area after the phlebotomy procedure. If the patient is homebound, the phlebotomist must be sure that the patient is no longer bleeding, the puncture site has been appropriately bandaged, and that the patient is able to stay by him- or herself.

verbal confirmation from the patient. If a hospitalized patient does not have an armband, a positive confirmation must be made by a unit nurse who knows the patient. This process should be well documented by the phlebotomist. Special identification procedures should also be well documented for ambulatory patients, especially in cases of homebound patients, mobile vans, and other off-site locations. Armbands are not commonly used in ambulatory settings; however, an identification card usually is. It may include some demographic data and other identifying information, such as the patient's identification number, date of birth (DOB), address, or a combination of these. This information should be confirmed by the patient prior to blood collection.

Some health care facilities insist that the health care worker ask for the patient's complete address, whereas others require the mention of the patient's hometown, birthdate, or street name to reinforce and confirm identity. Some prefer that patients spell out an unusual last name. This portion of the specimen collection procedure ensures that the remainder of the diagnostic testing protocol provides information on the correct person.

NONVERBAL COMMUNICATION

Some theories suggest that communication consists of 10 to 20 percent verbal and 80 to 90 percent nonverbal messages. Nonverbal cues, or body language, can be positive—and facilitate understanding—or negative—and hinder effective communication. These are summarized in Table 1-5.

Positive Body Language

SMILING.   A simple, compassionate smile can set the stage for open lines of communication. It can make each patient feel that he or she is the most important person at that moment. In addition, most people look better with smiles on their faces than they do with frowns. It takes fewer muscle movements to smile than it does to frown.

EYE CONTACT AND EYE LEVEL.   The most expressive parts of the human face are the eyes. Therefore eye contact is important in effective communication. Eye contact promotes a sense of trust and honesty between the patient and phlebotomist. It can make the entire

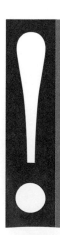

Clinical Alert

The patient should always be asked, "What is your name?" not "Are you Ms. Smith?" The first question is a more reliable and direct way of confirming identity. The second question is inappropriate and less reliable because a patient who is heavily medicated will often agree with anything that he or she is asked.

TABLE 1–5. Nonverbal Communication/Body Language

Positive Body Language
- Aids communication
- Can make interactions more pleasant

Face to face positioning
Relaxed hands, arms, shoulders
Erect posture
Eye contact, eye level (avoid looking down on someone)
Smiling
Appropriate "zone of comfort"

Negative Body Language
- Is distracting
- Prevents effective communication
- Causes discomfort, uneasiness

Slouching, shrugged shoulders
Rolling eyes, wandering eyes
Staring blankly or at ceiling
Rubbing eyes, excessive blinking
Squirming, tapping foot, pencil, etc.
Deep sighing, groaning
Crossing arms, clenching fists
Wrinkling forehead
Thumbing through books or papers
Stretching, yawning
Peering over eyeglasses
Pointing finger at someone

Figure 1–3. Maintaining a Professional Appearance

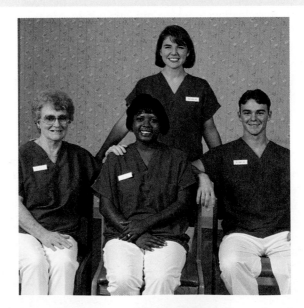

A smile, erect posture, and good grooming promote a sense of professionalism.

Figure 1–4. Negative Body Language

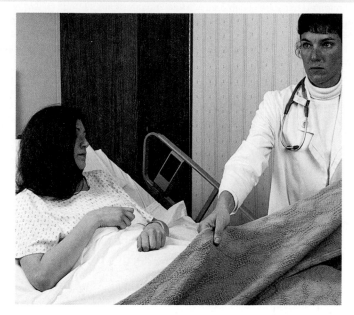

Notice the unpleasant effect of this stern look!

procedure less traumatic for the patient if he or she sees a compassionate expression in the phlebotomist's eyes. There is an expression: "The eyes are the windows of the soul."

Eye level is also a consideration. Bedridden patients must always look up to those in the room, including the health care team members. This can create a feeling of intimidation, of being "looked down on," or of weakness. Most of the time, phlebotomists do not have the extra time to spend finding a chair to sit in so that they are at eye level; however, if a health care worker must explain a lengthy procedure or if it is noted that the patient is particularly nervous about the procedure, the explanation should be done while seated at eye level with the patient.

A word of caution about eye contact is needed when dealing with patients of certain cultures. Generally speaking, Americans view eye contact as a positive aspect of human nature, and avoidance of eye contact might mean that someone is not being truthful. However, some Asian and Native American cultures believe that prolonged eye contact is rude and an invasion of privacy. Muslim women may avoid eye contact due to modesty.[3] Patients may not appreciate direct eye contact with a health care provider because it may make them feel self-conscious; it may be unacceptable in their culture, or may not be acceptable with the opposite gender. The health care worker should take cues from the patient. If the patient does not look at the health care worker when she is speaking, perhaps she or he would feel more comfortable with more space between them or less direct eye contact. The phlebotomist can take the interaction at a slower pace to monitor the patient's comfort level. The more secure and comfortable that the patient feels, the easier the procedure will become for the phlebotomist.

Box 1–14	Practice Exercise for Developing Sensitivity to Bedridden Patients

Health care workers should strive to be as compassionate as possible. Bedridden patients often feel intimidated because health care workers must repeatedly "look down" on them to provide care. Sometimes these patients are depressed because of their condition or prognosis. This exercise will help you imagine yourself in the patient's condition and can make you a more compassionate member of the health care team. Practice the exercise with a coworker that you do not know very well.

1. Lie on a bed while your coworker stands directly over you, looking down.

2. Have the coworker go through the motions of a venipuncture procedure, including the greeting and identification process. Try to imagine the anticipation of the needle stick. Have the coworker maintain eye contact with you while conversing.

3. Repeat step 2, without eye contact.

4. Mentally note the positive and negative aspects of this procedure.

FACE-TO-FACE COMMUNICATION.   Phlebotomists should face patients directly. Otherwise, the patient may feel neglected, that he or she is being avoided, or that information is being withheld. If a patient turns away from a phlebotomist, however, it should be taken as a cue that the patient is uncomfortable for some reason. The phlebotomist should do everything possible to make the patient feel more comfortable during the phlebotomy procedure.

ZONE OF COMFORT.   Most individuals begin to feel uncomfortable when strangers get too close to them physically. A zone of comfort is the area of space around a patient that is private territory, so to speak, where they feel comfortable with an interaction. If that zone is crossed, feelings of uneasiness may occur.

For most western cultures, there are four zones of interpersonal space:

- **Intimate space (direct contact up to 18 inches)**—for close relationships and health care workers who bathe, feed, dress, and perform venipunctures
- **Personal space (18 inches to 4 feet)**—for interactions among friends and for many patient encounters
- **Social space (4 feet to 12 feet)**—for most interactions of everyday life
- **Public space (more than 12 feet)**—for lectures, speeches, etc.

When a stranger gets too close, it can cause the patient to feel nervous, fearful, or anxious. Health care workers must be understanding and approach nervous patients slowly and gently to avoid causing feelings of being threatened. This is particularly true with children, many of whom have a wide zone of comfort; that is, they do not like anyone to approach them except close relatives or friends. A skilled health care worker must be aware of his or her threat to a patient and use a calm, professional, and confident manner. It is helpful to slowly approach the patient while crossing the zone of comfort, not to be too hasty, and to talk to patients during the process.

Cultural Sensitivity

Culture is a system of values, beliefs, and practices that stem from one's concept of reality. Culture influences decisions and behaviors in many aspects of life. Learning about various

Box 1-15   What Is Culture?

Culture is variable among groups of individuals, but it usually encompasses the following traits:

Values—the accepted principles of a group, i.e., individualism versus socialism, importance of education and financial security, competition versus cooperation, sanctity of life, etc.

Beliefs—doctrine or faith of a person or group, i.e., spiritual orientation, family bonds, etc.

Traditions and practices—customs and behaviors associated with groups, i.e., holidays, foods, music, dance, health care practices, etc.

ethnic groups and cultures is important for health care professionals so as to understand the reasons for patients' behaviors during times of health and illness.

Specific traits that vary among cultures have been addressed previously (e.g., eye contact and zone of comfort). However, with the changing demographics of the U.S. population, it is vital for all health care workers to become more sensitive and compassionate about accepting cultural practices that vary from our own. When a health care worker is unsure or unaware of acceptable patterns of behavior for a patient, the recommended action is to "follow the patient's lead." For example, if a patient speaks softly and slowly, speak the same way. If the patient turns to a family member when speaking to you, include the family member in the conversation. If a patient moves closer to you during the conversation, try not to back away from the patient's zone of comfort. The best way to become more culturally competent is to allow patients to teach us, to become active observers of how culturally diverse patients interact with each other and with health professionals. Becoming keen observers of mannerisms, gestures, and facial expressions of group members, reading about cultural groups, watching films and videos, reading novels that depict different cultures, and reading newspapers published by cultural groups will make health care workers better and more informed at what they do.[3]

Box 1-16   Role Reversal Exercise

Having respect for an individual's personal space, or zone of comfort, is part of being a compassionate health care worker. The comfort zone of each person varies with gender, culture, and situation. However, most people feel uneasy when strangers are touching them or are "too close for comfort." An example of this uncomfortable sensation is standing in a crowded elevator. People take great measures to move so that they are not touching strangers, and as people exit the elevator, the remaining people move and shift to provide more space around themselves. This same sense of uneasiness is felt by patients who are approached by unfamiliar health care workers.

To simulate a real patient–health care worker interaction, practice the following exercise with a coworker who is not a close friend. Eye contact should be made during this exercise.

1. Lie on a bed as if you are a patient.

2. Have the coworker slowly approach you. He or she should begin 10 feet away and pause between steps.

3. Note at what distance you begin to feel awkward or uncomfortable. (Usually, this distance is about 2 to 4 feet from the bed.) This distance is the boundary of your zone of comfort.

4. Repeat the exercise with the same coworker. You will probably require a smaller zone of comfort because a person becomes a little more at ease after initial contact with an unfamiliar person.

In some cultures, the zone of comfort may be wide, and in others, people naturally speak more closely to each other. How much at ease a person feels with physical closeness can also vary with gender. Some women feel very uncomfortable having a male health care worker standing over them preparing to draw a blood specimen, and vice versa. It is particularly considerate if a phlebotomist recognizes this and responds accordingly. Again, respect for the patient's needs and dignity must be considered. Phlebotomists can practice having the sensation that someone is "too close for comfort" by using role reversal.

Negative Body Language and Distracting Behaviors

WANDERING EYES. When people roll their eyes upward, they convey the sense of being bored, inattentive, or unwilling to perform a duty. Because this behavior is distracting, it should be avoided when a phlebotomist is communicating with, listening to, or observing patients, coworkers, or supervisors.

The same can be said about gazing out the window or looking up at the ceiling. If a phlebotomist enters a patient's room and begins addressing the patient while looking out the window, the patient will feel neglected, and the phlebotomist will appear unconcerned. If

Figure 1–5. Examples of Negative Body Language

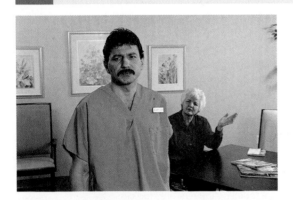
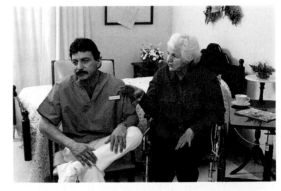
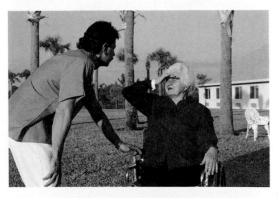
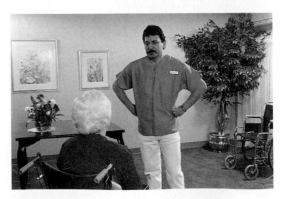

Identify the barriers to effective communication.

the window is too tempting to avoid a glance at, the phlebotomist can include the patient in his or her observations. A friendly comment about the weather might be appropriate; then the phlebotomy procedure can be continued when full attention can be given to the patient. The objective is to make the patient feel at ease through good communication techniques so that the procedure can be successful.

NERVOUS BEHAVIORS.   Behaviors such as squirming or tapping a pencil or a foot can be very distracting. They can make a patient feel nervous, hurried, or anxious about the venipuncture. A calm and confident image maximizes the patient's comfort and trust. It is also helpful to recognize these behaviors in patients, especially children, so that efforts can be made to reduce fear. Allowing a few extra moments of conversation or preparation may help.

BREATHING PATTERN.   A deep sigh can convey a feeling of being bored or a reluctance to do the job. Phlebotomists should avoid sighing, especially when communicating with an angry, uncooperative patient. Likewise, if a patient sighs deeply or moans at the mere sight of the phlebotomist, this should be a cue that a little extra attention, conversation, or a smile might ease the patient's reluctance for the procedure.

OTHER DISTRACTING BEHAVIORS.   Many other actions can convey negative or defensive emotions. Among these are crossed arms, a wrinkled forehead, frequent glances at a clock or watch, rapid thumbing through papers, chewing gum, yawning, or stretching. Health care workers should realize that these behaviors can detract from their professional image when they are communicating with patients, families, visitors, coworkers, and supervisors. It is also important to realize what these cues mean if a patient exhibits them. Regular in-services or continuing education programs can be directed at reminding phlebotomists to be aware of positive and negative body language, both in their own behavior and that of patients.

ACTIVE LISTENING

Another component of effective communication is the art of listening. Active listening helps close the communication loop by ensuring that the message sent can indeed be repeated and understood. Listening skills do not depend on intellect or educational background; they can be learned and practiced. Table 1–6 provides tips for becoming an active listener.

Listening carefully to the patient can have important ramifications in the test results. For example, the nursing staff may have instructed the inpatient that he or she will be fasting or will have "nothing by mouth" until after the early morning blood collections. The phlebotomist should listen to patients' comments, such as, "I didn't have breakfast yet," and "they won't feed me." Even a question or comment about food may inspire a response to confirm that the patient was truly fasting. When in doubt, the phlebotomist can confirm that the patient has been fasting by simply asking the patient if they have eaten or had anything to drink other than water.

APPEARANCE, GROOMING, AND PHYSICAL FITNESS
Posture

Phlebotomists usually perform their work while standing. There are occasions, however, particularly with ambulatory patients, when it is more effective to sit adjacent to the patient for the blood collection procedure. Erect posture conveys a sense of confidence and pride in job performance. Slouching conveys a sense of laziness and apathy. Good posture is

TABLE 1–6.   Steps for Active Listening

The following steps are presented as a starting point for the development of listening skills by health care workers. Because individuals can mentally process words faster than they can speak them, a good listener must concentrate and focus on the speaker to keep his or her mind from wandering. Development of these skills can help an individual in professional life as well as in personal life.

Get ready	Concentrate on the speaker by "getting ready" to listen. Take a moment to clear your mind of distracting thoughts. Begin the interaction with an open, objective mind. Sometimes taking a deep breath can help clear your mind and prepare it to receive more information.
Pause occasionally	Use silent pauses in the conversation wisely to mentally summarize what has been said.
Verify that you are listening	Let the speaker know that someone is listening by using simple phrases, such as "I see," "Oh," "Very interesting," and "How about that," to reassure the speaker and communicate understanding and acceptance.
Avoid making hasty judgments	Keep personal judgments to yourself until the speaker finishes relaying his or her idea. Listen for true meaning in the message, not just the literal words.
Provide feedback	Verify the conversation with feedback. Make sure that everything was clear to the receiver. Ask for more explanation if necessary. Mentally review the key words to summarize the overall idea being communicated. Paraphrase the idea or conversation to ensure complete understanding.
Notice body language	Pay attention to body language and ask for clarification. Simple prompts, such as "You look sad," and "You seem upset or nervous," can add more meaning to the conversation and encourage the speaker to verbalize feelings.
Maintain eye contact	Eye contact communicates interest or concern.
Use encouragement	Encourage the listener to expand his or her thoughts by using simple phrases, such as "Let's discuss it further," "Tell me more about it," and "Really?"
Practice, practice, practice	Practice active listening at work and at home.

helpful for both the phlebotomist and the patient. It minimizes the health care worker's back and neck strain and eases the patient's mind about the confidence of the phlebotomist. Relaxed hands, arms, and shoulders enable the health care worker to work more freely and to show the patient how to relax their arms and shoulders as well.

Grooming and Personal Hygiene

Physical appearance communicates a strong impression about an individual. Neatly combed hair, clean fingernails, a clean, pressed uniform, protective garb, and an overall tidy appearance communicate a commitment to cleanliness and infection control, and they instill confidence in a person. This is particularly important in today's health care environment, where patients and employees are deeply concerned about the spread of infectious diseases. Employers of health care workers are legally required to provide personal protective equipment (PPE) or barrier protection for workers handling biohazardous, infectious substances. This type of garb includes gowns, gloves, masks, laboratory coats or aprons, and face shields. Due to latex sensitivities and allergies, employers must provide an array of sizes and styles of gloves and gowns in order to protect their employees. Careful compliance with safety standards minimizes the risk of occupational exposures to bloodborne pathogens. Safety considerations are covered in more detail in Chapter 5. A daily bath or shower followed by the use of deodorant is also recommended. Table 1–7 illustrates a dress code policy.

TABLE 1–7.   Sample of a Dress Code Policy

Purpose: Presenting a professional and positive image to all patients, customers, and members of the community is a goal of this health care organization. Professional dress, good grooming, and personal cleanliness are important aspects of the overall effectiveness and morale of all employees. To establish a standard appearance, the following guidelines will be enforced. Employees who appear inappropriately dressed or groomed will be sent home. Please note that these are minimum guidelines and that individual departments may have more rigid requirements due to safety, infection control, or patient preferences. Consult your supervisor regarding any questions you may have regarding these guidelines.

Identification	Name badges will be visibly worn at all times. Stickers, pins, or other types of tokens should not cover the employee or department name.
Daily Hygiene	Having clean teeth, hair, clothes, and body are basic daily requirements. Clean, wrinkle-free clothes, scrubs, or uniforms that are in good condition should be worn.
Hair	Hair should be clean, neat, and trimmed. Conservative styles are recommended. Well-groomed, closely trimmed beards, sideburns, and mustaches are allowed. Shoulder-length hair should be pulled back and secured.
Nails	Nails should be clean and neatly manicured, conservative in color of nail polish, and not more than ¼ inch past the fingertip. Artificial nails are not recommended.
Fragrances/Scents	Perfumes and fragrances can be offensive and/or nauseating to patients who are ill. It is recommended that the use of fragrances be minimized or eliminated.
Make-up	Make-up should be conservative and lightly applied. Extreme or excessive make-up is not allowed.
Clothing	Denim clothing of any type or style will not be allowed except on special occasions announced by the hospital administration. Tight-fitting clothing or clothes that are revealing or distracting are not permitted. Shirts should be buttoned up to the second button. Shirttails should be tucked in and T-shirts with logos or athletic prints will not be allowed. Proper undergarments should be worn at all times. Skirts and dresses should not be shorter than 3 inches above the knee. Shorts are not permitted. Pants/slacks should be worn with a belt if they have belt loops. Tight-fitting leggings are not permitted. It is recommended that male employees who are not involved in patient care wear ties.
Shoes	Shoes should be comfortable, safe in the work environment, clean, and polished. Consideration should be made to minimizing noise when walking. Socks and/or proper hosiery should be worn. Sandals and flip-flops are not permitted.
Jewelry	Excessive jewelry is not allowed. Since safety is a major concern, chains must be worn inside the collar, and long dangling earrings are not acceptable. Other types of exposed jewelry (facial piercings) may also pose hazards and/or may become irritated with the use of personal protective equipment, therefore they are not recommended.

NUTRITION, REST, AND EXERCISE

The role of a health care worker requires physical stamina. Good health improves the health care worker's appearance, attitude, job performance, and ability to cope with stress. Appropriate eating habits, rest during lunch and break periods, and off-duty exercising are essential to an individual's well-being. Practicing a healthy lifestyle while on and off duty will facilitate a return to work with a refreshed and more productive attitude. In most health care environments, the pace is hectic, and overtime work is common. Therefore, it is also helpful to know how to deal with stress.

ROLE OF FAMILY, VISITORS, AND SIGNIFICANT OTHERS

Family members and friends of patients are often present when phlebotomists need to acquire specimens. It is important to realize that their presence can make the patient more secure and comfortable. Sometimes, however, families and visitors are much more difficult to deal with than the patients. They may make requests that are beyond the phlebotomist's scope of acceptable or authorized responsibilities, and it is better then to inform the appropriate health care team member of the family member's request. If several visitors are in the hospital room with the patient, they may be asked to step into the hall while the blood specimen is being drawn. If the health care worker believes that assistance is required (to give emotional support, etc.) and the patient agrees, a family member may be asked to stay during the procedure. Children should be accompanied by a parent or guardian. This can make the family members feel helpful and provides reassurance to patients.

Physicians, priests, and chaplains have the right to visit privately with patients. Unless the blood specimen is "timed," the health care worker should respect that privacy and return to the patient after completing the other draws in the unit or area. If the procedure is timed or STAT, the health care worker can apologize for the interruption, explain the nature of the request, and ask permission to collect the specimen.

Families and visitors of patients except for parents of pediatric patients should not be permitted in the clinical laboratory or provided with patient information, except by prior arrangement and permission of the patient. The patient's privacy and safety and the confidentiality of patient records must be considered.

Box 1–17   Tips for Dealing with Stress

Find time for privacy.

Plan rest/relaxation periods (short naps, meditate, listen to relaxing music, read poetry, yoga).

Associate with gentle people and share feelings with them.

Devote time to physical exercise (10 minutes at three different times a day is better than none).

Eat more nutritious foods (Imagine your plate with 50% vegetables/fruits, 25% protein, and 25% carbohydrates).

Engage in satisfying hobbies and social activities.

Rearrange your schedule to make it work more effectively.

Keep a journal.

Read interesting books and articles to get new ideas.

■■■■ QUALITY IMPROVEMENT AND ASSESSMENT

PERCEPTIONS OF QUALITY

Stakeholders are individuals, groups, organizations, or communities that have an interest in, or are influenced by, the quality of health care services. Stakeholders are also considered to be "customers." Internal stakeholders are individuals or groups within a health care organization itself; external stakeholders are individuals or groups outside the organization.

Health care workers, including phlebotomists themselves, are concerned about the quality of their work as evidenced by the following:

- Educational programs have been established to teach basic skills.
- Certification examinations have been implemented to certify basic knowledge.
- Associations have been established to voice and publicize the issues related to phlebotomy practice.
- Codes of ethics have been designed.
- Competencies have been identified.

The concept of "quality" can be described in a variety of ways. Scientific or technical aspects of care entail how well clinical skills are applied to the situation; for example, whether the correct procedures and therapies are used for the patient. The nontechnical or interpersonal aspects of care involve how well the personal needs of the patient are satisfied; for example, whether communication skills are adequate, the services convenient and timely, the patients

---

Box 1–18	Examples of Stakeholders (Customers) in Health Care

External stakeholders (outside the health care organization)

- Local community
- Insurance companies that pay for services
- Employers who pay for services for their employees
- Grant agencies and/or foundations that provide funding
- Federal agencies—OSHA, CDC, etc.
- State agencies
- Accrediting agencies—JCAHO, CAP
- Advocacy groups—AARP

Internal stakeholders (within the health care organization and/or specimen collection services)

- Inpatients and outpatients
- Patient's families and friends
- Patient's support groups
- Blood donors
- Clinical laboratory staff
- Secretaries and clerks
- Pathologists
- Nurses
- Administrators
- Students
- Research staff
- Volunteers

satisfied with the comfort and safety of the environment, and the health care workers professional and careful.[4] Another way to describe quality in health care uses three major concepts: efficacy—the health care services provided have a positive impact on the patient's health, that is, the health outcome is that the patient improves or gets well; appropriateness—procedures performed on the patient were the correct ones for that particular condition or illness; and caring functions—services provided to the patient are available, timely, effective, safe, efficient, respectful, and sensitive to the patient's needs. The quality of phlebotomy services focuses not only on meeting a minimum standard but also on the processes and assessments to constantly improve the services that are provided to customers.

Quality improvement efforts for phlebotomy services often involve evaluating the following:

- The health care worker's technique
- Complications such as hematomas
- Recollection rates resulting from contamination
- Multiple sticks on the same patient

All these issues have the potential to result in a negative outcome for the patient. Thus, continuous improvement in minimizing these problems would be most beneficial to the patient and the health care worker.

Box 1-19	Components of a Quality Plan for Phlebotomy Services

Factors related to structure—Physical or organizational properties of the settings where care is provided. Assessments of structural components include:

- **Physical structure**—Facilities where services are provided, adequacy of supplies and equipment, safety devices, safety procedures, and availability and condition of equipment, e.g., computers, sterilizers, refrigerators, thermometers, centrifuges, autoclaves, and glucose-monitoring devices.
- **Personnel structure**—Adequate numbers of personnel and support staff, ratios of staff to patients, qualifications of staff, and availability of the medical director or supervisors.
- **Management or administrative structure**—Updated, available procedure manuals, adequacy of systems for secure record keeping, and open lines of communication throughout the organization.

Quality assessments of structural components may reveal potential problems that other assessments cannot. For example, the use of outdated blood collection tubes may cause faulty laboratory test results, even though the blood collection, testing, and reporting processes are perfect and the treatment plan for the patient is appropriate.

Assessment of processes—what is done to the patient or client. Process assessments are common throughout the specimen collection and clinical testing arenas and include procedures and skill assessment. This is where traditional quality control (QC) measures are applicable. In addition to the normal laboratory data collection routines, however, other methods are effective for monitoring processes. These include evaluation of patient records for complications, correct technical skills, and correct documentation procedures; direct observation of practices; videotaping of health care interactions and practices; patient interviews; and questionnaires.

Assessments of outcomes—what is accomplished for the patient. Most outcomes assessments rely on information in the patient's medical record. Chart reviews usually evaluate the health status after services are provided. Timing is usually an important component of these measures. Outcomes assessments are typically the most difficult to measure and often relate to recovery rates, nosocomial infection rates, return to normal functions, and so on. Poor patient outcomes have been described as the "5 Ds": death, disease, disability, discomfort, dissatisfaction.

Clinical Alert

Unfortunately, phlebotomists can have a negative impact on quality. For example, misidentification of a patient can result in an erroneous cross-match and blood transfusion, which could be fatal to a patient (death). Inappropriate cleansing techniques or hand washing could result in transmitting nosocomial infections (hospital-acquired disease). Poor venipuncture techniques, such as improper needle insertion or excessive probing, could result in nerve damage (disability) or severe pain (discomfort). And lengthy waiting times, rude behavior, or messy work sites can contribute to an overall feeling of patient dissatisfaction.

CUSTOMER SATISFACTION

The study of satisfaction among patients and health care workers is usually accomplished by using questionnaires, mail-outs, and telephone or personal interviews. Although the information gathered using these techniques may be subjective, knowing why customers are dissatisfied and which customers are unhappy is extremely valuable. This information can be used to improve targeted services or aspects of a service.

TOOLS AND TRENDS FOR PERFORMANCE ASSESSMENT

In a laboratory, check sheets, run charts, and statistical tests can be used to review both the analytic and nonanalytic parts of the laboratory. In an analytic sense, clinical laboratory scientists and technicians use data collection to ensure test sensitivity, specificity, precision, and accuracy. In a nonanalytic sense, data can be used to assess the timeliness of responses to requests, turnaround time for reporting test results, and effective communication. Tools for implementing **continuous quality improvement** (CQI) include the following:[3]

- **Flowcharts.** Useful for breaking a process into its components so that people can understand how it works (refer to Figure 1–6 ■).
- **Pareto charts.** Bar charts that show the frequency of problematic events; the Pareto principle says that "80 percent of the trouble comes from 20 percent of the problems" (refer to Figure 1–7 ■).
- **Cause-and-effect (Ishikawa) diagrams.** Diagrams that identify interactions between equipment, methods, people, supplies, and reagents (Figure 1–8 ■).
- **Plan-Do-Check-Act cycle (PDCA).** A cycle for assessing and making positive changes, then reassessing.
- **Line graphs, histograms, scatter diagrams.** Pictorial images representing performance trends.
- **Brainstorming.** Method used to stimulate creative solutions in a group.

There are many varied strategies for assessing performance of laboratories, most of which are highly effective. The phlebotomist should be a routine part of quality and performance assessments.

Figure 1–6. Flowchart

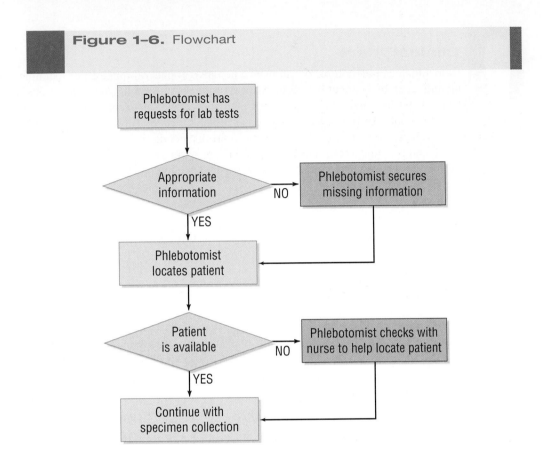

Flowcharts demonstrate steps in a process.

QUALITY IN SPECIMEN COLLECTION SERVICES

Phlebotomists can consider the clinical laboratory testing process in several phases, with the primary goal of specimen collection being to obtain an accurate sample for analysis. Many variables exist, however, before the specimen is actually analyzed. Preanalytic, analytic, and postanalytic phases in specimen collection, processing, and testing are part of every laboratory's operation. For purposes of this text, the quality assessment discussion focuses on the preanalytic phases, where the phlebotomist has the most impact. Analytic and postanalytic phases involve rigorous quality control procedures and other types of quality assessment procedures, including proficiency testing using specimens from outside approved sources and periodic inspections from authorized agencies. Box 1–21 summarizes the phases in specimen collection and processing, and Box 1–22 indicates examples of preanalytic processes that are subject to quality reviews and monitoring. A monthly review of the laboratory's collection procedures and policies is recommended to reduce collection errors. The clinical laboratory should also provide the nursing staff with a floor book (online or paper version) that describes laboratory services, preparation of the patient, and special handling of patients' specimens. In

Figure 1–7. Pareto Chart

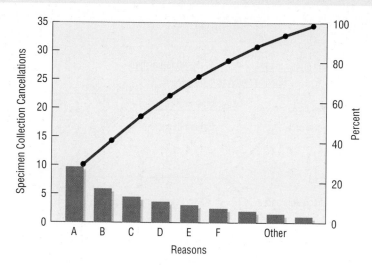

Pareto charts tally the number of times each specified problem occurs. Letters across the bottom indicate reasons for cancellations, e.g., the patient was unavailable, supplies were not accessible, documentation was not complete, etc.

addition, the phlebotomist should have access to a pocket-sized collection booklet or ready access to online information that contains the same information as found in the floor book, along with other useful information for specimen handling, transporting, and processing.

IMPORTANT FACTORS AFFECTING QUALITY

Anticoagulants and Preservatives

Phlebotomists use anticoagulants and preservatives in the collection of blood specimens. (A more thorough discussion is presented in Chapters 7 and 9.) Phlebotomists are responsible for filling the tubes in the correct order so that carryover of anticoagulants to other tubes will not occur and for mixing the specimens with the anticoagulant promptly after blood is drawn. The anticoagulants and preservatives used must also meet requirements established by the National Committee for Clinical Laboratory Standards (NCCLS). The manufacturer of the anticoagulants and preservatives must provide the shelf life or expiration date of these additives on the packages so that the user will know how long these additives are effective. When restocking the supply of collection tubes, phlebotomists should place the tubes with a shelf life (expiration date) nearest the current date at the front of the shelf so that these tubes are used first. Manufacturers of collection tubes must test and verify draw and fill accuracy until the stated expiration date. The health care worker should be cognizant of expiration dates on any item used in specimen collection. Accreditation standards require health care institutions to establish procedures for proper inspection of new lot numbers of evacuated blood collection tubes. In addition, quality can be obtained in specimen collection only with fresh specimens. If the blood specimen is not to be tested immediately, the health care worker must make certain that it is preserved and stored properly until the analysis can be performed.

Figure 1-8. Cause-and-Effect Diagram

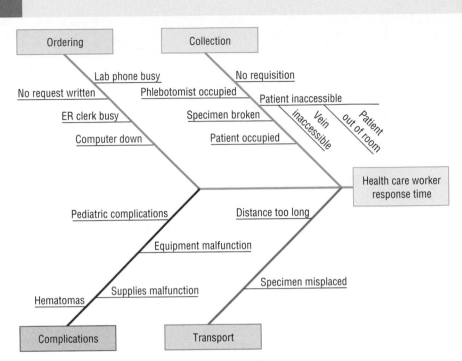

Cause-and-effect diagrams demonstrate interactions or factors that influence an outcome. For example, this cause-and-effect diagram demonstrates the issues affecting response time.

Number of Blood Collection Attempts

Another way to provide quality services to patients is by monitoring and reducing the number of unsuccessful collection attempts. If the phlebotomist has had consecutively unsuccessful phlebotomy attempts on different patients, the problem in the blood collection technique must be identified and solved to prevent harm to patients.

| Box 1-20 | Brainstorming Exercise |

This exercise can be used in groups of no more than three or four people or by individuals. Groups are preferred because they tend to come up with a greater number and more creative ideas.

One group should take the viewpoint of a new phlebotomist and the other group should take the viewpoint of the patient. (There are no "wrong" answers!)

Consider the idea of "excellence" or "perfection" in a phlebotomy encounter. What factors are important from your point of view? List/discuss as many and all ideas as you can in about 10 minutes.

Next, come to a consensus about the order of importance of the factors. Make sure everyone in the group has a chance to participate and give their opinions about the order of importance. Compare and discuss the lists from each group's viewpoint.

Box 1-21   Examples of Preanalytic, Analytic, and Postanalytic Factors in the Phases of Specimen Collection, Processing, Testing, and Reporting

Even though clinical laboratories differ in their operating procedures, the nature of their services include the phases listed below. Phlebotomists have the greatest impact on laboratory testing in the preanalytic phases. These variables are discussed in greater detail throughout this text.

Preanalytic Phase outside the Laboratory

Patient identification and information

Isolation techniques

Universal precautions

Correct venipuncture or skin puncture technique

Appropriate use of supplies and equipment

Appropriate transportation and handling

Preanalytic Phase inside the Laboratory

Sample treatment

Specimen registration and distribution

Centrifugation

Identification of aliquots

Appropriate storage

Analytic Phase

Testing the specimen

Postanalytic Phase

Reporting results

Appropriate follow-up or repeat testing

Box 1-22   Continuous Quality Improvement Assessments for Specimen Collection Services

- Health care worker response time (for inpatients).
- Patient waiting time (for outpatients).
- Time required for completion of the phlebotomy procedure.
- Percentage of successful blood collections taken on the first attempt.
- Number of successful blood collections on the second attempt.
- Volume of daily blood loss per patient due to venipunctures.
- Number and size of hematomas.
- Number of patients who faint.
- Amount of time spent and number of telephone calls needed to acquire appropriate identification.
- Number of redraws requested because of inadequate specimens.
- Contribution of health care worker to turnaround times of designated laboratory tests.
- Number of incomplete forms, documents, logs, and so forth.
- Number of therapeutic drug-monitoring tests that have incorrect documentation or timing.
- Number of specimens received in incorrect tubes.
- Contamination rate for blood cultures.
- Results of patient satisfaction questionnaires or focus groups.
- Frequency of complaints

Blood Loss Due to Phlebotomy

For adults, blood loss due to venipuncture is usually well tolerated physiologically because the volume constitutes a small percentage of the total blood volume in the body. However, in some cases, patients are very ill and need to be closely monitored, so the frequency of blood collection and volumes needed may increase to a clinically significant level. Patients in intensive care units, those with arterial lines, and those with poor prognoses tend to have more total blood collected and more often. The same is true for neonates and infants where even a small volume of blood may represent a large portion of the total blood volume. In these cases phlebotomists must realize that blood conservation is a priority to avoid anemia and other complications.

EQUIPMENT AND PREVENTIVE MAINTENANCE

Phlebotomists may also participate in quality control checks and preventive maintenance of laboratory instruments including thermometers, sphygmomanometers (blood pressure cuffs), and centrifuges. For example, a centrifuge that is used to "spin down" the blood must be checked for accurate speed.

In summary, the basic requirements for a *quality* specimen include the following:

1. Using universal standard precautions, the patient is identified, assessed, and prepared properly, and medication interference is avoided if possible.
2. Collecting specimens from the correct patients and labeling appropriately. Because the policy of most clinical laboratories is to discard specimens that are unlabeled or labeled incorrectly, the health care worker must abide by the written laboratory policy describing acceptable identification of specimens. The potential errors in after-the-fact reidentification of a specimen by floor personnel can be extremely detrimental to the patient in question and must be avoided. (See Chapter 9 for identification and labeling procedures.)
3. Using correct anticoagulants and preservatives with a sufficient amount of blood collected. Devices that minimize needle sticks should be used.
4. Specimens should be handled carefully so as not cause damage and/or hemolysis.
5. Fasting specimens should be collected in a timely fashion and should actually be fasting samples. If they are not, the condition should be noted.
6. Timed specimens should be correctly timed and documented.

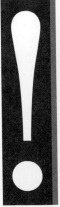

Clinical Alert: Inability to Collect a Blood Specimen

Clinical laboratories should have a written procedure on the inability to draw specimens that describes the steps that should be taken by the phlebotomist when (1) collection attempts are unsuccessful (no more than two sticks), (2) the patient is unavailable, or (3) the patient refuses to have blood drawn.

Box 1–23   Why Does the Laboratory Need So Much Blood for Testing?

In the laboratory, analytical variables that influence minimum blood volume requirements include the following:

- Analytical instruments require a minimum volume to aspirate for testing
- Analytical instruments may require a standard test tube size to function automatically
- Special handling procedures for separating plasma or serum into sample aliquots for testing in different areas of the laboratory or for sending to a reference laboratory
- Repeat testing after a quality control failure
- Add-on testing ordered by a physician after the initial specimen is drawn
- Volume requirements by the tube manufacturers to ensure adequate dilution with an anticoagulant or other additive

Strategies to reduce phlebotomy volume losses usually focus on organizing and coordinating blood draws. More specifically, phlebotomists can have an impact by assisting with the following:[5]

- Coordinating all requests into a single phlebotomy event daily or by shift
- Schedule blood draws on a regular and frequent basis to eliminate the need for random STAT requests
- Ask for a review of duplicate requests for tests that are already pending
- Maintain a daily tally of blood loss in the cases where it is clinically indicated and for neonates
- Suggest a review of standing orders that may no longer be needed because the patient has improved
- Assist the laboratory in reducing turnaround time for test results through efficient, accurate, and timely preanalytical processes

---

7. Specimens without anticoagulants should be allowed to stand a minimum of 30 minutes so that clot formation can be completed. (Gel separator tubes, depending upon the manufacturer, may shorten the time of clot formation.)
8. Specimens should be transported to the clinical laboratory in a timely fashion (within 45 minutes) to maintain freshness. A list of the specimens that are delivered after the designated time limits should be documented so as to help detect the source of the problem if needed.

All phlebotomists should aspire to provide the highest quality patient specimens in a professional and safe environment 100 percent of the time.

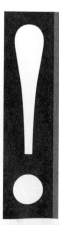

Clinical Alert

If too much blood is withdrawn in a short period of time, a patient may require a blood transfusion. Therefore it is important to monitor daily blood loss if patients are neonates, have poor prognoses, or are being tested frequently. In these cases, the use of smaller test tubes and/or microcollection techniques might be warranted.

KEY TERMS

active listening

acute care

ambulatory care

American Hospital Association (AHA)

American Nurses Association (ANA)

American Society for Clinical
  Laboratory Science (ASCLS)

American Society for Clinical Pathology
  (ASCP)

anatomic pathology

Clinical Laboratory Improvement
  Amendments of 1988 (CLIA 1988)

clinical pathology

competency statement

culture

home health care services

inpatients

long-term care

Medicaid

Medicare

National Phlebotomy Association
  (NPA)

nosocomial infections

Patient's Bill of Rights

personal protective equipment (PPE)

phlebotomist

physician's office laboratories (POLs)

point-of-care

quality

zone of comfort

STUDY QUESTIONS

The following questions may have more than one answer.

1. Which of the following are common categorizations for health care organizations?
   a. ambulatory care
   b. anatomical pathology
   c. inpatient care
   d. clinical care

2. Examples of nonverbal, distracting behaviors include which of the following:
   a. chewing gum
   b. gazing outside the window
   c. direct eye contact
   d. glancing at the clock

3. Which of the following statement(s) is inappropriate during a phlebotomy procedure?
   a. "This won't hurt a bit!"
   b. "Your name is Mrs. Jones, isn't it?"
   c. "You are required to cooperate
      with this."
   d. "Could you please spell your last
      name for me?"

4. Which of the following are key elements in effective communication?
   a. active listening
   b. nonverbal cues
   c. verbal skills
   d. point-of-care procedures

5. Which of the following is the main area of responsibility for every phlebotomist?
   a. analytic testing
   b. data collection
   c. reporting results
   d. preanalytic processes

6. Slouching posture, a nonverbal behavior, conveys what message?
   a. confidence
   b. pride
   c. laziness
   d. apathy

7. What feelings does one experience when a stranger gets "too close for comfort"?
   a. anxiety
   b. fear
   c. confidence
   d. security

8. Hospitals differ according to which of the following?
   a. bed size
   b. length of stay
   c. mission
   d. ownership

9. Culture is composed of which of the following aspects?
   a. beliefs
   b. spirituality
   c. traditions
   d. values

10. Why is the attention to grooming and personal hygiene important for phlebotomists?
    a. provides a professional appearance
    b. cleanliness reduces the spread of infections
    c. keeps employees looking stylish
    d. provides a safer work environment

11. Of the following, which are examples of customers for phlebotomy services?
    a. outpatients
    b. patient's family members
    c. attending physicians
    d. nursing staff

12. Examples of unfavorable patient outcomes include which of the following?
    a. excessive probing for a vein
    b. multiple sticks on the same patient
    c. nosocomial infections
    d. hematomas

13. Which of the following are examples of process components of quality that should be checked?
    a. documentation procedures
    b. hematomas
    c. multiple sticks
    d. use of incorrect anticoagulants

References

1. Wright, D: *The Ultimate Guide to Competency Assessment in Healthcare,* 2nd ed. Minneapolis, MN: Creative Healthcare Management, 1998.

2. Johnson, DW, Johnson, RT: *Joining Together, Group Theory and Group Skills,* 6th ed. Boston: Allyn & Bacon, 2000.

3. Luckman, J: *Transcultural Communication in Health Care.* Albany, NY: Delmar, 2000.

4. Graham, NO: *Quality in Health Care: Theory, Applications, and Evolution.* Gaithersburg, MD: Aspen Publishers, 1995.

5. McPherson, RA: Blood sample volumes: Emerging trends in clinical practice and laboratory medicine. *Clin Leader Manage Rev,* Jan/Feb 2001; 3–10.

Ethical, Legal, and Regulatory Issues

2

CHAPTER OBJECTIVES

Upon completion of Chapter 2, the learner is responsible for the following:

1. Define basic ethical and legal terms and explain how they differ.
2. Describe the basic functions of the medical record.
3. Define **informed consent.**
4. Describe how to avoid litigation as it relates to blood collection.
5. Identify key elements of the Health Insurance Portability and Accountability Act (HIPAA).

 MediaLINK

Access the accompanying CD-ROM to explore a wide variety of review questions and interactive activities for this chapter, including multiple choice, true/false, and video exercises.

The topics of law, ethics, and bioethics are all interrelated and difficult to discuss without referring to one another.

- "Laws are societal rules or regulations that are advisable or obligatory to observe. Laws protect the welfare and safety of society, resolve conflicts in an orderly and nonviolent manner, and constantly evolve in accordance with an increasingly pluralistic society."[1]
- Ethics are the moral standards of behavior or conduct that govern an individual's actions. Bioethics (*bio* refers to life) are the moral issues or problems that have resulted because of modern medicine, clinical research, and/or technology. Usually, bioethics refers to "life-and-death" issues such as abortion, when a patient should be allowed to die, and who receives organ donations.

ETHICS OVERVIEW

All health care workers are faced with ethical decisions at one time or another. Each individual should reflect on their own standards of behavior and those of their professional affiliations. The simple set of questions listed below can serve as an "ethics check" for individuals facing an ethical dilemma or decision. To evaluate a difficult situation it involves simply asking oneself:[1]

- Is this legal and does it comply with institutional policy?
- Does it foster a "win-win" situation with the patient/supervisor or other individuals?
- How would I feel about myself if I read about this decision in the newspaper? How would my family feel?
- Can I live with myself after making this decision?
- Is it right?

Box 2-1   Example of Ethical Behavior for a Phlebotomist

If the phlebotomist realizes that he or she has made a mistake in identifying a patient and specimens, the phlebotomist faces an ethical decision about whether or not to report his/her own mistake. Reporting it may result in disciplinary action against him or her.

- Each phlebotomist should go through the ethics check questions to see that the right ethical decision would be to report his or her own mistake as soon as possible in order to avoid any clinical and/or treatment decisions based on the wrong test results.
- This is the right decision because it complies with policy, it fosters a "win-win" situation for the patient and doctor, the alternative would be embarrassing to see reported in the newspaper, and above all, it is just the right thing to do. In addition, legal risk is minimized for the phlebotomist and the health care facility if the error is appropriately corrected and documented.

GOVERNMENTAL LAWS

The legislative, executive, and judicial branches of government control laws. The legislative written laws are called statutes and are made at the federal, state, and county levels. The executive branch makes administrative laws, and the judicial branch establishes case law that is based on legal cases from lower-level judicial branches.

■■■■■ BASIC LEGAL PRINCIPLES

The laws governing medicine and medical ethics complement and overlap one another. For many years, even centuries, the decision of the physician or health care professional was unquestioned. This has changed. Health care consumers and patients have become more aware, more critical, and much more willing to sue anyone that their lawyer believes has been at fault, including health care workers who are collecting blood specimens.

LEGAL TERMINOLOGY

If a health care worker understands basic legal concepts, this understanding can help to define how personnel involved in the specimen collection process can be liable for activities that may occur in this field of health care. Such understanding can also reduce the conflicts between law and the health care workers.

Liability for the lack of a proper standard of health care may be imposed on any health care worker, including health care institutions, physicians, nurses, laboratorians, patient care technicians, and phlebotomists. The number of substantial awards against health care workers as a result of improper care has grown in recent years as patients have become more sensitive to treatment complications.

To grasp the legal implication of health care, the health care provider must have some knowledge of basic legal terminology. A few major definitions with health care examples can be found in Box 2–2.

NEGLIGENCE

In the past decade, the number of legal cases in which the laboratory has been directly or indirectly involved has increased noticeably. Negligence is "a violation of a duty to exercise reasonable skill and care in performing a task."[2]

Four factors, or key points, must be considered in alleged negligence cases.[2]

1. **Duty**—relates to what duties or responsibilities the hospital or health care worker had toward the patient; it also includes all the individuals who had a duty toward the patient to use the appropriate standard of care.
2. **Breach of duty**—relates to whether the duty was breached and if it was avoidable. The plaintiff must be able to show what actually happened and that the defendant acted unreasonably.
3. **Proximate causation**—relates to whether the breach of duty actually contributed to or caused injury; also concerns all the parties involved in contributing to the alleged injury. There must be a direct line from the conduct to the injury.
4. **Damages**—relates to whether the plaintiff was actually injured and when these injuries were discovered. Once negligence and causation are established, plaintiffs must be able to show that they were actually damaged by the negligent act.

Many circumstances could be considered negligence if health care workers are not extremely careful. For example, there have been legal cases in which the confusion of patient samples led to a patient's death.[3]

Box 2-2   Legal Terminology

- **Assault.** The unjustifiable attempt to touch another person or the threat to do so in such circumstances as to cause the other to believe that it will be carried out, or to cause fear. An assault may be permissible if proper consent has been given (e.g., consent to obtain a blood specimen).
- **Battery.** The intentional touching of another person without consent; also, the unlawful beating of another or carrying out of threatened physical harm. Because battery always includes an assault, the two are commonly combined in the phrase *assault and battery*. Liability of hospitals, physicians, and other health care workers for acts of battery is most common in situations involving lack of or improper consent to medical procedures, such as blood collecting.
  - For example, a small boy who refused to have his blood drawn was locked in the blood collection room by the health care worker and was forced to have his blood drawn by the health care worker. The patient's parents sued and won.
  - If a patient is feeling stressed because of pain and not knowing what medical procedures will be occurring and a health care professional displays behavior in a threatening manner, this can lead to legal intervention. The health care worker must obviously avoid using threatening language (e.g., "If you don't let me collect your blood, your illness will probably become critical").
- **Breach (neglect) of duty.** An infraction, violation, or failure to perform.
- **Civil law.** Not a criminal action; the plaintiff sues for monetary damages.
- **Criminal actions.** Legal recourse for acts or offenses against the public welfare; these actions can lead to imprisonment of the offender.
- **Defendant.** The health care worker or institution against whom the action or lawsuit is filed.
- **False imprisonment.** The unjustifiable detention of a person without a legal warrant.
- **Felony.** Varies by state but generally is defined as public offenses; if the defendant is convicted, he or she will spend time in jail.
- **Liable.** Under legal obligation, as far as damages are concerned.
- **Litigation process.** The process of legal action to determine a decision in court. Many malpractice cases are negotiated and settled out of court.
- **Malice.** Knowing that a statement is false or making a statement with reckless disregard of the truth.
- **Malpractice.** Defined as professional negligence. Improper or unskillful care of a patient by a member of the health care team, or any professional misconduct or unreasonable lack of skill.
- **Misdemeanor.** The general term for all sorts of criminal offenses not serious enough to be classified as felonies.
- **Misrepresentation.** Use of misleading information or omission of important facts.
- **Negligence.** Failure to act or to perform duties according to the standards of the profession.
- **Plaintiff.** The claimant who brings a lawsuit or an action.
- **Respondeat superior.** Under this concept, supervisors and directors may be held liable for the negligent actions of their employees.
- **Subpoena.** Court order for a person and documents (e.g., phlebotomist and phlebotomy technical procedures) to be brought to court proceedings.
- **Tort.** A legal wrong for which one is liable for damages in civil action.

MALPRACTICE

Malpractice, or professional negligence, is defined as improper or unskillful care of a patient by a member of the health care team, or any professional misconduct or unreasonable lack of skill.

If the physician is the medical director overseeing clinical laboratory testing, in most cases he or she is responsible under the law for the standard of care and the performance of all aspects of laboratory testing. Therefore, a breach of standard on the part of the health care worker collecting blood for laboratory assays could place both the physician and the health care worker at risk.

PATIENT CONFIDENTIALITY

Negligence cases can also arise out of violation of the right to privacy or of patient confidentiality. "No one except the patient may release patient results without a clinical need to know." Patient or employee laboratory test results must be considered strictly confidential. Negligence can be claimed if employees' or patients' drug abuse test results are released to anyone other than the attending physician or other authorized individuals. This is particularly true regarding employee or athlete drug or alcohol abuse screening and human immunodeficiency virus (HIV) testing. Confidential materials include communications between the physician and the patient, the patient's verbal statements, medical computer entries on patients, and nonverbal communications, such as laboratory test results.

CONFIDENTIALITY AND HIV EXPOSURE

An increasing concern for health care workers collecting blood from patients who are homebound is the health care worker's rights in relation to accidental exposure to blood or body fluids, whether by a needle stick or some other means. In some states, laws allow health care workers to know the identity of a patient who has acquired immunodeficiency syndrome (AIDS) or who is HIV positive. Many states, however, do not provide for the easy acquisition of this sensitive patient information. A home health care worker who routinely collects blood specimens from homebound patients should obtain information on the state's law regarding confidentiality and HIV status.[4] It can be obtained from the health care worker's employer, from legal counsel, or from a national or state health professional organization.

It is important to use the proper blood collection techniques with safety precautions and required infection control procedures for homebound patients. If exposure to the blood occurs through a needle stick, a lancet, or another means, the home health care worker needs to be certain of obtaining the patient's HIV status and other potential infectious diseases (e.g., Hepatitis C) to ensure that the proper immediate and long-term self-protective procedural steps can be taken.

If employed by a health care facility, the health care worker should follow the guidelines established by the facility. If he or she is self-employed, it is important to monitor his or her own HIV status. Also, counseling should be sought to obtain emotional support during this stressful time.

STANDARD OF CARE

If a patient has suffered injury due to blood collection for laboratory testing, the patient must show that the health care worker who collected the blood failed to meet the prevailing standard of care. All health care workers must conform to a specific standard of care to protect patients. It is a measuring stick representing the conduct of the average health care worker in the community. The community has been expanded to be a national community as a result of national laboratory standards and requirements. Examples of setting the standard of care include statutes, licensing requirements, rules and regulations of regulatory or professional organizations (e.g., American Hospital Association, Joint Commission for Accreditation of Healthcare Organizations [JCAHO], etc.), internal health care facility rules and regulations, and professional publications.

INFORMED CONSENT

Informed consent is voluntary permission by a patient to allow touching, examination, and/or treatment by health care providers. It allows patients to determine what will be performed on or to their bodies. Without informed consent, intentional touching can be considered a criminal offense. In the health care environment, patients must be informed of the possible consequences of having or not having particular medical treatments. An informed consent form is then signed by the patient for approval of medical treatment(s), including blood collection. Integral to consent is the patient's belief that the health care worker to whom the consent is given has the knowledge, skills, and technical ability to perform such tasks. Thus, the patient can expect the blood collector to know the proper blood collection techniques and procedures.

INFORMED CONSENT FOR RESEARCH PURPOSES

Due to unethical treatment of humans in the past for research purposes, the United States passed a law in 1974, the National Research Act, which established Institutional Research Boards (IRBs) at institutions (e.g., hospitals, universities) that perform research. These IRBs were established to review and approve only those research proposals with research protocol that would protect the human subjects involved. The IRB ensures that human subjects do not bear any inappropriate risk and have properly consented to their involvement.

Frequently, in hospitals, health care facilities, and health science universities, health care workers become involved in collecting blood from research participants for research projects. The National Research Act states that any research project utilizing human subjects requires the informed consent of those subjects. In order to collect blood for a research project, the participant must understand the nature of the research study and the risks and benefits involved if they are to make an informed decision about their participation.

Clinical Alert

- Minors must have the informed consent of their parents or legal guardians for medical care, including blood collections.
- Since language can be a barrier to informed consent, an interpreter may be necessary so that information for consent may be given in the native tongue.
- States have enacted legislation requiring that informed consent be obtained before most HIV specimen collection and testing is performed. The statutes indicate the type of information that must be given for the patient to be considered informed. This information includes:
  - An explanation of the test;
  - Potential uses of the HIV test; and
  - Testing limitations and the meaning of its results

Box 2-3   Informed Consent

Informed consent for research requires a "consent document" that:

- Explains the nature of the research and any risks (e.g., blood collection problems) and benefits to the participant
- Describes the level of confidentiality of the research data
- Describes the measures that the researcher will take to ensure that confidentiality is maintained

---

This information must be presented and signed by the participant in the research before any blood collection can occur for the research activities. In addition, working as a blood collector in the research project requires attending a course on the protection of human subjects in research projects.

IMPLIED CONSENT

Implied consent exists when immediate action is required to save a patient's life or to prevent permanent impairment of the patient's health. In other words, an emergency removes the need for consent. Implied consent differs legally from one state to another. Health care providers need to know the legal boundaries of implied consent because they someday may need to decide whether to perform a vital emergency procedure (e.g., cardiopulmonary resuscitation).

STATUTE OF LIMITATIONS

The statute of limitations is a law that defines how soon after an injury (e.g., due to malpractice) a plaintiff must file the lawsuit or be forever barred from doing so. The purpose of this law is to prevent the threat of a lawsuit from hanging over a possible defendant's (e.g., health care worker's) head forever and to force legal action while memories are fresh, records are available, and witnesses are still living.

Box 2-4   Statute of Limitations

The statute of limitations for professional negligence in most states is 2 years. A complete and accurate medical record with laboratory testing results is the best defense in these cases because the attending physician and health care workers for the patient may have little recollection of the events in question.

◼◼◼◼ LEGAL CLAIMS AND DEFENSE

In a malpractice lawsuit, the first statement of a case by the plaintiff(s) against the defendant(s) is the complaint. It states a cause of action, notifying the defendant(s) of the reason for the lawsuit (Figure 2–1 ◼).

A health care worker who receives a summons to provide a deposition before a trial and/or testimony during a trial for a lawsuit will find the following guidelines helpful:

- Answer only the questions asked.
- Be organized in your recollection of the facts regarding the incident.
- Do not be antagonistic in answering the questions.
- Explain the laboratory and/or blood collection procedures and policies in simple terminology for the jury.
- Do not overdramatize the facts that you are presenting.
- Dress neatly and be groomed appropriately.
- Be polite, sincere, and courteous.
- Be sure to ask for clarification of questions that you did not clearly hear and questions that you did not understand.
- If you are not sure of an answer, indicate that you do not know the answer or that you are not sure.
- Above all, be truthful.

EXPERT WITNESS

Expert testimony, as well as scientific or medical data, is sometimes used to assist in establishing the standard of care required in any given situation. An expert witness may be used to assist a plaintiff in proving the wrongful act of a defendant or to assist a defendant in refuting such evidence. At the time of testifying, each expert's training, experience, and special qualifications will be explained during the deposition and later to the jury during the trial.

EVIDENCE

Evidence during the trial is used to prove or disprove the lawsuit. Evidence must be competent, relevant, and material. It may include such items as vacuum tubes and tube holders, needles, safety apparatuses such as biohazardous waste containers, infection control logs and reports, JCAHO standards, board certification standards for health care workers, and laboratory policies and procedures.

Box 2-5   Procedures for a Malpractice Lawsuit

Several steps follow the beginning of a malpractice lawsuit:

- If the case is not dismissed before trial, the parties to a lawsuit have the right to discovery—to examine the witnesses before the trial. Examination before trial is a method used to enable the plaintiff(s) and defendant(s) to learn more regarding the nature and substance of each other's case.
- This discovery process consists of oral testimony under oath and includes cross-examination by the lawyers.
- The deposition is the testimony of a witness that has been recorded in a written legal format. Either party in the lawsuit—plaintiff or defendant—may obtain a court order permitting examination and copying of laboratory reports, incident reports from personnel files, medical records, phlebotomy and laboratory policies and procedures, training manuals and so forth, and other facts and information that may help in the discovery.
- In addition to the deposition, the parties may undergo cross-examination at the time of the trial. They will provide testimony regarding the cause for the case that will be recorded and filed with the court.

Figure 2-1. Giving Testimony in a Lawsuit

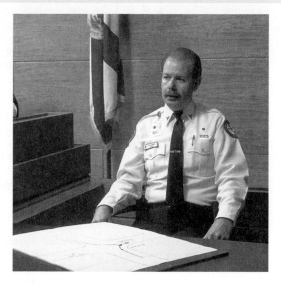

Being involved in a lawsuit can be very unsettling for both the plaintiff and defendant.

ADVICE TO AVOID LAWSUITS

Justice is expensive in the United States. Lawyers' fees typically range from $200 to $600 per hour, and associated costs can lead to thousands of dollars in legal fees. Also, legal proceedings are time consuming, expensive, and most of all, emotionally devastating to both the plaintiff(s) and the defendant(s). Thus, to avoid a malpractice lawsuit, the health care provider should heed the advice in Box 2–6.

RESPONDEAT SUPERIOR

Respondeat superior (a Latin term meaning "let the master answer") is a legal doctrine that holds employers responsible for acts of their employees within the scope of the employment relationship. Not only may the injured party sue the employee directly, but the employer, if sued, may also seek indemnification from the employee. Indemnification is compensation for the financial loss suffered from the employee's act.

▬▬▬ MEDICAL RECORDS

Medical records are vital. A health care worker cannot be expected to remember a patient from whom blood was drawn three to four years ago. The medical records must be neat, legible, and accurate. They are extremely important if a medical malpractice case goes to court.

Medical records are also used for nonmedical reasons that are not directly tied to medical services, such as billing, utilization review, quality improvement, and so on.

Box 2-6	Lawsuit Prevention Tips for Minimizing Risks

COMMON ISSUES IN LAWSUITS AGAINST HEALTH CARE PROVIDERS	PREVENTION TIPS FOR PHLEBOTOMISTS, NURSES, AND OTHERS INVOLVED IN BLOOD COLLECTION
Documentation	Always document the time, date, and blood collector's initials on the blood collection containers.
Reporting of incidents	Document the information legibly and spell correctly. If an adverse incident occurs to the patient and/or the blood collector before, during, or after blood collection, report the incident to your immediate supervisor and complete the appropriate documentation in a legible manner.
Failure to follow health care facility's procedure	Be knowledgeable of the health care facility's and clinical laboratory's policies and procedures.
	If you must deviate from a policy or a procedure, discuss the incident with your immediate supervisor and decide on the appropriate action.
Failure to ensure patient's safety	Monitor the patient in an appropriate, timely manner during and after blood collection.
	Return bed rails to the raised position if the bed rails were raised prior to blood collection.
	Lock the patient in the blood collection chair for the duration of the blood collection procedure.
	If an outpatient says that he or she faints during blood collection, place the patient in a supine position to collect blood, and monitor the patient for at least 20 minutes after collection before allowing him or her to stand up and leave the facility.
	Remove all supplies and equipment after the procedure.
Improper treatment and performance of treatment	Use proper technique and equipment (e.g., gloves) when performing procedures.
	Follow the health care facility's and clinical laboratory's procedures when performing treatments.
	Update your collection skills and techniques through continuing education classes.
Failure to monitor and to report	Report any significant changes in a patient's condition (e.g., patient continues to bleed from puncture site after blood collection).
Equipment use	Learn how to use blood collection equipment as designed.
	Use biohazardous waste containers as indicated in procedures.
	If involved in off-site blood collections, carry biohazardous waste containers.
	If involved in off-site collections, have the correct types and amounts of insurance coverages to address liability exposures with respect to transporting biohazardous specimens.
Patients with HIV	Be conscious of actions that could result in a lawsuit:
	Discrimination in treatment Nosocomial transmission of the virus Breach of confidentiality
	Follow health care facility's procedures for blood collection and disposal of biohazardous waste.

Box 2-7   Purpose of Medical Records

Medical records have four basic purposes:

1. To allow for continuity of the patient's care plan

2. To provide documentation of the patient's illness and treatment

3. To document communication between the physician and the health care team

4. To provide a legal document that can be used by patients and hospital or health care workers to protect their legal interests

Health care workers and their supervisors have a legal duty to keep records, documentation, and laboratory test results confidential. This duty may be waived only if a patient has given express permission for the information to be released, if the patient is in the process of suing the institution or its health care personnel, or if the health care worker is specifically obligated to release patient information (e.g., to the CDC). But even in these situations, the confidentiality of patient records and reports cannot be breached while they are communicated or in transit.

 ## HIPAA

The use of electronic transfer of patient's medical information is regulated by the federal Health Insurance Portability and Accountability Act (HIPAA) (Figure 2–2 ■).[5] HIPAA requires that health care providers obtain a patient's written consent before disclosing

Figure 2–2. Proper Documentation

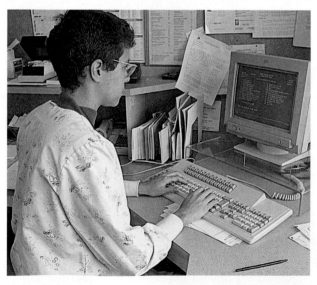

Proper electronic or written documentation of laboratory test results into medical records is extremely important.

medical information for the routine uses of diagnosis, treatment, payment, or health care operations (e.g., laboratory data collection for quality assurance). Thus, each laboratory must give patients information on their rights and on the ways their laboratory test results will be used.[6] Phlebotomists must review and sign a confidentiality and nondisclosure agreement that describes the sensitivity of patient information.

This signature verifies that they will:

- maintain the confidentiality of all patients' information;
- keep the computer sign-on code for entering the laboratory patients' database secure from others' knowledge; and
- maintain the confidentiality of patients' information when looking at the computer database of patients' medical record information.

■■■■ ■ LEGAL CASES RELATED TO CLINICAL LABORATORY ACTIVITIES

Most phlebotomy cases are settled after a lawsuit is filed but before the court renders a judgment. It is important to remember that many cases are not cited in the literature because often health care institutions or health care workers negotiate, arbitrate, and settle out of court. The following sections discuss cases that are of interest to health care workers involved in blood collection.

SCHMERBER V. STATE OF CALIFORNIA

Nurses, technologists, and health care workers are concerned about drawing a blood sample from an unconscious patient or lacking the patient's consent when requested by police. The U.S. Supreme Court ruled in *Schmerber* v. *State of California* that tests performed on a blood sample drawn by a hospital physician from a person arrested by the police were admissible in a court action. This may vary by state.

LAZERNICK V. GENERAL HOSPITAL OF MONROE COUNTY (PA 1977)

A patient who was pregnant for the first time had her blood typed in January 1971. The report sent to her physician indicated that her blood type was A-positive. The patient gave birth to her second child on June 1977. The child was brain damaged and paralyzed on the right side of the body as a result of hemolytic blood disease. The laboratory records in 1971 and 1977 showed that the mother's blood type was O-negative. In a malpractice suit, the parents charged that the physician's and his employee's negligence caused the child's injuries. The physician, who was chief of the laboratory when the blood test was performed, was found liable, as was the health care worker.

WALTON V. PROVIDENCE HOSPITAL

A patient was admitted to Providence Hospital for treatment of pneumonia. On the second day, the patient complained of coldness and numbness in his right hand. On the fourth day, a vascular surgeon examined the hand and ordered 4000 U of heparin in hopes of restoring blood flow. The hand had to be amputated. In court, the expert witness testified that a blood pressure cuff had been left on for an extended period. The patient was awarded $40,000.

HELMANN V. SACRED HEART HOSPITAL

Failure to follow proper isolation techniques, such as proper hand washing and prevention of cross-contamination, is a major area of concern for hospitals. The patient in *Helmann* v. *Sacred Heart Hospital* (62 Wash. 2d 136, 381 P. 2d 605 [1963]) had multiple fractures in the area of the left hip socket. After surgery on his hip, he was returned to a semiprivate room. His roommate complained of a boil under his right arm. Eight days later, a culture was taken of the roommate's wound drainage. Three days later, the laboratory identified the wound infection as *Staphylococcus aureus.* The infected roommate was immediately placed in isolation for the wound. For the preceding 11 days, however, the hospital attendants had administered care to both patients without washing their hands between patient care.

The patient with the hip injury developed a *S. aureus* infection at the site of his hip incision. The infection penetrated into the hip socket, destroying tissue and leading to additional surgery and the hip being fused into a nearly immovable position. Negligence on the part of the hospital personnel was identified as the cause of the injury and a deviation from the accepted standard of care.

CASES RESULTING FROM IMPROPER TECHNIQUE AND NEGLIGENCE

Health care workers who collect blood by venipuncture must be thoroughly trained and skilled in proper technique, safety, and the use of collection equipment. Problems that can arise include:

- Wristband or identification error
- Hematoma
- Abscess at the puncture site
- Patient falling
- Fainting
- Nerve damage
- Emotional distress

In one case settled out of court, a health care worker had not received proper blood collection training. She performed a venipuncture by inserting the needle approximately 2 inches above the antecubital fold. The needle went through the vein, through muscle, and into the nerve, severely injuring the patient's arm, which remained permanently damaged even after three surgeries to repair the damage from the resultant hematoma and nerve injury.

Another case involved a medical technologist under pressure to collect specimens from ambulatory patients as quickly as possible. One of the patients stated prior to blood collection that she had fainted during blood collection at a previous time. The phlebotomist, however, took no precautions to avoid syncope, collected the patient's blood, and allowed the patient to leave immediately. The patient fainted at the elevator and suffered permanent loss of smell and a permanent "ringing sound" in her ears.

In another case, a health care worker collecting bedside glucose results misread the glucometer and caused the deaths of three patients with diabetes. The errors might have been avoided with better training, supervision, and quality monitoring.

In another case, a phlebotomist collected blood at an excessive angle of needle insertion from the patient's basilic vein when the median cubital vein was clearly an option for collection. The blood collection resulted in injury to the patient's median nerve and a malpractice lawsuit. In addition, documentation errors were evident for the collection. In all, the patient was awarded thousands of dollars for the health care worker's violations regarding proper standard of care.[7]

HIV-RELATED ISSUES

If a health care worker becomes infected with HIV during employment at a health care facility, workers' compensation benefits are usually available. The health care worker must, however, demonstrate a causal connection between his or her HIV infection and his or her employment. This causal connection includes having a documented incident report at the health care facility involving a needle-stick injury, a puncture wound, or other exposure to HIV-contaminated blood or body fluids. In addition, the health care worker's lifestyle will be investigated to determine whether the exposure occurred elsewhere. Preemployment health evaluations may prove useful later should the health care worker allege contraction of infection during the time of employment. Employers are legally responsible for monitoring postexposure follow-up.

If a health care worker resigns because of contracting AIDS, unemployment benefits may be available if the worker can show that he or she believed in good faith that continued employment would jeopardize his or her health.

MALPRACTICE INSURANCE

Because hospitals are places where seriously ill patients are admitted and treated with highly sophisticated medical technology, the likelihood for problems is greater there than in other health care settings. Often, the health care staff in the hospital or clinical laboratory is on a blanket malpractice insurance policy. If, however, the health care worker is employed by a pathologist who has a contract with an institution or owns a clinic, the staff may be protected by the pathologist's malpractice insurance policy.

The health care worker, having less money than a hospital or no insurance, in the past has not been a target for suit. The advances in technology and increased complexity of health care have, however, increased legal exposure for allied health and nursing professionals. The health care worker that routinely deals with the public in patient–health care worker relationships is indeed liable. Therefore, each individual should examine the possibility of malpractice suits and the need for malpractice insurance from a personal standpoint.[8] (See Box 2–8.)

With the purchase of malpractice professional liability insurance, the attorney's fee and court costs are usually covered. Some professional organizations offer professional liability insurance at a reasonable or reduced rate. A genuine concern for others and careful attention to technique are good investments of the health care worker's time. A record of continuing education courses, seminars, workshops, and academic credits should be a part of each health care worker's personal file.

Box 2-8	Purchasing Malpractice Insurance

If the health care worker decides to purchase malpractice insurance, the following factors should be carefully considered:[9]

1. Does the employer carry liability insurance?

2. Is adequate dollar value coverage provided? In recent lawsuits, total damages of $1 million or more have been awarded against physicians.

3. What are the coverage limitations? How much does one have to lose if sued?

4. What are the procedures that must be followed for the policy to provide coverage? Some policies state that divulging the amount of coverage or the fact of coverage voids the policy.

5. The health care worker should not assume that the lawyers representing the hospital, laboratory, or clinic will have his or her best interests at heart. The attorney's first obligation is to serve those who have hired him or her. There have been cases in which the hospital was cleared of all charges but the health care professional was held liable for damages.

6. Is a job change expected soon?

7. Are specimen collecting services provided off-site or in patient's homes?

CLINICAL LABORATORY IMPROVEMENT AMENDMENTS (CLIA)

In October 1988, the U.S. Congress passed Public Law 100-578, Clinical Laboratory Improvement Amendments (CLIA). These regulations are enforced to ensure the quality and accuracy of laboratory testing.[10] CLIA '88 essentially applies to every clinical laboratory testing facility in the United States and requires laboratory certification by the federal government. The certification requires an inspection by federal and/or state agencies to determine whether the laboratory testing facility uses methods to test patients' specimens that lead to accurate, reliable, and quality test results. Only laboratories or clinics that perform "waived" laboratory tests (e.g., simple tests such as dipstick urinalysis) are not required to undergo an inspection. If the laboratory test is not categorized as waived by the CLIA '88 federal regulations, it falls into the category of "moderately complex" or "highly complex," depending on the difficulty of conducting the test and the risk of harm to the patient if the test is not performed correctly. For the moderately complex or highly complex testing, the inspection considers all procedural steps in laboratory testing—preanalytic, analytic, and postanalytic. Thus, the blood collection procedures area is a major part of CLIA inspections.

KEY TERMS

assault

battery

bioethics

breach of duty

civil law

Clinical Laboratory Improvement
Amendments (CLIA)

criminal actions

defendant

deposition

discovery

ethics

evidence

expert witness

felony

HIPAA

implied consent

informed consent

liable

litigation process

malpractice

medical records

misdemeanor

negligence

patient confidentiality

plaintiff

respondeat superior

standard of care

statute of limitations

tort

STUDY QUESTIONS

For the following, choose the one best answer.

1. What is the legal term for improper or unskillful care of a patient by a member of the health care team, or any professional misconduct, unreasonable lack of skill, or infidelity in professional or judiciary duties?

   a. a misdemeanor

   b. malpractice

   c. litigation

   d. liability

2. What are the factors, or key points, that must be considered in alleged negligence cases?

   1. duty
   2. breach of duty
   3. proximate causation
   4. damages

   Select one choice:

   a. 1, 2, and 3 are correct

   b. 1 and 3 are correct

   c. 2 and 4 are correct

   d. only 4 is correct

   e. all are correct

3. Which of the following legal branches writes regulations that enforce the laws?

   a. legislative branch

   b. judicial branch

   c. U.S. Supreme Court

   d. executive branch

4. A child who refused to have his blood collected was locked in a room by a phlebotomist and was forced to have his blood collected. This is an example of which legal concept?
   a. invasion of privacy
   b. informed consent
   c. a misdemeanor
   d. assault and battery

5. The standard of care currently used in malpractice legal cases involving health care providers is based on the conduct of the average health care provider in which area?
   a. state
   b. city
   c. national community
   d. local community

6. Which legal concept refers to the voluntary permission by a patient to allow touching, examination, and/or treatment by health care providers?
   a. implied consent
   b. assault and battery
   c. battery
   d. informed consent

7. When should incident reports involving accidental HIV exposures be reported?
   a. at the end of the work shift
   b. immediately
   c. after 24 hours
   d. after seeing the employee health physician

References

1. Lewis, MA, Tamparo, CD: *Medical Law, Ethics, and Bioethics for Ambulatory Care,* 4th ed. Philadelphia: F.A. Davis Company, 1998.
2. Rakich, JS, Longest, BB, Darr, K: *Managing Health Services Organizations.* Baltimore: Health Professions Press, 1992.
3. *Parker* v. *Port Huron Hospital,* 105, N.W. 2d 854 (1981).
4. Brent, NJ: Confidentiality and HIV status: The nurse's right to know. *Home Healthcare Nurse,* 1990; 8(3): 6–8.
5. Health Insurance Portability and Accountability Act of 1996, 18 USC S264.
6. Travis J: Complying with HIPAA: Are you ready? *ADVANCE for Medical Laboratory Professionals,* February 10, 2003; 15 (4): 16–18, 25.
7. Ernst, D: Phlebotomy on trial. *MLO,* April 1999: 46–50.
8. Pozgar, GD: *Legal Aspects of Health Care Administration.* Gaithersburg, MD: Aspen Publishers, 1993.
9. Markus, K: Your legal risk in giving advice or care. *Healthweek,* October 6, 1997: 5.
10. Department of Health and Human Services (DHHS), Health Care Financing Administration (HCFA), Public Health Service: 42 CFR 405 et seq, 57 FR 7002–7186, February 28, 1992.

Basic Anatomy and Physiology of Organ Systems

3

CHAPTER OBJECTIVES

Upon completion of Chapter 3, the learner is responsible for the following:

1. Define the terms *anatomy, physiology,* and *pathology.*
2. Describe the directional terms, anatomic surface regions, and cavities of the body.
3. Describe the role of homeostasis in normal body functioning.
4. Describe the purpose, function, and structural components of the 11 body systems.
5. Identify examples of disorders associated with each organ system.
6. List common diagnostic tests associated with each organ system.

 MediaLINK

Access the accompanying CD-ROM to explore a wide variety of review questions and interactive activities for this chapter, including multiple choice, true/false, and video exercises.

ANATOMIC REGIONS

The human body has distinctive characteristics: a backbone, bisymmetry, body cavities, and 11 major organ systems.

This chapter highlights the basic anatomy (structural components of the body) and physiology (functional components) of each system except the circulatory, or cardiovascular, system, which is covered in Chapter 4. This chapter also identifies common disorders of the major organ systems and laboratory tests to detect abnormalities. Phlebotomists should have a general understanding of organ systems and their role in bodily functioning.

Body regions can be categorized in various ways. One way is to begin at the top and work down in large regions as in Figure 3–1 ■. Another way is to define the four major body cavities where vital organs, glands, blood vessels, and nerves are housed, as depicted in Figure 3–2 ■. Figure 3—3 ■ shows the approximate placement of major organs and tissues in the body. By mentally visualizing the location of major organs and structures, phlebotomists can begin an understanding of human anatomy, which be-

Figure 3–1. Body Regions

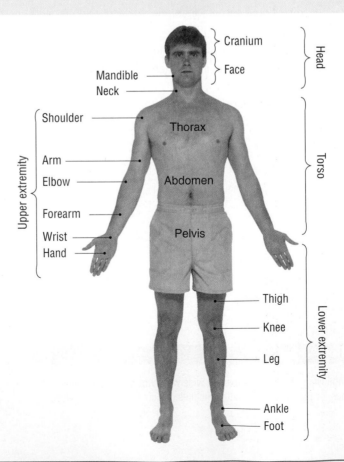

Box 3-1	Organ Systems

NORMAL BODY FUNCTIONS	ORGAN SYSTEMS
Protection	Integumentary
Support	Skeletal
Movement	Muscular
Control	Nervous
Regulation	Endocrine
Fluid Regulation	Cardiovascular
Transport	Lymphatic
Environmental Control and Exchange	Respiratory
	Digestive
	Urinary
Birth	Reproductive

comes more important when dealing with the delicate anatomy of the arms, hands, and legs.

The human body can also be described according to imaginary planes or transecting lines as in Figure 3–4 ■. The front, anterior, or ventral, surface of the body contains the thoracic and abdominopelvic cavities. The back, posterior, or dorsal, surface contains the cra-

Figure 3–2. Body Cavities

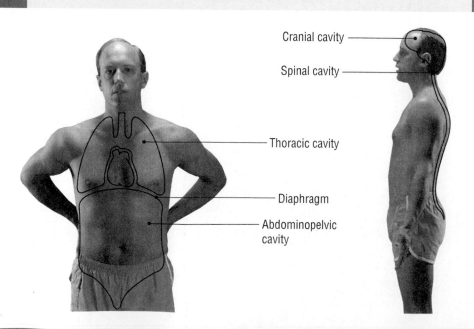

Cranial cavity

Spinal cavity

Thoracic cavity

Diaphragm

Abdominopelvic cavity

Figure 3–3. Location of Major Body Organs

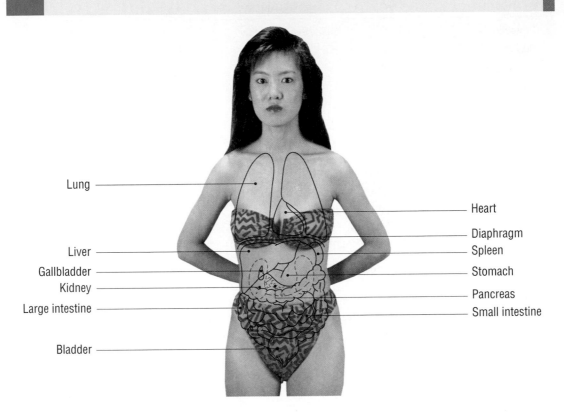

Lung

Heart

Diaphragm

Spleen

Liver

Gallbladder

Stomach

Kidney

Pancreas

Large intestine

Small intestine

Bladder

SOLID ORGANS

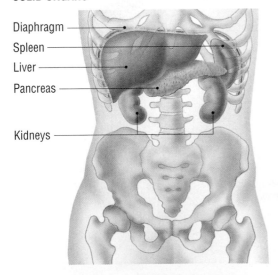

Diaphragm

Spleen

Liver

Pancreas

Kidneys

HOLLOW ORGANS

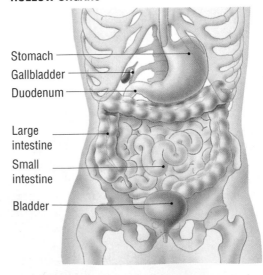

Stomach

Gallbladder

Duodenum

Large
intestine

Small
intestine

Bladder

Figure 3-4. Body Planes

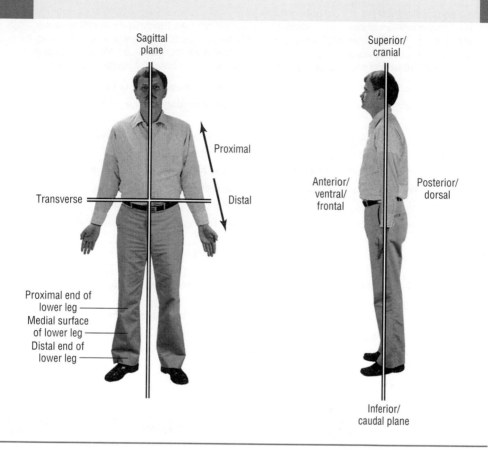

nial and spinal cavities. Areas and directions of the body can be described by their distance from or proximity to one of these body planes.

STRUCTURAL ORGANIZATION

The design of the human body is elaborate and sophisticated. A human body can be divided into eight structural levels: atoms; molecules (chemical constituents); small structures within cells, or organelles; cells (the basic living units of all plants and animals); tissues (groups of similar cells); organs (two or more tissues); organ systems (groups of organs); and the organism (the human body) itself. Trillions of cells make up each individual. Similar groups of cells are combined into tissues, such as muscles or nerves, and tissues are combined into systems, such as the circulatory or reproductive system. These organ systems work simultaneously to serve the needs of the body. No one system works independently of the others.

Survival is the primary function of the human body, and many complex processes work independently and together to achieve this function. In human physiology, the body strives for a steady state, or homeostasis. Literally, homeostasis means "remaining the same." It is

Box 3-2   Terms Related to Body Planes

Anatomical terms provide a description of the body's landmarks. These terms are helpful to health care workers during an assessment of a patient to make the patient's condition understandable to others, especially if the patient is in a remote location. The following terms may be useful for phlebotomists when describing or evaluating a venipuncture complication, an interfering surgical wound site, the location of a vein or artery, or a potential venipuncture site.

Anterior—in front of (Example: I will draw blood from the *anterior* side of the arm.)

Posterior—toward the back (Example: There is a large bandage on the *posterior* side of the arm.)

Transverse plane—crosswise or horizontally, dividing the body into upper and lower sections

Medial—toward the midline (Example: The heart is *medial* to the right shoulder.)

Lateral—toward the sides of the body (Example: The hip is *lateral* to the navel.)

Dorsal—backside (Example: The mole was on the *dorsal* side of her shoulder.)

Ventral—frontside (Example: The scrape was on the *ventral* side of the knee.)

Proximal—near the point of attachment (Example: The leg broke on the *proximal* side of the knee.)

Distal—distant or away from point of attachment (Example: The birthmark was *distal* to the wrist.)

Superficial—near the surface of the body (Example: *Superficial* veins show up easily on her skin.)

Deep—far from the surface of the body (Example: Major arteries are in the *deep* tissues.)

Sagittal plane—lengthwise from front to back, dividing the body into right and left halves

Frontal plane—lengthwise from side to side, dividing the body into anterior and posterior sections

Box 3-3   Terms Related to Body Positions

Normal anatomic position—erect standing position with arms at rest and palms forward

Supine position—lying face-up on his/her back (good position for performing phlebotomy from patients who are in bed)

Prone position—lying face-down on his/her stomach

Lateral recumbent position—lying on left or right side, also known as recovery position

Box 3-4   Right and Left Sides

When speaking with patients, phlebotomists should refer to the *patient's right* and the *patient's left* sides. This often comes up when the phlebotomist asks to see a patient's right or left arm prior to vein selection for venipuncture. Even though the task seems rather basic, some phlebotomists confuse right and left arms when they are face to face with a patient. Phlebotomists should practice using the terms by directly facing a friend and pointing to the friend's right and left side until it is done correctly each time. It is important that the phlebotomist not confuse his or her own right and left side with the patient's right or left side. This becomes particularly critical when there are specific instructions to draw blood from only one side of a patient due to some clinical conditions.

Box 3–5   Cells of the Body

The size and shape of a cell depend on its function. Some cells fight disease-causing viruses and bacteria; some transport gases, such as oxygen (O_2) and carbon dioxide (CO_2); some produce movement, store nutrients, or manufacture proteins, chemicals, or liquids; and others, such as the egg and the sperm, can create a new life. At the same time, other cells contribute to thoughts and emotions. Despite such diverse functions, several cells have basic structural elements in common. The **cell membrane** encloses the contents of the cell. This membrane serves as a protective barrier that selectively allows certain substances to move in or out. Nutrients and O_2 are taken in through the membrane only when needed, and wastes are eliminated as they build up. Most cells also have a nucleus, which is enclosed inside a nuclear membrane. The **nucleus** (*nuclei* for two or more) is commonly thought of as the control mechanism of the cell that governs the functions of the individual cell (i.e., growth, repair, reproduction, and metabolism). Inside the nucleus is a **nucleolus** and threadlike chromatin, which also aid in cell metabolism and reproduction. The nucleus contains a blueprint of itself in the genetic material so that it can reproduce itself when necessary. If the nucleus of a cell is damaged or destroyed, in most cases the cell will die; however, even though **red blood cells (RBCs)** lose their nuclei when they mature, the cells continue to live and carry O_2 for several months. Another component of the cell, the **cytoplasm**, contains mostly water with dissolved nutrients and fills up the rest of the cell membrane. Within the cytoplasm are smaller structures called organelles such as **mitochondria** (produce energy for the cell), **ribosomes** (assemble amino acids into proteins), **endoplasmic reticulum** (acts as transport channel between the cell membrane and the nuclear membrane), **lysosomes** (release digestive enzymes into vacuoles, or small pouches, for digestion of food particles), **Golgi apparatus** (stores proteins), and the **centriole** (plays a role in cell division).

Cells communicate with each other in sophisticated reactions using electrical impulses (such as from one nerve cell to another) or in chemical reactions that result in the release of hormones or other enzymes and proteins to stimulate a particular function.

Within each cell, **deoxyribonucleic acid (DNA)** is a molecule containing thousands of genes, commonly described as a double helix or twisted ladder. DNA carries the code, or blueprint, for an individual's genetic makeup, such as eye color, sex, and height. DNA directs the development, growth, and functioning of all body systems and can create exact copies of itself.

a condition in which a healthy body, although constantly changing and functioning, remains in a normal, healthy condition. Homeostasis, or a steady-state condition, allows the normal body to stay in balance by compensating with changes. For example, if the body is taking in too much water, it responds to this imbalance by excreting water from the kidneys (urine), skin (perspiration), intestines (feces), and lungs (water in expiration). A healthy body maintains constancy of its chemical components and processes in order to survive. Each organ system and body structure plays a part in maintaining homeostasis.

Box 3–6   How Does the Body Make and Use Energy?

Metabolism is the process of making necessary substances or breaking down chemical substances in order to use energy. Catabolism is a series of chemical reactions produced in cells to change complex substances into simpler ones while simultaneously *releasing* energy for the body to use in order to function, whether for moving a chair or for allowing its heart to beat. Conversely, anabolism is a process by which cells use energy to make complex compounds from simpler ones. It allows synthesis of body fluids, such as sweat, tears, saliva, and chemical constituents (enzymes, hormones, and antibodies). Both phases are required to maintain metabolic functions in a healthy individual.

Figure 3–5. Basic Cellular Structure with Examples of Human Cells

Basic cell structures

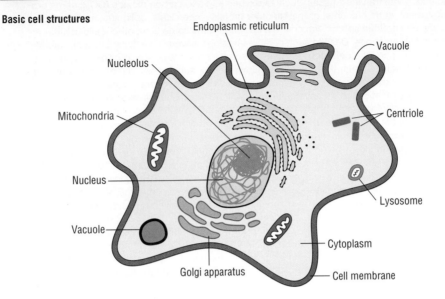

Endoplasmic reticulum
Vacuole
Nucleolus
Centriole
Mitochondria
Nucleus
Lysosome
Vacuole
Cytoplasm
Golgi apparatus
Cell membrane

Human cells

Blood cells

Red blood cell

Lymphocyte

Monocyte

Neutrophil

Eosinophil

Basophil

Muscle cells

Striated (voluntary)

Smooth (involuntary)

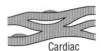
Cardiac

Reproductive cells

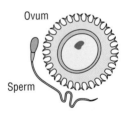
Ovum
Sperm

Box 3-7   **Laboratory Specimens**

Laboratory testing can provide a wealth of information about the individual organ systems and the integrated processes. Specimens, such as blood, bone marrow, urine, cerebrospinal fluid (CSF), synovial or joint fluid, pleural fluid (from around the lungs), biopsy tissue, semen, and others, can be microscopically analyzed, assayed, and cultured to determine pathogenesis (the origin of the disease). Phlebotomists may have a part in the collection, processing, or testing of these specimens.

Health care workers can assess homeostasis, or normal functioning, by taking "vital signs," for example, temperature, **pulse rate**, and respiration rate (together known as TPR) and blood pressure. Methods for taking vital signs are described in Appendix 2.

In a normal, healthy body, structural and functional aspects work together. Organization of all the body structures, such as cells, tissues, organs, and systems, together with proper functioning, such as digestion, respiration, circulation, nerve sensitivity, movement, and secretion, provide for a healthy individual. Systems working together can keep a body metabolizing properly and in homeostasis, which is the basis of survival.

MAJOR ORGAN SYSTEMS

Figures 3–6 ■ to 3–15 ■ depict 10 of the 11 major organ systems. For each system, there is a summary of the structure, function, disorders, and a few common laboratory tests.

INTEGUMENTARY SYSTEM

Structure and Function

The **integumentary system** consists of the skin, hair, sweat and oil glands, teeth, and fingernails. It serves for protection and regulatory functions like insulation, thermal regulation, excretion, and the production of vitamin D. Skin is the largest organ of the body (covering about 3,000 square inches and weighing about 6 pounds) protecting the deeper tissues by providing a barrier to entering microorganisms and foreign bodies and by protecting from hazardous exposures such as heat and cold. The skin also prevents water loss or allows for perspiration as needed by the body during exercise or fever or due to weather conditions. Sebaceous glands in the skin produce oils for hair and skin protection, and sweat glands produce perspiration, which helps cool the body as needed and eliminates some waste. **Melanin** in the skin provides skin color and protects underlying tissues from absorbing ultraviolet rays. Ultraviolet light stimulates production of inactive vitamin D in the skin. The liver and kidneys then activate vitamin D so that it is beneficial to the body. Other functions of the skin are to store fat in the layers next to the underlying tissues and to allow an individual to experience sensations such as touch, temperature, pain, and pressure. Hair on the head provides protection by acting as a heat insulator; eyebrows keep perspiration out of the eyes; eyelashes protect eyes from foreign objects; and hairs in the nasal passages filter out dust and harmful microorganisms. Likewise, fingernails protect the tips of the hands. Teeth aid in breaking up food to begin the digestive process.

Disorders

Bacterial infections, such as acne, impetigo (caused by *Staphylococcus aureus*), and decubitis ulcers; viral infections, such as fever blisters or cold sores, rubeola, rubella, chickenpox, and herpes zoster (shingles); fungal infections, such as ringworm and athlete's foot; allergic reactions, such as dermatitis and eczema; psoriasis; and skin cancers, such as malignant melanoma.

Laboratory Tests

For many of these conditions, involve skin scrapings; bacteriologic, viral, or fungal tissue cultures; potassium hydroxide (KOH) preparations; or biopsy staining procedures.

Figure 3–6. Integumentary System

Integumentary System

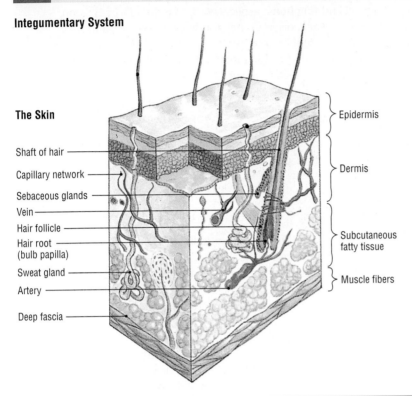

The Skin

- Shaft of hair
- Capillary network
- Sebaceous glands
- Vein
- Hair follicle
- Hair root (bulb papilla)
- Sweat gland
- Artery
- Deep fascia

- Epidermis
- Dermis
- Subcutaneous fatty tissue
- Muscle fibers

On the cross-section of the skin, note that the capillary network extends almost to the top layers of the skin as do some of the nerve endings. This superficial layer is the area that is punctured during a skin puncture procedure or "fingerstick."

SKELETAL SYSTEM

Structure and Function

The **skeletal system** refers to all bones and joints of the body. This system comprises primarily two types of tissue: bone and cartilage. Bone is composed of cells surrounded by calcified intercellular substances that allow for a rigid structure. **Cartilage** is composed of similar cells, but these cells are surrounded by a gelatinous material, instead of calcified substances, that allows for more flexibility. Likewise, tendons and ligaments provide flexibility and leverage. The skeletal system serves the body in five major ways: support, protection for softer tissues (brain and lungs), movement and leverage, **hematopoiesis** (blood cell formation) in the bone marrow, and mineral storage.

More than 200 bones are contained in the human body, and they are classified into four groups based on shape. Long bones include leg bones (e.g., femur, tibia, fibula) and arm and hand bones (e.g., humerus, radius, ulna, phalanges). Short bones include carpals and tarsals, or wrist and ankle bones, respectively. Among flat bones are several cranial bones, the ribs, and the scapulae (or shoulder blades). Finally, irregular bones include cranial bones (e.g., sphenoid, ethmoid) and bones of the vertebral column (e.g., vertebrae, sacrum, coccyx).

Bones are connected to each other by a variety of joints that permit flexion, extension, abduction (away from median), adduction (toward median), rotation, and combinations of these movements. Bone structure differs between male and female skeletons. Besides being somewhat larger and heavier, the male has a pelvis that is deeper, with a narrow pubic arch. In contrast, the female pelvis is shallow and broad and has a wider pubic arch to facilitate childbirth.

In general, bones consist of several layers covered by a membrane, the periosteum. The periosteum contains blood vessels that bring blood from inside the bone to the outer layer. The outer layer, or compact bone, is more rigid and heavier than the inner layer, which is like a honeycomb. The inner layer is spongy bone but is just as strong as compact bone. In the center of a bone is the marrow, which produces most blood cells. Approximately 5 billion red blood cells (RBCs) are produced daily by about ½ pound (227 g) of bone marrow. Marrow is located in all the bones of an infant, but in adults it is in the skull, sternum (or breastbone), vertebrae, hipbones, and ends of the long bones.[1] Minerals stored in bones include calcium and phosphorus. When these minerals are needed in other parts of the body, they are released from the bone through the bloodstream.

Disorders

Inflammatory conditions such as arthritis and bursitis; gout; bacterial infections such as **osteomyelitis**; porous bone conditions such as osteoporosis; developmental conditions such as gigantism, dwarfism, and rickets; and bone tumors.

Laboratory Tests

Serum calcium and phosphate levels, serum alkaline phosphatase (ALP) levels, uric acid, vitamin D, erythrocyte sedimentation rate (ESR), complete blood cell (CBC) counts, microscopic analysis, and microbial cultures of the bone marrow and synovial fluid (fluid between joints and bones).

MUSCULAR SYSTEM
Structure and Function

The muscular system refers to all muscles of the body, including those attached to bones and those along walls of internal structures, such as the heart. On the basis of location, microscopic structure, and neural control, muscles are classified as follows: (1) skeletal (striated voluntary) muscles—attached to bones; (2) visceral (nonstriated [smooth] involuntary) muscles—lining the walls of internal structures, such as veins and arteries; and (3) cardiac (striated involuntary) muscles—which make up the wall of the heart. Muscles provide movement, maintain posture, and produce heat. Movement takes place not only during locomotion, but also during body movements, changes in the size of openings, and propulsion of substances (e.g., propulsion of blood through veins or passage of food through intestines). Posture is maintained during sitting and standing by continued partial

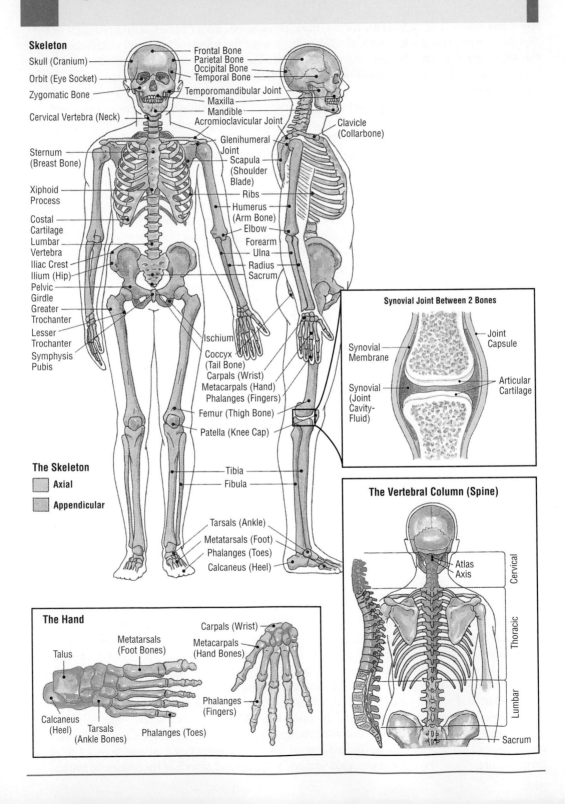

Figure 3–7. Skeletal System

Skeleton

Skull (Cranium)
Orbit (Eye Socket)
Zygomatic Bone
Cervical Vertebra (Neck)

Sternum (Breast Bone)

Xiphoid Process
Costal Cartilage
Lumbar Vertebra
Iliac Crest
Ilium (Hip)
Pelvic Girdle
Greater Trochanter
Lesser Trochanter
Symphysis Pubis

Frontal Bone
Parietal Bone
Occipital Bone
Temporal Bone
Temporomandibular Joint
Maxilla
Mandible
Acromioclavicular Joint
Glenihumeral Joint
Scapula (Shoulder Blade)
Ribs
Humerus (Arm Bone)
Elbow
Forearm
Ulna
Radius
Sacrum

Ischium
Coccyx (Tail Bone)
Carpals (Wrist)
Metacarpals (Hand)
Phalanges (Fingers)
Femur (Thigh Bone)
Patella (Knee Cap)

Clavicle (Collarbone)

The Skeleton

Axial

Appendicular

Tibia
Fibula

Tarsals (Ankle)
Metatarsals (Foot)
Phalanges (Toes)
Calcaneus (Heel)

Synovial Joint Between 2 Bones

Synovial Membrane
Synovial (Joint Cavity-Fluid)
Joint Capsule
Articular Cartilage

The Vertebral Column (Spine)

Atlas
Axis

Cervical
Thoracic
Lumbar
Sacrum

The Hand

Talus
Metatarsals (Foot Bones)
Calcaneus (Heel)
Tarsals (Ankle Bones)
Phalanges (Toes)

Carpals (Wrist)
Metacarpals (Hand Bones)
Phalanges (Fingers)

contraction of specific muscles. Muscle cells that provide mechanical energy for movement also release energy in the form of heat. All three muscle types work by extending, contracting, conducting, and being easily stimulated.

Skeletal muscles (more than 400 in humans) compose approximately 40 percent of a man's body. In contrast, women have less muscle and more fat than men. Muscles are strongest at about age 25, but with proper nutrition and exercise, they can remain strong throughout life. Without sufficient exercise, muscles become smaller and weaker. Glycogen is the form of stored glucose in muscles. Without stores of glycogen, muscles must wait for glucose, which is transported through the bloodstream. Exercise increases the amount of glycogen available for muscles, which in turn allows them to function more easily.

Disorders

Muscular dystrophy (MD), conditions that disrupt nerve stimulation (as in severe accidents or myasthenia gravis), muscle cramps and tendinitis, and viral infections, such as multiple sclerosis (MS) and polio.

Laboratory Testing

Clinical assays of specific muscle enzymes, such as creatine phosphokinase (CK) and lactate dehydrogenase (LDH), analysis of autoimmune antibodies, microscopic examination, or culturing of biopsy tissue.

NERVOUS SYSTEM

Structure and Function

The **nervous system** provides communication in the body, sensations, thoughts, emotions, and memories. Nerve impulses and chemical substances regulate, control, integrate, and organize body functions. The nervous system is composed of specialized nerve cells (neurons), the brain, the spinal cord, brain and cord coverings, fluid, and the nerve impulse itself. An estimated 10 billion neurons or more reside in the human body, most of which are in the brain. Sensory neurons transmit nerve impulses to the spinal cord or the brain from muscle tissues. Motor neurons transmit impulses to muscles from the spinal cord or the brain. Both the brain and the spinal cord are covered by protective membranes (**meninges**). Between these protective membrane layers are spaces filled with **cerebrospinal fluid (CSF)** that provide a cushion for the brain and the spinal cord. Furthermore, the brain and spinal cord are protected by the skull and vertebral column respectively. The bony segments of the vertebral canal are divided into regions as shown in the figure (cervical, thoracic, and lumbar vertebrae). There are seven cervical vertebrae (C1–C7) that extend from the head to the thorax, twelve thoracic vertebrae (T1–T12) that extend from the chest to the back, and five lumbar vertebrae (L1–L5) that extend to the lower back. At the lower end of the vertebral column the sacrum (S1–S5) and coccyx are fused elements of the sacral and coccygeal vertebrae.

The brain, along with the cranial nerves, functions in all mental processes and many essential motor, sensory, and visceral responses. The spinal cord and the spinal nerves control sensory (touch), motor (voluntary movement), and reflex (knee-jerk) functions. Reflexes are responses to stimuli that do not require communication with the brain. A simple reflex, such as moving a finger from something hot, occurs even before the brain

Figure 3–8. Muscular System

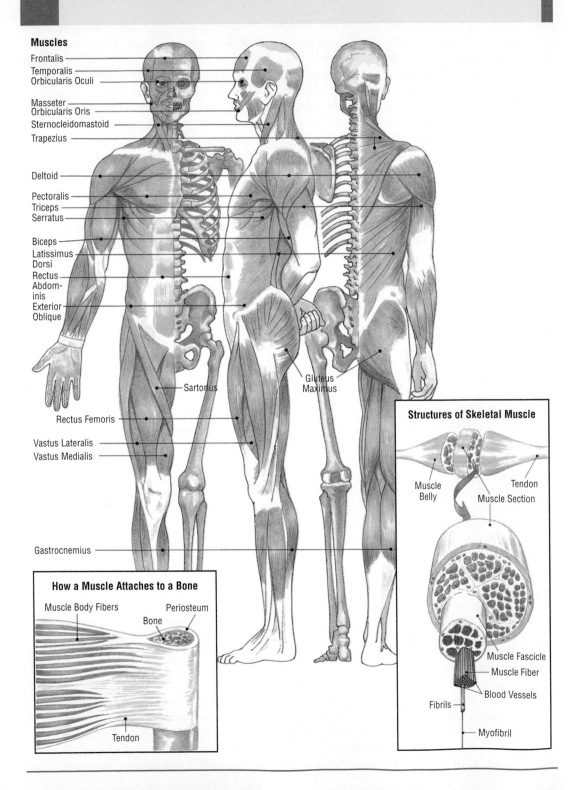

Muscles

Frontalis
Temporalis
Orbicularis Oculi

Masseter
Orbicularis Oris
Sternocleidomastoid
Trapezius

Deltoid

Pectoralis
Triceps
Serratus

Biceps
Latissimus Dorsi
Rectus Abdominis
Exterior Oblique

Sartorius

Gluteus Maximus

Rectus Femoris

Vastus Lateralis
Vastus Medialis

Gastrocnemius

Structures of Skeletal Muscle

Muscle Belly
Tendon
Muscle Section

Muscle Fascicle
Muscle Fiber
Blood Vessels
Fibrils
Myofibril

How a Muscle Attaches to a Bone

Muscle Body Fibers
Periosteum
Bone
Tendon

realizes the pain. Specific cranial and spinal nerves control all complex or simple action processes in the body. There are 31 pairs of spinal nerves (nerves that branch off of the spinal cord), each of which is identified by its location to the nearest vertebrae. Nerves that branch from the spinal cord (C5 through T1) and extend into the arm region (the brachial plexus) are the axillary, radial, musculocutaneous, median, and ulnar nerves. These nerves control all muscle movement of the shoulder, arm, and hand, and also control sensations of the skin of the entire shoulder, arm, and hand. In summary, the nervous system is the primary communication and regulatory system in the body. The autonomic nervous system entails the functions that work without voluntary control of an individual, such as, heartbeat, rate of breathing, tear and saliva production, and bladder constrictions.

Disorders

Infectious conditions such as encephalitis, meningitis, tetanus, herpes, and poliomyelitis, and conditions such as amyotrophic lateral sclerosis (ALS), multiple sclerosis (MS), Parkinson's disease, cerebral palsy (CP), tumors, epilepsy, hydrocephaly, neuralgia, and headaches.

Clinical Alert

Nerve damage can occur as a result of accidental injury during phlebotomy procedures. Injury may be the result of excessive probing with the needle, sticking the needle in a poor site for venipuncture, deep needle penetration all the way into the nerve, and/or if the patient suddenly jerks his or her arm during the venipuncture procedure, causing the needle to puncture a nerve. Phlebotomists should choose sites that are least likely to cause nerve damage and take precautions to have the patient's movements stabilized as much as possible. Under no circumstances should phlebotomists use the anterior or palmar side of the wrist to collect a blood specimen because the risk of hitting a nerve is high due to nerve locations close to the skin's surface.

Laboratory Testing

Chemical assays can reveal drug interactions, as well as hormonal, protein, and enzyme alterations. Infections can be detected by bacterial, viral, or fungal cultures or by the presence of specific antibodies in the CSF.

RESPIRATORY SYSTEM

Structure and Function

Respiration allows for the exchange of gases between blood and air. Once gases (oxygen, O_2, and carbon dioxide, CO_2) enter the blood, the circulatory system transports them between lungs and tissues. Together, the respiratory and circulatory systems carry O_2 to the cells and remove CO_2 from the tissue cells. Oxygen allows the body to burn its fuel from the nutrients eaten. It makes up about one fifth of the air around us. The average person inhales and exhales about 15 times per minute or approximately 20,000 times per day. As a

Figure 3-9. Nervous System

**Nervous System
Divisions of the Spinal Cord**

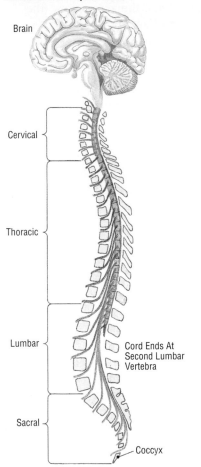

Brain

Cervical

Thoracic

Lumbar

Cord Ends At
Second Lumbar
Vertebra

Sacral

Coccyx

Section of the Spinal Cord

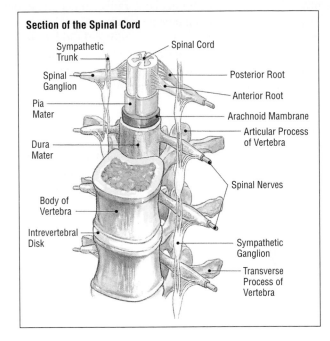

Sympathetic Trunk

Spinal Ganglion

Pia Mater

Dura Mater

Body of Vertebra

Intrevertebral Disk

Spinal Cord

Posterior Root

Anterior Root

Arachnoid Mambrane

Articular Process of Vertebra

Spinal Nerves

Sympathetic Ganglion

Transverse Process of Vertebra

Brachial Plexus

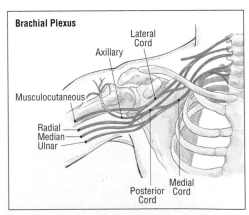

Lateral Cord

Axillary

Musculocutaneous

Radial
Median
Ulnar

Posterior Cord

Medial Cord

Sympathetic (partial representation) **Parasympathetic**

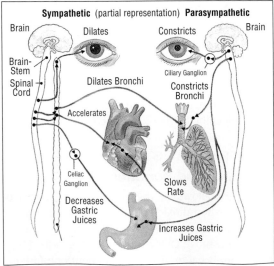

Brain

Brain-Stem

Spinal Cord

Dilates

Dilates Bronchi

Accelerates

Celiac Ganglion

Decreases Gastric Juices

Constricts

Brain

Ciliary Ganglion

Constricts Bronchi

Slows Rate

Increases Gastric Juices

Figure 3–10. Respiratory System

Respiratory System

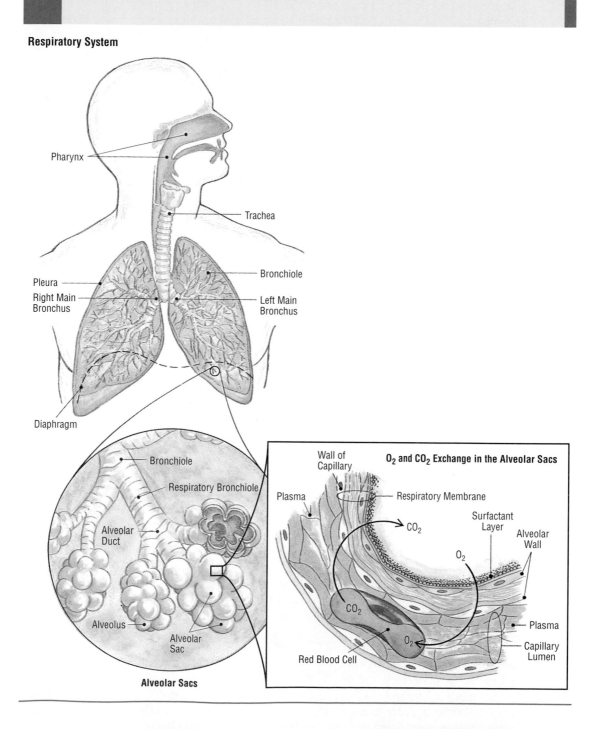

Pharynx

Trachea

Bronchiole

Pleura

Right Main Bronchus

Left Main Bronchus

Diaphragm

Bronchiole

Respiratory Bronchiole

Alveolar Duct

Alveolus

Alveolar Sac

Alveolar Sacs

Wall of Capillary

O_2 and CO_2 Exchange in the Alveolar Sacs

Plasma

Respiratory Membrane

CO_2

Surfactant Layer

Alveolar Wall

O_2

CO_2

O_2

Plasma

Red Blood Cell

Capillary Lumen

person breathes in, the O_2 travels through air passages to the lungs. In the lungs, the exchange of gases occurs. Oxygen is exchanged for CO_2, which is then breathed out as the person exhales. The main components of the respiratory system are in the head, the neck, and the thoracic cavity and include the nose, the pharynx, the larynx, the trachea, the bronchi, and the lungs.

Receptors in the nose provide the sense of smell and allow for changes in voice. The nose is also the primary filter for air entering the body. In the nose, the throat, and the bronchial tree, mucus is continuously produced to trap unwanted particles and prevent them from entering the lungs or vocal cords. Tiny hairlike cilia line the passageways and sweep the mucus to the nose and mouth so that it can be coughed up, sneezed, or swallowed. The pharynx is a tubelike passageway for both food and air. Along with the larynx (voice box), it determines the quality of voice. The trachea and the bronchial passages provide openings for outside air to reach the lungs. Within the bronchi are grapelike **alveolar sacs** that are enveloped by capillaries and allow diffusion between air and blood.

The lungs are structured into millions of branches of alveoli with surrounding capillaries and therefore can quickly take in large amounts of O_2 and release large amounts of CO_2 if they are functioning properly. The lungs are soft and spongy and reach from just above the collarbone down to the diaphragm. They have no muscles; consequently, the diaphragm and other surrounding muscles help enlarge and contract the chest cavity as respiration occurs. Humans have two lungs: the right lung has three lobes, and the left lung has only two, to allow room for the heart. An adult's lungs hold 3 to 4 quarts (approximately 3 to 4 L) of air, depending on how vigorously the person is moving or exercising. In patients with pneumonia, the alveolar sacs become inflamed, and fluid or waste products block the minute air spaces, thus normal O_2 and CO_2 exchange is difficult.

Red blood cells (RBCs) transport O_2 and CO_2 as part of a molecule called hemoglobin. After O_2 crosses the respiratory membranes (in the lung) into the blood, about 97 percent of the O_2 combines with the iron-containing heme portion of **hemoglobin** inside the RBCs. The remaining 3 percent dissolves in **plasma**. O_2 goes from the alveolar capillaries through the blood vessels to the tissue capillaries. Oxygen and CO_2 rapidly combine with hemoglobin in RBCs to form oxyhemoglobin and carbaminohemoglobin, respectively. Association (chemical combination) and dissociation (chemical release) with hemoglobin depends on the gaseous pressure. In lung capillaries, O_2 pressure (partial pressure of oxygen [Po_2]) increases and CO_2 (partial pressure of carbon dioxide [Pco_2]) decreases, which allows O_2 to rapidly associate, or combine chemically, with hemoglobin, and CO_2 to dissociate, or be released, from carbaminohemoglobin. Thus, humans inhale O_2 into the lungs and exhale CO_2 from the lungs. In tissue capillaries, the opposite occurs: O_2 pressure decreases and CO_2 pressure increases, which allows O_2 to dissociate from oxyhemoglobin and CO_2 to combine with hemoglobin. Thus, O_2 is released into tissues and muscles, and CO_2 is picked up, taken to the lungs, and exhaled.

Carbon dioxide has an important effect on the pH (acidity) of the blood. Normal body pH has a narrow range of between 7.35 and 7.45. Deviations from the normal or reference range can be dangerous and deadly. As CO_2 levels increase, the blood pH decreases (becomes more acidic) and chemoreceptors in the brain cause a faster rate of respiration (hyperventilation) in order to blow off excess CO_2 from the body. (The urinary system also plays a role in maintaining body pH, as described later in this chapter.)

Disorders

Infectious conditions, such as tuberculosis, laryngitis, bronchitis, colds, sore throat, whooping cough, tonsillitis, rhinitis, coughs, sneezing, runny noses, bronchitis, pneumonia, *Pneumocystis carinii* pneumonia, Legionnaires' disease, pleurisy, respiratory distress syndrome, respiratory syncytial virus and influenza; conditions such as asthma, emphysema, and cystic fibrosis; and tumors. In cases of pneumonia, the air sacs in the lungs fill with fluid, and gaseous exchanges cannot occur. Pneumocystis infections are considered opportunistic infections (i.e., they become pathogenic when the patient is immunosuppressed) and are associated with acquired immunodeficiency syndrome (AIDS).

Laboratory Tests

Blood gases (CO_2 and O_2), blood pH, chemical constituents (sodium, chloride, bicarbonate, and potassium) often indicate respiratory abnormalities. Lung biopsies, throat swabs, sputum cultures, and bronchial washings can be examined microscopically or cultured for pathogenic microorganisms. Procedures for collecting specimens for a throat culture and a sputum specimen are included Chapter 14.

DIGESTIVE SYSTEM

Structure and Function

The **digestive system** functions, first, to break down food chemically and physically into nutrients that can be absorbed and used by body cells and, second, to eliminate the waste products of digestion. The gastrointestinal (GI) tract is made up of the following components: mouth, pharynx, esophagus, stomach, intestines, and some vital accessory organs, such as salivary glands, teeth, liver, gallbladder, pancreas, and appendix. Many proteins, enzymes, and juices are released by these components to facilitate digestion, absorption, and movement through the GI tract. The food passageway, or alimentary canal, which begins at the mouth and ends at the anus, has an average length of 27 feet in adults. (One meal can take 15 hours to 2 days to pass through.) Circular muscles surround the intestines to assist the movement of food through the body using wavelike contractions called **peristalsis**. (Peristalsis is such an effective process that a person can even swallow upside down!) If the process is reversed, vomiting enables the body to reject food.

Saliva produced in the mouth moistens food and contains an enzyme that helps begin the breakdown of carbohydrates into simple sugars such as glucose. (If a salt cracker is chewed a long time, saliva begins the breakdown process so it may taste sweet.) Also, the liver secretes bile, which aids in fat digestion and absorption. In addition, it is involved in carbohydrate **metabolism**, protein and fat **catabolism**, and synthesis of many vital blood proteins for clotting and regulatory purposes. Each component functions either mechanically or chemically to keep the body in **homeostasis**.

The digestive system helps regulate the intake and output of essential proteins, carbohydrates, fats, minerals, vitamins, and water. The body can then use these substances by catabolizing them for stored energy or by anabolizing them to build other complex compounds, such as hormones, other tissue proteins, and enzymes. Materials that are not digested in the alimentary canal are eliminated from the body as fecal material or urine.

Figure 3–11. Digestive System

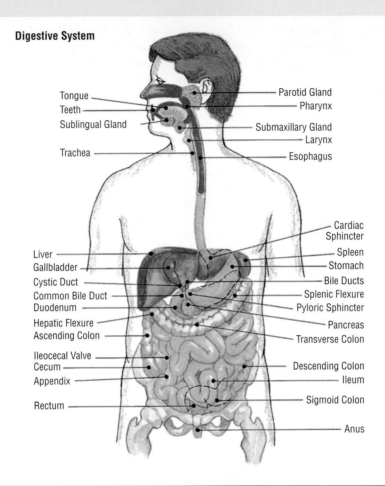

Digestive System

Disorders

The oral cavity can contain dental caries, or tooth decay, and periodontal disease, which is an inflammation and degeneration of the gums, ligaments, and bone around the teeth. Stomach disorders can include acid reflux, hiatial hernias (protrusion through the diaphragm), vomiting, and ulcers. Intestinal disorders (affecting small and large intestines) include polyps, maldigestion, malabsorption, cancer, appendicitis, constipation, diarrhea, dysentery, and hemorrhoids. Liver inflammation is referred to as hepatitis and can be caused by various agents, such as excessive alcohol consumption and viral hepatitis. A common disorder of the gallbladder is gallstones, which can cause blockage of the bile duct, pain, and inflammation. Numerous bacterial and parasitic infections can also affect the digestive tract. Examples include staphylococcal food poisoning, salmonellosis, typhoid fever, cholera, giardiasis, tapeworms, pinworms, hookworms, and ascariasis (roundworm).

Laboratory Tests

Tissue biopsies, occult blood test (testing for blood in feces), bacterial cultures, and analysis for ova and parasites. Procedures for performing an occult blood test are included in Chapter 14.

URINARY SYSTEM

Structure and Function

The primary purpose of the **urinary system** is to produce and eliminate urine. This system consists of two kidneys, two ureters, one bladder, and one urethra. The kidneys' main function is to regulate the amount of water, electrolytes (sodium, potassium, chloride, calcium, phosphate, magnesium), and nitrogenous waste products (urea) from protein metabolism. The proper concentration of these blood constituents is vital to life. Electrolytes function to maintain the body's acid–base balance. The normal ratio of acid (carbonic acid) to base (bicarbonate) is 1:20. Blood pH and blood gas determinations provide useful information about acid–base balance in the body. Normal blood pH is within a range of 7.35 to 7.45. The kidneys help correct the body's acid–base imbalances. As blood passes through the specialized kidney cells, called glomeruli, water and solutes are filtered out. Only the necessary amounts of these substances are reabsorbed into the blood. The rest are excreted as waste products in the urine. Ureters collect urine as it forms and transport it to the bladder, which serves as a reservoir until the urine can be voided. The urethra is the terminal component of the urinary system. In women, it is merely a passageway from the bladder, whereas in men, it eliminates both urine and semen from the body.

Two thirds of human body weight is water. About 60 percent of the body's water is inside cells, and the rest is in the bloodstream or tissue fluids. The salt content of the body's water is extremely important for survival. When excess salt is in the tissues, the kidneys eliminate it; if there is excess water, the kidneys eliminate it.

Disorders

Acidosis occurs when the blood pH decreases to less than 7.35, thus the bloodstream becomes acidic. If the condition worsens, the individual can become comatose. Respiratory acidosis is a serious condition that results when the respiratory system is unable to eliminate adequate amounts of CO_2 (in conditions such as a collapsed lung or blockage of respiratory passages). Metabolic acidosis results when the body retains acids or loses bicarbonate buffers or the kidneys eliminate acidic substances. There are several causes of metabolic acidosis and they can result in kidney (renal) failure and/or death.

Alkalosis results when plasma bicarbonate increases, thereby increasing the blood pH to more than 7.45. Respiratory alkalosis results from hyperventilation or the loss of too much CO_2 from the lungs. Metabolic alkalosis usually results from excessive vomiting or an abnormal secretion of certain hormones that cause excess elimination of acid from the stomach or kidneys.

The kidneys are vitally important in compensating for respiratory acidosis or alkalosis. Conversely, the respiratory system is vitally important in compensating for metabolic and respiratory acidosis or alkalosis. If the kidneys are not functioning properly, a mechanical filtering process (dialysis) must be used or one of the kidneys must be replaced with a transplant.

Figure 3–12. Urinary System

Urinary System

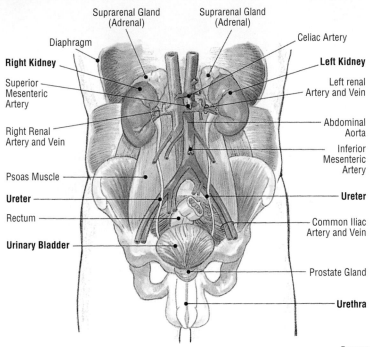

- Suprarenal Gland (Adrenal)
- Suprarenal Gland (Adrenal)
- Diaphragm
- Celiac Artery
- **Right Kidney**
- **Left Kidney**
- Superior Mesenteric Artery
- Left renal Artery and Vein
- Right Renal Artery and Vein
- Abdominal Aorta
- Inferior Mesenteric Artery
- Psoas Muscle
- **Ureter**
- **Ureter**
- Rectum
- Common Iliac Artery and Vein
- **Urinary Bladder**
- Prostate Gland
- **Urethra**

Cross-section of Kidney

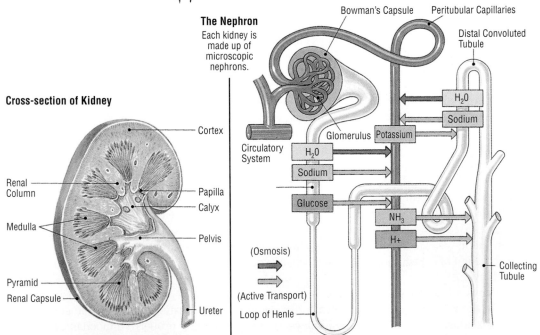

The Nephron
Each kidney is made up of microscopic nephrons.

- Bowman's Capsule
- Peritubular Capillaries
- Distal Convoluted Tubule
- Cortex
- Glomerulus
- H_2O
- Sodium
- Circulatory System
- Potassium
- Renal Column
- Papilla
- H_2O
- Calyx
- Sodium
- Medulla
- Glucose
- Pelvis
- NH_3
- $H+$
- (Osmosis)
- Collecting Tubule
- Pyramid
- Renal Capsule
- (Active Transport)
- Ureter
- Loop of Henle

Laboratory Tests

Detection of osmolality and constituents, such as proteins, glucose blood, microorganisms, and cells in the urine, as well as chemical analysis of albumin, ammonia, creatinine, total protein, blood urea nitrogen (BUN), blood pH, blood gases, and electrolytes in the blood. The creatinine clearance test evaluates the degree to which kidneys are filtering out waste products of metabolism.

ENDOCRINE SYSTEM

Structure and Function

The human body has two types of glands: exocrine glands secrete fluids, such as sweat, saliva, mucus, and digestive juices, which are transported through channels or ducts; and endocrine glands, or ductless glands, release their secretions (hormones) directly into the bloodstream. This glandular system has the same functions as those of the nervous system: communication, control, and integration. Hormones play an important role in metabolic regulation that influences growth and development, in fluid and electrolyte balance, in energy balance, and in acid–base balance. **Endocrine glands** include pituitary, thyroid, parathyroid, thymus, and adrenal glands, as well as ovaries and testes.

The **pituitary gland**, or master gland, as it is sometimes called, stimulates the other glands to produce hormones as needed. It controls and regulates hormone production through chemical feedback. The pituitary hormones also regulate retention of water by the

Figure 3–13. Endocrine System

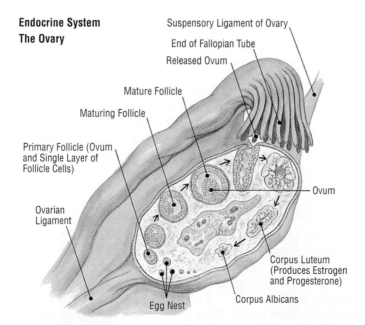

kidneys, cause uterine contractions during childbirth, stimulate breast milk production, and produce growth hormone (GH). This hormone controls growth by regulating the nutrients that are taken into cells. It also works with insulin to control blood sugar levels. The thyroid gland produces a hormone that affects cell metabolism and growth rate. Parathyroid glands regulate calcium and phosphorus in the blood and the bones. The thymus gland affects the lymphoid system. The **adrenals** (two glands) produce hormones as a result of emotions like fright or anger. This hormone production causes an increase in blood pressure, widened pupils, and heart stimulation. The adrenals also produce hormones that regulate carbohydrate metabolism and electrolyte balance.[1] As mentioned earlier, ovaries and testes produce estrogens and progesterone, and testosterone, respectively. The pineal gland secretes melatonin, a regulatory hormone. The pancreas contains exocrine tissue, which secretes pancreatic juice to aid in digestion, and endocrine tissue to secrete hormones, such as insulin and glucagon.

Disorders

Many are inherited and result in excessive or insufficient hormone production. Diseases of this system include Addison's disease, Cushing's syndrome, dwarfism, acromegaly, gigantism, diabetes insipidus, diabetes mellitus, hypo- or hyperthyroidism, hyperinsulinism, hypoglycemia, goiter, and creatinism.

Laboratory Tests

Since hormones are transported by the bloodstream, abnormalities are easily detected by analyzing blood samples. Chemical assays are available for all types of constituents that are regulated by the endocrine system, including glucose, insulin, renin, serotonin, erythropoietin, cortisol, and others. In addition, specific thyroid function tests (triiodothyronine [T3], thyroxine [T4], and thyroid-stimulating hormone [TSH]) are available.

REPRODUCTIVE SYSTEM

Structure and Function

Male reproductive structures include the testes, the seminal vesicles, the prostate gland, the epididymis, the ejaculatory ducts, the urethra, the penis, and the spermatic cords. The primary functions of this system are spermatogenesis (sperm production); storage, maintenance, and excretion of seminal fluid; and secretion of hormones (the most important of which is testosterone). Female reproductive structures include the ovaries, the fallopian tubes, the uterus, the vagina, the labia, and the mammary glands. These structures play a role in ovulation, fertilization, menstruation, pregnancy, labor, lactation, and secretion of hormones (estrogens and progesterone).

A sperm is one of the smallest cells in the body, whereas the mature egg is the largest. Each of these cells contains a nucleus with 23 chromosomes. Because a mother's egg and a father's sperm contain different sets of DNA, various genetic characteristics are paired. One of the pairs of chromosomes determines the sex of the fetus. The egg contains only an X chromosome; however, the sperm may contain an X or a Y chromosome. Therefore, if an X sperm fertilizes the egg, an XX pair of chromosomes forms, and the neonate will be a girl; if a Y sperm fertilizes the egg, an XY pair forms, and it will be a boy. The 46 combined chromosomes contain the DNA-coded blueprint for the newborn.

Figure 3-14. Reproductive System

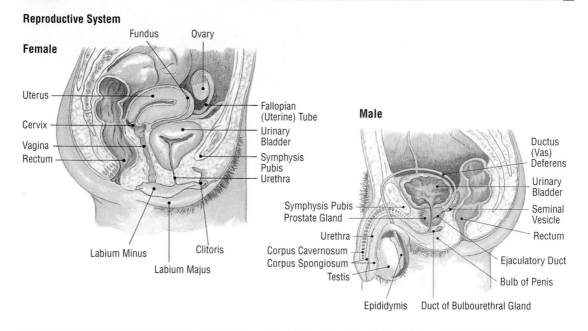

Reproductive System

Female

- Fundus
- Ovary
- Uterus
- Cervix
- Vagina
- Rectum
- Fallopian (Uterine) Tube
- Urinary Bladder
- Symphysis Pubis
- Urethra
- Labium Minus
- Labium Majus
- Clitoris

Male

- Symphysis Pubis
- Prostate Gland
- Urethra
- Corpus Cavernosum
- Corpus Spongiosum
- Testis
- Epididymis
- Duct of Bulbourethral Gland
- Ductus (Vas) Deferens
- Urinary Bladder
- Seminal Vesicle
- Rectum
- Ejaculatory Duct
- Bulb of Penis

Disorders

Cancerous tumors, infertility, cysts, and sexually transmitted diseases (STDs), such as gonorrhea, genital herpes, syphilis, and human immunodeficiency virus (HIV).

Laboratory Tests

Semen, cytogenetic analysis, tissue biopsies, Pap smears, and microbiological and viral cultures of infected areas. Blood tests include hormonal analysis (of, e.g., estrogen, follicle-stimulating hormone [FSH], luteinizing hormone [LH], human chorionic gonadotropin [HCG], testosterone), the rapid plasma reagin (RPR) test for syphilis, and acid phosphatase and prostatic specific antigen (PSA) for diagnosing and monitoring of prostate cancer.

LYMPHATIC SYSTEM

Structure and Function

The **lymphatic system** consists of lymph, **lymphocytes**, lymph vessels, lymph nodes, tonsils, the spleen, bone marrow, and the thymus gland. Three main functions of the system are to maintain fluid balance in the tissues by filtering blood and lymph fluid, to provide a defense against disease, and to absorb fats and other substances from the digestive tract. About 30 liters of fluid passes from the blood to the tissue spaces each day. If more than 3 liters were retained in the tissue, edema (swelling) would result. The lymph nodes filter lymph fluid, and the spleen filters blood, removing microorganisms or other foreign sub-

Figure 3-15. Lymphatic System

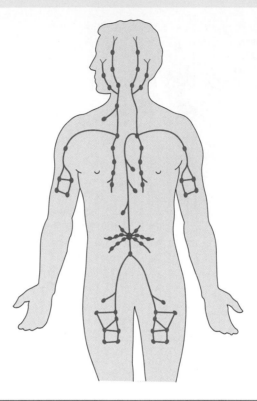

stances. Enlarged or swollen lymph nodes are common after infections. Lymphatic organs contain lymphocytes, macrophages, and other cells that provide immunity and protection against infections from microorganisms.

Disorders

Tumors (such as lymphoma and Hodgkin's disease), immune disorders, and infectious processes.

Laboratory Tests

Some immune disorders can be analyzed from blood samples, bone marrow, or both. Lymph nodes, however, are often surgically removed or aspirated so that cells can be analyzed or cultures performed. Analysis of markers on the surface of the cellular material is also diagnostically valuable.

CARDIOVASCULAR SYSTEM

Since knowledge of the cardiovascular system is important for phlebotomists, it is described separately in greater depth and scope in Chapter 4.

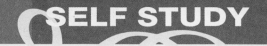

SELF STUDY

KEY TERMS

acidosis

adrenals

alkalosis

alveolar sacs

anabolism

anatomy

anterior

body planes

cardiac (striated involuntary) muscles

cartilage

catabolism

centriole

circulatory system

cytoplasm

deoxyribonucleic acid (DNA)

digestive system

dorsal

endocrine glands

endoplasmic reticulum

exocrine glands

frontal plane

genes

Golgi apparatus

hematopoiesis

homeostasis

hormones

human immunodeficiency virus (HIV)

hyperventilation

integumentary system

lateral

lymphatic system

lysosomes

medial

melanin

meninges

metabolic acidosis

metabolic alkalosis

metabolism

mitochondria

muscular system

nervous system

neurons

nucleolus

nucleus

pathology

peristalsis

physiology

pituitary gland

posterior

reproductive system

respiratory acidosis

respiratory alkalosis

respiratory system

ribosomes

sagittal plane

sexually transmitted diseases (STDs)

skeletal (striated voluntary) muscles

skeletal system

steady state

transverse plane

urinary system

ventral

visceral (nonstriated, smooth, involuntary) muscles

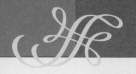

STUDY QUESTIONS

The following may have more than one answer.

1. Which of the following body systems provide protection and support, and allow the body to move?
   - a. integumentary
   - b. skeletal
   - c. muscular
   - d. lymphatic
   - e. digestive

2. Which of the following body systems provides for CO_2 and O_2 exchange?
   - a. nervous
   - b. muscular
   - c. respiratory
   - d. reproductive
   - e. endocrine

3. Which of the following body systems is the primary regulator of hormones?
   - a. digestive
   - b. endocrine
   - c. urinary
   - d. integumentary
   - e. nervous

4. The skeletal system provides which of the body's functions?
   - a. support
   - b. protection of tissues
   - c. calcium storage
   - d. blood cell formation
   - e. leverage and movement

5. Germ cells are defined as
   - a. sperm
   - b. ova
   - c. mammary glands
   - d. neurons
   - e. hair follicles

6. Which of the following pairs of words describe opposite regions or planes of the body?
   - a. anterior/posterior
   - b. distal/proximal
   - c. anterior/ventral
   - d. lateral/medial

7. The pituitary gland is often referred to as which of the following?
   - a. respiratory control gland
   - b. master gland
   - c. lymph tissue
   - d. germ cells

8. How many chromosomes are contained in human cells?
   - a. 25
   - b. 50
   - c. 46
   - d. 100
   - e. 1000

9. What portion of human body weight is water?
   - a. ninety percent
   - b. one half
   - c. one fourth
   - d. two thirds

10. Homeostasis refers to which of the following?
    a. chemical imbalance
    b. steady-state condition
    c. balanced chemistry
    d. thousands of genes
    e. anabolism

11. What role does DNA play in the human body?
    a. allows for hormone changes
    b. provides a genetic blueprint
    c. catabolism
    d. assists in the aging process

12. The lymphatic system assists in providing which of the following?
    a. immunity
    b. structure/support
    c. reproduction
    d. digestion

References

1. Guy, JF: *Learning Human Anatomy: A Laboratory Text and Workbook.* Norwalk, CT: Appleton & Lange, 1992.

The Cardiovascular System

4

CHAPTER OBJECTIVES

Upon completion of Chapter 4, the learner is responsible for the following:

1. Identify and describe the structures and functions of the heart.
2. Trace the flow of blood through the cardiovascular system.
3. Identify and describe the structures and functions of different types of blood vessels.
4. Identify and describe the cellular and noncellular components of blood.
5. Locate and name the veins most commonly used for phlebotomy procedures.

 MediaLINK

Access the accompanying CD-ROM to explore a wide variety of review questions and interactive activities for this chapter, including multiple choice, true/false, and video exercises.

All body systems are linked by the cardiovascular system, a transport network that affects every part of the body within seconds. To maintain homeostasis, the cardiovascular system must provide for the rapid transport of water, nutrients, electrolytes, hormones, enzymes, antibodies, cells, and gases to all cells. In addition, it contributes to body defenses and the coagulation process and controls body temperature. This chapter discusses the three primary components of the cardiovascular system: the heart, the circulating blood, and numerous connected blood vessels (the circulatory system).

■■■■■ THE HEART

The human **heart** is a muscular organ about the size of a man's closed fist. Refer to Figure 4–1 ■. The heart contains four chambers and is located slightly left of the midline in the thoracic cavity. The two atria are separated by the interatrial septum (wall), and the interventricular septum divides the two ventricles. Heart valves are positioned between each atrium and ventricle so that blood can flow in one direction only, thereby preventing backflow.

Tracing the flow of blood as in Figure 4–2 ■, the right atrium of the heart receives O_2-poor blood from two large veins, the superior vena cava and the inferior vena cava. The superior vena cava brings blood from the head, neck, arms, and chest; the inferior vena cava carries blood from the rest of the trunk and the legs. Once the blood enters the right atrium, it passes through the heart valve (right atrioventricular, or tricuspid, valve) into the right ventricle. When blood exits the right ventricle, it begins the **pulmonary circuit**, where it enters the right and left pulmonary arteries. Arteries of the pulmonary circuit differ from those of the **systemic circuit** because they carry deoxygenated blood. Like veins, they are usually shown in blue on color-coded charts. (Refer to Figure 4–3 ■.) These vessels branch into smaller arterioles and capillaries within the lungs, where gaseous exchange occurs (O_2 is picked up and CO_2 is released). From the respiratory capillaries, blood flows into the left and right pulmonary veins and then into the left atrium. The left atrium also has a valve (left atrioventricular, or bicuspid, or mitral, valve). Blood flows through the mitral valve into the left ventricle. When blood exits the left ventricle, it passes through the aortic semilunar valve and into the systemic circuit by means of the ascending aorta. The systemic circuit carries blood to the tissues of the body. If a valve malfunctions, blood flows backward and a heart murmur results. The right side of the heart pumps O_2-poor blood to the lungs to pick up more O_2; the left side pumps O_2-rich blood toward the legs, head, and organs.

The heart's function is to pump sufficient amounts of blood to all cells of the body by contraction (systole) and relaxation (diastole). Because the lungs are close to the heart, and the pulmonary arteries and veins are short and wide, the right ventricle does not need to pump very hard to propel blood through the pulmonary circuit. Thus, the heart wall of the right ventricle is relatively thin. On the other hand, the left ventricle must push blood around the systemic circuit, which covers the entire body. As a result, the left ventricle has a thick, muscular wall and a powerful contraction.

Blood pressure increases during ventricular systole and decreases during ventricular diastole. Blood pressure not only forces blood through vessels, but also pushes it against the walls of the vessels like air in a balloon. Therefore, it can be measured by how forcefully it presses against vascular walls. Refer to Appendix 2 for detailed information about taking blood pressure measurements and other vital signs.

Figure 4–1. Superficial Anatomy of the Heart

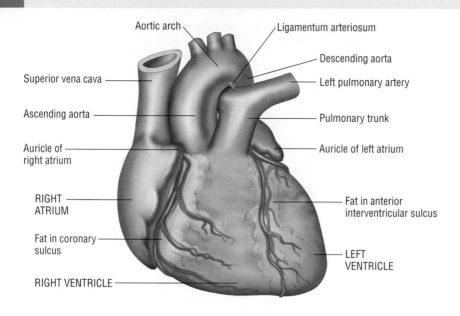

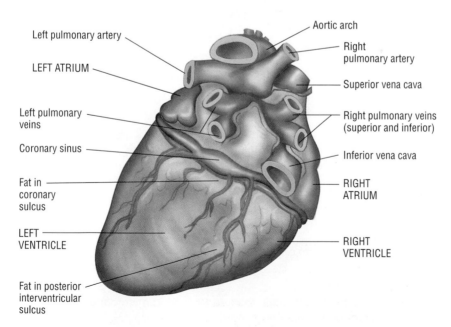

(Top) Anterior (sternocostal) view of the heart showing major anatomic features. (Bottom) Posterior (diaphragmatic) surface of the heart. (Coronary arteries are shown in red, coronary veins in blue.)

Figure 4–2. Sectional Anatomy of the Heart

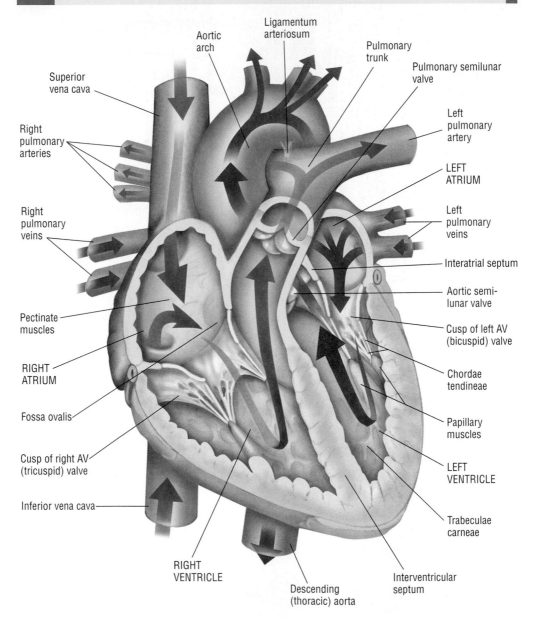

A diagrammatic frontal section through the heart showing major landmarks and the path of blood flow through the atria and ventricles.

Figure 4–3. The Pulmonary Circuit

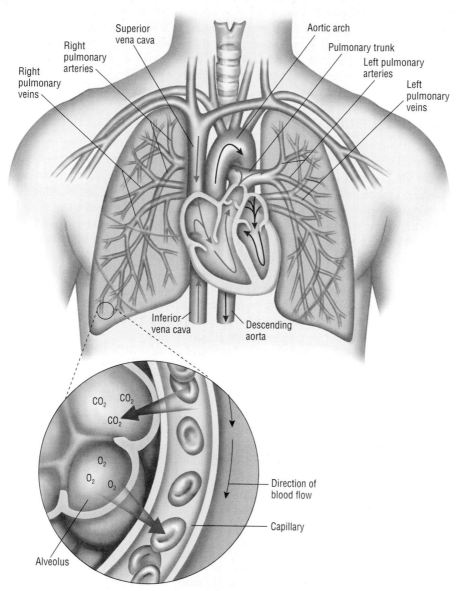

Superior vena cava

Right pulmonary arteries

Right pulmonary veins

Aortic arch

Pulmonary trunk

Left pulmonary arteries

Left pulmonary veins

Inferior vena cava

Descending aorta

CO$_2$ CO$_2$

CO$_2$

O$_2$

O$_2$ O$_2$

Direction of blood flow

Capillary

Alveolus

The right ventricle of the heart pumps blood into the pulmonary artery (pulmonary trunk), which divides into the right and left pulmonary arteries that go to each lung. In the lungs the arteries branch extensively into small arteries and arterioles, then to capillaries. The capillaries surround the alveoli so that exchange of oxygen and carbon dioxide can take place. The capillaries flow into veins and finally into the two pulmonary veins that return blood to the heart through the left atrium. This oxygenated blood will then travel to the rest of the body. (Note that the pulmonary veins contain oxygenated blood. They are the only veins that carry blood with a high oxygen content. All other veins of the body carry blood with a low oxygen content.)

The average heart beats 60 to 80 times per minute. Children have faster heart rates than adults, and athletes have slower rates because more blood can be pumped with each beat. During exercise the heart beats faster to supply muscles with more blood. During and after meals it also beats faster to pump blood to the digestive system. During fever the heart pumps more blood to the skin surface to release heat. The heart rate (pulse rate) is measured by feeling for a pulse and counting the pulses per minute.

THE BLOOD

Circulating blood provides nutrients, oxygen, chemical substances, and waste removal for each of the billions of individual cells in the body and is essential to homeostasis and to sustaining life. Any region of the body that is deprived of blood may die within minutes.

Human bodies contain approximately 5 quarts (4.73 L) of whole blood, which is composed of water, solutes (dissolved substances), and cells. The volume of blood in an individual varies according to body weight; for instance, adult men usually have 5 to 6 L of whole blood, whereas adult women usually have 4 to 5 L. Abnormally low or high blood volumes can seriously affect other parts of the cardiovascular system. Whole blood is composed of approximately 3 quarts (2.84 L, or about 60 percent) of plasma and 2 quarts (1.89 L, or about 40 percent) of cells. Plasma contains 92 percent water and 8 percent solutes. Solutes include proteins, such as albumin, globulins, and fibrinogen; metabolites, such as lipids, glucose, nitrogen wastes, and amino acids; and ions, such as sodium (Na), potassium (K), calcium (Ca), magnesium (Mg), and chloride (Cl).

Circulating blood cells are classified as **red blood cells** (RBCs, or erythrocytes), **white blood cells** (WBCs, or leukocytes), and **platelets** (thrombocytes). Approximately 99 percent of the circulating cells are RBCs. White blood cells are divided further into cell lines called granulocytes (basophils, neutrophils, eosinophils), lymphocytes, and monocytes.

Box 4–1	Functions of the Blood
Transportation	Carry gases
	Carry oxygen from the lungs to the tissues
	Carry carbon dioxide from the tissues to the lungs
	Transport waste products to sites such as the kidneys for excretion
	Transport antibodies and white blood cells to defend against pathogenic microbes and viruses
Disbursement of nutrients	Distribute nutrients absorbed in the digestive tract to all organs of the body
	Take nutrients released from fat, muscle, and tissues for use in other parts of the body
Regulation	Regulate the blood pH in all parts of the body
	Regulate electrolyte balance to maintain a "steady state" condition
	Control body temperature by redistribution of heat
Hemostasis	Restrict fluid loss when blood vessels are damaged
	Formation of blood clots to prevent bleeding

All blood cells develop from undifferentiated stem cells in the hematopoietic (blood-forming) tissues, such as the bone marrow. Stem cells are considered immature cells because they have not developed into their functional state. As the stem cells mature, they differentiate into the different cell lines mentioned in Table 4–1. The cells undergo changes in the nucleus and cytoplasm so that when they reach the circulating blood they will have developed into a specific cell type that is fully mature and functional. The distinguishing features of each blood cell type are clearly visible when staining techniques and light microscopy are used, and they can also be categorized by specialized hematology instruments. Common laboratory tests to assess the blood and cells are listed in Table 3–2. Phlebotomists should be familiar with these blood tests.

ERYTHROCYTES

Red blood cells measure about 7 μm in diameter with a thickness of 2 μm. Prior to reaching maturity in the bone marrow, normal RBCs lose their nuclei and simultaneously become biconcaved disks. Their unique and flexible shape enables them to pass through very narrow capillaries and provides for maximum surface area to transfer oxygen and carbon dioxide. Within each mature RBC are millions of hemoglobin molecules, each capable of carrying four oxygen (O_2) and carbon dioxide (CO_2) molecules. Refer to Figure 4–4 ■ for details on gas exchange in the capillaries.

The process of maturing from a stem cell to a circulating RBC takes several days, and the stages are called rubriblast, prorubricyte, rubricyte, metarubricyte, reticulocyte, and mature RBC. Because nomenclature differs among laboratories, however, the terms pronormoblast, basophilic normoblast, polychromatic normoblast, and orthochromatic normoblast can also be used for the first four stages. The life span of RBCs is approximately 120 days in the circulating bloodstream. Then they begin to fragment and are finally removed and destroyed in the liver, spleen, and bone marrow. As hemoglobin breaks down into iron-containing pigments (hemosiderin) and bile pigments (bilirubin and biliverdin), the bone marrow reuses the iron for new RBCs, and the liver excretes the bile pigments into the intestines.[1]

TABLE 4–1.   Blood Cells

CELLS	NUMBER/ SIZE	FUNCTION	FORMATION	DESTRUCTION
Erythrocytes (RBCs)	4.5–5.5 million/mm³; size 6–7 μm	Transport O_2 and CO_2	Bone marrow	Fragmentation and removal in spleen, liver, and bone marrow; life span— 120 days
Leukocytes (WBCs)	5000–9000/mm³; size 9–16 μm	Defense	Granulocytes in bone marrow; nongranular WBCs in all lymphatic tissue	Removed in spleen, liver, bone marrow; life span—1 day to 1 year
Thrombocytes (platelets)	250,000–450,000/mm³; size 1–4 μm	Clotting	Bone marrow	Removed in spleen; life span—9 to 12 days

Abbreviations: RBCs, red blood cells; WBCs, white blood cells.

Figure 4–4. Exchange of Gases in Systemic and Pulmonary Capillaries

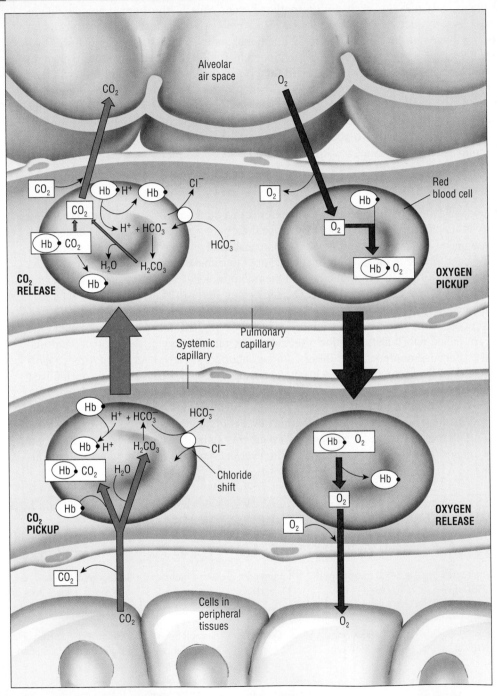

Oxygen (O_2) and carbon dioxide (CO_2) molecules are carried in red blood cells by hemoglobin (Hb) molecules. In the systemic or tissue capillaries, O_2 is released and CO_2 is picked up. When the red cell returns to the pulmonary capillaries in the lungs, CO_2 is released and O_2 is picked up.

Box 4-2   What Triggers the Production of Blood Cells?

Erythropoiesis means the production of red blood cells, millions of which normally are formed and destroyed daily. Erythropoietin is the hormone (produced in the kidney) that triggers erythropoiesis. When the body is not receiving enough O_2 (hypoxia), the kidneys are stimulated to produce erythropoietin, which in turn activates the bone marrow to begin producing more RBCs. The bone marrow also needs an adequate supply of amino acids, vitamin B complexes, and minerals such as iron to produce RBCs. Deficiencies of any of these substances or failure of the bone marrow to function properly may result in anemia.

Box 4-3   Blood Typing: Antibodies and Antigens

All humans have one of the four blood types: A, B, AB, or O; this is known as the the ABO blood group system. Type O is the most common blood type (46 percent of the U.S. population), followed by types A (40 percent), B (10 percent), and AB (4 percent). On the surface of RBCs there are antigens that designate one's blood type. Refer to Figure 4-5 ■.

ABO antibodies (also called agglutinins) are present in plasma and provide protection and cross-reactions with opposing antigens. For example, type A blood contains anti-B, which will attack type B RBCs. Conversely, type B blood contains anti-A, which will cross-react with type A blood cells. Type O whole blood contains anti-A and anti-B, and type AB does not contain A or B antibodies. Type O individuals are called universal donors. Their RBCs can be transfused into a person with any ABO type because their RBCs do not contain A or B antigens to react with either the anti-A or the anti-B present in type B or type A blood, respectively.

Another blood group system contains the Rh factor, in which Rh-positive individuals have the antigen for Rh factor on their RBCs, and Rh-negative people do not. In contrast to the ABO system, Rh antibodies are present *only* if the body has been exposed to Rh-positive RBCs, either accidentally by transfusion, or during childbirth when an Rh-negative mother is carrying an Rh-positive fetus (the Rh-positive gene came from the father). During delivery when the placenta separates and bleeding occurs, the mother is exposed and develops Rh antibodies. If she becomes pregnant again, the Rh antibodies will cross-react with the Rh-positive blood of the fetus. This condition can result in hemolytic disease of the newborn (HDN), but is preventable by the administration of RhoGam (anti-Rh agglutinins) during and after the first pregnancy.

Figure 4-5. Blood Antigens

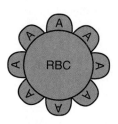

Type A
A antigen is present
(a)

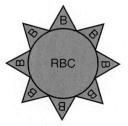

Type B
B antigen is present
(b)

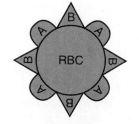

Type AB
A and B antigens
are present
(c)

Type O
A or B antigens
are not present
(d)

LEUKOCYTES

White blood cells (WBCs or leukocytes) differ in color, size, shape, and nuclear formation, and they are divided into two major groups: granular (with granules in the cytoplasm) and agranular (without cytoplasmic granules). Neutrophils, eosinophils, and basophils are granulocytes. Neutrophilic granules stain bluish with neutral dyes, and their nuclei generally have two or more lobes. These granulocytes are often referred to as polymorphonuclear (PMN) leukocytes. Eosinophilic granules stain orange-red with acidic dyes. Their nuclei normally have two lobes. Basophilic granules stain dark purple or black with basic dyes, and their nuclei are often S-shaped. Agranular leukocytes, lymphocytes, and monocytes have relatively large nuclei (see Figure 4–6 ■). Leukocytes serve as part of the body's defense mechanism. The cells phagocytize (ingest) pathogenic microorganisms. Consequently, lymphocytes play a role in immunity and in the production of antibodies.

WBCs are formed in bone marrow and lymphatic tissues. The exact life span of a cell varies with cell type from one day to several years. Normally, blood contains 5,000 to 9,000 leukocytes/mm^3, with designated percentages for each cell line (refer to Table 4–2). The morphological characteristics of WBCs and RBCs are observed by using special laboratory staining techniques, which can be performed manually or by using specialized instrumentation and viewing the cells under the microscope, called a differential. Hematology instruments are able to produce automated differentials at a high speed in a cost-effective manner, whereas manual readings require significant expertise and time to interpret microscopic analysis.

WBCs also have specific cell surface antigens that are expressed at certain times during their development. These antigens can be identified by laboratory methods including flow cytometry and monoclonal antibodies. Using these laboratory techniques, clinicians can tell more precisely how mature or immature the WBCs in the bone marrow and/or peripheral blood are.

Clinical Alert

Blood transfusions can be life-saving procedures in many clinical cases. However, blood transfused into a patient should never contain RBC antigens to which the patient has antibodies. If mismatched blood (due to misidentified samples, etc.) is transfused into a patient, antibodies of the patient cross-react with specific RBC antigens on the donor's RBCs. RBCs can rupture (hemolyze), clump together (agglutinate), and cause clogging of small blood vessels and/or damage to the kidneys, liver, lungs, heart, or brain. These reactions can lead to death. To prevent adverse reactions, physicians request cross-match testing, which involves exposing a blood donor's blood to the patient's (recipient) blood. This procedure detects incompatibility and cross-reactivity. In addition to ABO and Rh, at least 48 possible cross-reactions can occur because of numerous antigens on the blood cells and antibodies in sera.

Figure 4-6. Human Blood Cells

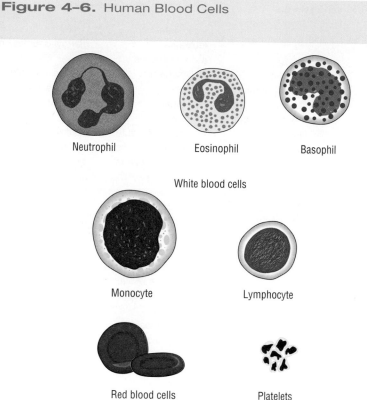

Neutrophil   Eosinophil   Basophil

White blood cells

Monocyte   Lymphocyte

Red blood cells   Platelets

THROMBOCYTES OR PLATELETS

Platelets are much smaller than other blood cells. They are fragments of megakaryocytes (*mega* means big), which are located in the bone. Normally, there are 250,000 to 450,000 platelets/mm^3. Platelets help in the clotting process by transporting needed chemicals for clotting, forming a temporary patch or plug to slow blood loss, and contracting after the blood clot has formed. Their life span is 9 to 12 days.

Abnormalities in the quality or quantity of platelets results in bleeding disorders, which are detected in the laboratory using the bleeding time tests for assessing platelet quality, and the platelet count for assessing the quantity of platelets in the blood.

PLASMA

The liquid portion of blood and lymph is called plasma. Blood cells, dissolved gases, proteins, and other chemical substances are suspended in plasma. Plasma is the medium for transporting constituents in the bloodstream. If a chemical agent called an anticoagulant is added to prevent clotting, a blood sample can be separated by centrifugation into the cells and the liquid plasma (Figure 4–7 ■).

TABLE 4–2. Common Blood Tests

Test	Abbreviation	Normal Range	EXAMPLES OF POSSIBLE DIAGNOSIS	
			Increase	**Decrease**
White blood cell count	WBC	5000-10,000 mm^3	Acute infection, leukemia, mononucleosis	Viral infections, bone marrow depression
Red blood cell count	RBC	Female: 4-5 million/mm^3 Male: 5-6 million/mm^3	Polycythemia, poisoning, pulmonary fibrosis	Anemia, multiple myeloma, lupus erythemia
Differential white blood cell count	Diff	Neutrophils 50-70%	*Neutrophilia:* acute bacterial infections, parasitic infections, liver disease	*Neutropenia:* acute viral infections, blood diseases, hormone diseases
		Eosinophils 1-4%	*Eosinophilia:* allergic conditions, parasitic infections, lung and bone cancer	*Eosinopenia:* infectious mononucleosis, congestive heart failure, aplastic and pernicious anemia
		Basophils 0-1%	*Basophilia:* Leukemia, hemolytic anemia, Hodgkin's disease	*Basopenia:* acute allergic reactions, hyperthyroidism, steroid therapy
		Lymphocytes 20-35%	*Lymphocytosis:* acute and chronic infections, carcinoma, hyperthyroidism	*Lymphopenia:* cardiac failure, Cushing's disease, Hodgkin's disease
		Monocytes 3-8%	*Monocytosis:* viral infections, bacterial and parasitic infections, collagen diseases, cirrhosis	*Monocytopenia:* prednisolone treatment, hairy cell leukemia
Hemoglobin	Hgb	Female, 12-16 g/100 mL Male: 14-18 g/100 mL	Congestive heart failure (CCHF), chronic obstructive pulmonary disease (COPD), severe burn	Hodgkin's disease, hyperthyroidism, cirrhosis
Hematocrit/microhematocrit	Hct, HCT	Female: 40-54% Male 37-47%	Shock, dehydration, burns	Anemia, leukemia, acute blood loss
Prothrombin time	PT	11-16 sec	Anticoagulant therapy, liver disease, biliary obstruction	Diuretics, pulmonary embolism, multiple myeloma
Erythrocyte sedimentation rate	ESR	(According to method used)	Collagen disease, inflammatory disease, rheumatoid arthritis	Sickle cell anemia, CHF, polycythemia
Platelet count		200,000-400,000/mm^3	Cancer, leukemia, splenectomy	Bone-marrow-depressant drug, pneumonia infection

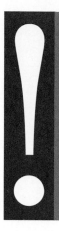

Clinical Alert

Phlebotomists should be on the alert for potential complications related to bleeding disorders. Platelet disorders involving low counts (thrombocytopenia) or dysfunctional platelets are often treated by platelet transfusions to restore normal blood-clotting capacity. Phlebotomists must be particularly cautious about patients on anticoagulant therapy such as aspirin, heparin, and coumadin, or the plasma expander dextran, because a simple venipuncture may cause excessive bleeding for these patients. On the contrary, thrombocytosis is a disease characterized by too many platelets. Patients with this condition may exhibit increased clot formation.

Plasma is composed of approximately 90 percent water and 10 percent dissolved solutes, which include nutrients such as glucose, amino acids, and fats, metabolic wastes (urea, uric acid, creatinine, and lactic acid), respiratory gases (O_2 and CO_2), regulatory substances (hormones, enzymes) electrolytes (sodium, potassium, calcium, and chloride) and protective substances (antibodies). The cellular portion of the specimen contains WBCs, platelets, and RBCs. If the specimen is centrifuged or allowed to settle, the RBCs (the heaviest) will sink to the bottom of the tube. The WBCs and platelets form a thin white layer above the RBCs, called the **buffy coat**. The thin fluid plasma portion is straw colored and remains on the

Figure 4–7. Centrifuged Blood Specimens With and Without Anticoagulant, Respectively

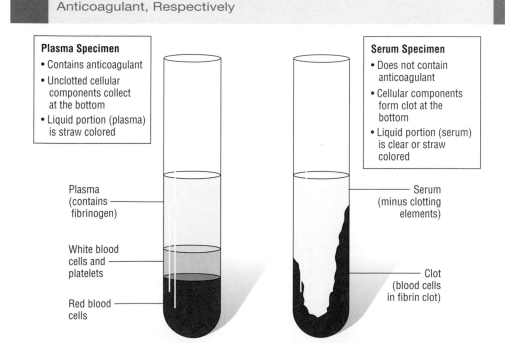

Plasma Specimen
- Contains anticoagulant
- Unclotted cellular components collect at the bottom
- Liquid portion (plasma) is straw colored

Serum Specimen
- Does not contain anticoagulant
- Cellular components form clot at the bottom
- Liquid portion (serum) is clear or straw colored

Plasma (contains fibrinogen)

White blood cells and platelets

Red blood cells

Serum (minus clotting elements)

Clot (blood cells in fibrin clot)

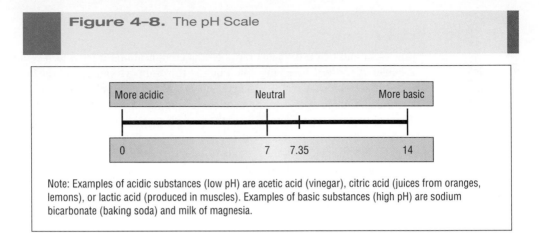

Figure 4–8. The pH Scale

More acidic   Neutral   More basic

0   7   7.35   14

Note: Examples of acidic substances (low pH) are acetic acid (vinegar), citric acid (juices from oranges, lemons), or lactic acid (produced in muscles). Examples of basic substances (high pH) are sodium bicarbonate (baking soda) and milk of magnesia.

top. However, if it is mixed or gently inverted, the cells will again become suspended and the entire sample tube will have the appearance of a freshly collected blood specimen.

Some of plasma's substances, such as proteins, cannot pass through the capillary pores because of their large molecular size. The majority of proteins stay in the vascular space, where they exert osmotic pressure. This pressure keeps fluid (blood volume) levels in balance. Proteins in the plasma perform other functions, such as providing energy when the body is not getting enough from regular food intake. In conjunction with electrolytes, proteins help "buffer" the blood. Buffering is a term used to describe the body's ability to control the pH of the blood. The pH describes the degree of acidity or alkalinity of a solution on a pH scale of 1 to 14. An "acidic" pH is low (1–7), and a "basic" pH is high (7–14). The normal range of blood pH is slightly basic, from 7.35 to 7.45. Refer to the pH scale in Figure 4–8 ■. If the pH in a patient's blood becomes too acidic or too basic serious complications can result for the patient. In acidosis, carbon dioxide (CO_2) and organic acids build up in the blood causing it to become acidic. If it is not detected by laboratory testing, blood and tissues can be damaged.

SERUM

If a blood specimen is allowed to clot, the result is **serum** (also straw color) plus blood cells meshed in a **fibrin** clot. Serum contains essentially the same chemical constituents as plasma, except the clotting factors and the blood cells are contained within the fibrin clot (see Figure 4–7).

■■■■■ THE VESSELS AND CIRCULATION

Three kinds of blood vessels exist in the human body: arteries, veins, and capillaries. This intricate system travels to every inch of the human body through repeatedly branching vessels that get smaller and smaller as they move away from the heart (arteries), and then get larger again as they return toward the heart (veins). Figures 4–9 ■ and 4–10 ■ provide an overview of the arterial and venous systems, showing the major branches of the vessels. The largest artery (aorta) and veins (venae cavae) are approximately 1 inch wide.

Figure 4-9. The Arterial System

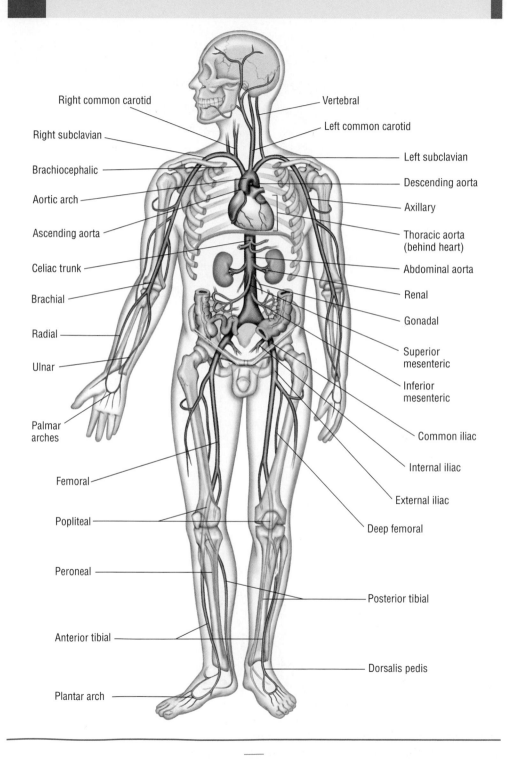

Right common carotid

Right subclavian

Brachiocephalic

Aortic arch

Ascending aorta

Celiac trunk

Brachial

Radial

Ulnar

Palmar arches

Femoral

Popliteal

Peroneal

Anterior tibial

Plantar arch

Vertebral

Left common carotid

Left subclavian

Descending aorta

Axillary

Thoracic aorta (behind heart)

Abdominal aorta

Renal

Gonadal

Superior mesenteric

Inferior mesenteric

Common iliac

Internal iliac

External iliac

Deep femoral

Posterior tibial

Dorsalis pedis

Figure 4–10. Venous System

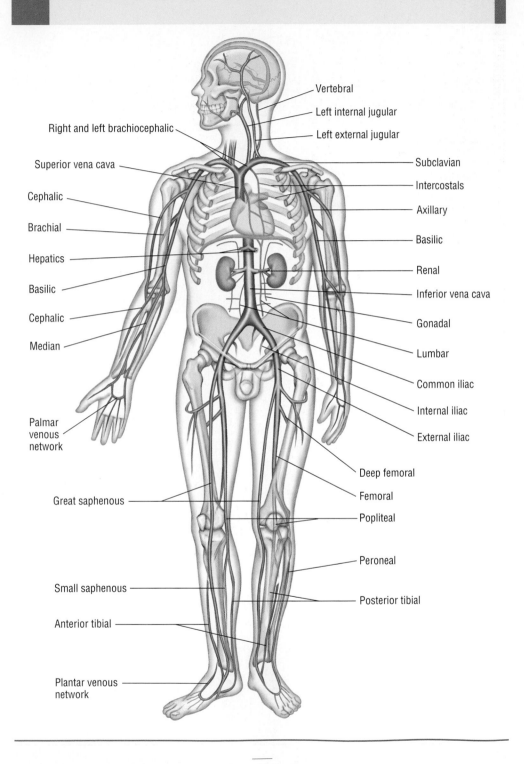

Vertebral

Left internal jugular

Left external jugular

Right and left brachiocephalic

Superior vena cava

Subclavian

Intercostals

Cephalic

Axillary

Brachial

Basilic

Hepatics

Renal

Basilic

Inferior vena cava

Cephalic

Gonadal

Median

Lumbar

Common iliac

Internal iliac

Palmar venous network

External iliac

Deep femoral

Femoral

Great saphenous

Popliteal

Peroneal

Small saphenous

Posterior tibial

Anterior tibial

Plantar venous network

Figure 4–11. Comparison of Arteries, Veins, and Capillaries

Capillaries: Thin walls permit exchange of blood and fluids from surrounding tissues. They are so small in diameter that only one RBC can pass through at a time.

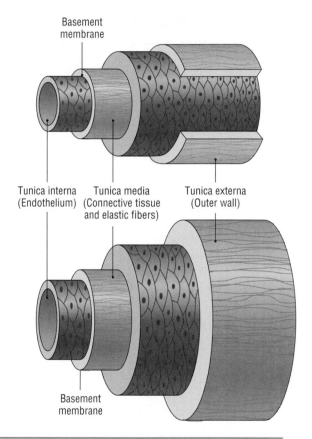

Endothelium

Basement membrane

Basement membrane

Veins: Thinner walls than arteries so they are more likely to collapse when blood is withdrawn.

Tunica interna (Endothelium)

Tunica media (Connective tissue and elastic fibers)

Tunica externa (Outer wall)

Arteries: Thicker walls (Tonica externa) than veins; resist the strong pressure of blood being pushed through.

Basement membrane

ARTERIES

Arteries are highly oxygenated vessels that carry blood away from the heart (efferent vessels). They branch into smaller vessels, called arterioles, and into capillaries. The principal arteries of the body are indicated in Figure 4–9. Arteries are normally bright red in color, have thicker elastic walls than veins do, and have a pulse. Refer to Figure 4–11 ■ for a comparison of capillaries, arteries, and veins.

Box 4–4	What Is "Hardening of the Arteries"?

With age, arterial walls may "harden" (called hardening of the arteries or arteriosclerosis). The inner walls of the vessels become rough because of cholesterol or calcium deposits. As the deposits (plaque) build, blood clots may form that clog the artery further, and the blood supply to tissues is reduced. In serious cases, this lack of blood results in a stroke (if the blood supply in the brain is reduced) or a heart attack (if the blood supply in the coronary [heart] vessels is reduced). Refer to Figure 4-12 ■.

VEINS

Blood is carried toward the heart by the **veins** (afferent vessels). It is remarkable that the blood in veins flows against gravity in many areas of the body, these vessels have one-way valves and rely on weak muscular action to move blood cells. The one-way valves prevent backflow of blood. All veins (except the pulmonary veins) contain deoxygenated blood

Figure 4–12. Plaque Build-Up Causing Partial Blockage of the Artery

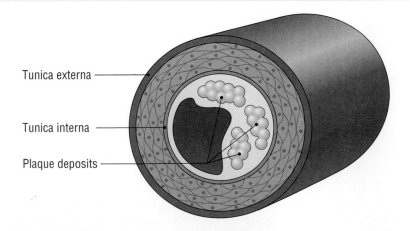

Tunica externa

Tunica interna

Plaque deposits

Figure 4–13. Venous System of the Upper Torso and Arm

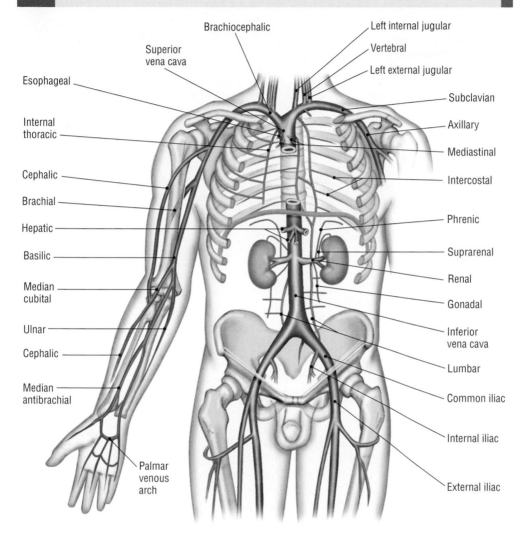

Note the antecubetal area of the arm where venipunctures are most often performed.

and are normally dark red in color and have thinner walls than arteries, as shown in Figure 4–11.

Phlebotomists should be familiar with the principal veins of the arms and legs (Figures 4–13 ■ to 4–16 ■). The antecubital area of the forearm is most commonly used for venipuncture. The median cubital vein is best for venipuncture because it is generally the largest and best anchored vein. Others in the antecubital area that are acceptable are the basilic vein and the cephalic vein.

Figure 4–14. Major Arm Veins

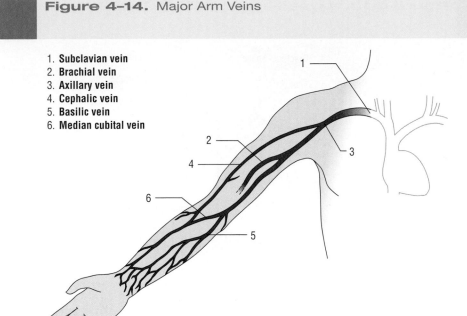

1. Subclavian vein
2. Brachial vein
3. Axillary vein
4. Cephalic vein
5. Basilic vein
6. Median cubital vein

Note that the *cephalic vein* extends almost the entire length of the arm. The superficial *median cubital vein* serves as a connection between the cephalic and basilic veins. The subclavian, brachial, and axillary veins are deeper veins.

CAPILLARIES

Capillaries are tiny microscopic vessels that connect or link arteries (arterioles) and veins (venules) and may be so small in diameter as to allow only one blood cell to pass through at any given time. They are the only vessels that permit the exchange of gases (O_2 and CO_2) and other molecules between blood and surrounding tissues. Capillaries do not work independently, but are a part of an interconnected network. Each arteriole ends in dozens of capillaries (capillary bed) that eventually feed back into a **venule** (when gas/nutrient exchange has been completed). Blood in the capillary bed is a mixture of arterial and venous blood. Refer to Figure 4–17 ■.

▄▄▄▄ HEMOSTASIS AND COAGULATION

Hemostasis (not to be confused with homeostasis) is the maintenance of circulating blood in the liquid state and retention of blood in the vascular system by preventing blood loss. When a small blood vessel is injured, the hemostatic process (clotting response) repairs the break and stops the hemorrhage by forming a plug or blood clot (refer to Figure 4–18 ■). The first (vascular) phase in this process is vasoconstriction, a rapid constriction of the vessel, which decreases the blood flow to the surrounding vascular bed. In the second (platelet) phase, platelets degranulate, clump together, and adhere to the injured ves-

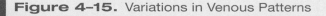

Figure 4–15. Variations in Venous Patterns

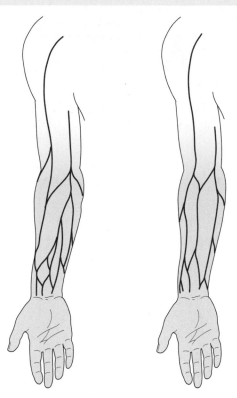

Since all individuals are unique, the exact location of veins may vary from one to another. This figure depicts variations in venous patterns in the arms of two individuals.

sel in order to form a plug and inhibit bleeding. In phase three (coagulation), many specific coagulation factors are released and interact to form a fibrin meshwork, or blood clot. This clot seals off the damaged portion of the vessel. Phase four (clot retraction) occurs when the bleeding has stopped. The entire clot retracts to bring torn edges closer together. In phase five (fibrinolysis), final repair and regeneration of the injured vessel occurs, and the clot slowly begins to break up (lysis) and dissolve as other cells carry out further repair.

The **coagulation** process (phase three) is a result of numerous coagulation factors. For simplicity, it is divided into two systems: intrinsic and extrinsic. All coagulation factors required for the intrinsic system are contained in the blood, whereas the extrinsic factors are stimulated when tissue damage occurs. For example, blood vessels are lined with a single layer of flat endothelial cells and are supported by collagen fibers. Normally, endothelial cells do not react or attract platelets; however, they do produce and store some clotting

Figure 4–16. Major Leg Veins

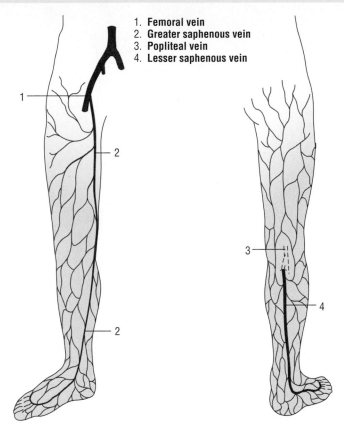

1. Femoral vein
2. Greater saphenous vein
3. Popliteal vein
4. Lesser saphenous vein

The *femoral vein* is a deep vein. Note that the *greater saphenous vein* is the longest vein in the body. It ascends up the medial side of the leg and the medial thigh and empties into the femoral vein in the groin area. The *lesser saphenous vein* comes up the lateral side of the ankle and enters the deeper *popliteal vein* behind the knee.

factors. When the clotting sequence begins due to a vessel injury, endothelial cells react with degranulated platelets in forming the fibrin plug.[1] Bleeding from small arteries and veins can be controlled by the hemostatic process; however, large- or medium-sized veins and arteries require rapid surgical intervention to prevent excessive bleeding.

◼◼ LABORATORY TESTS OF THE CARDIOVASCULAR SYSTEM

There are numerous laboratory tests that can be done to assess the cardiovascular system, some of which are described in Table 4–2. Most of them are performed in a hematology/coagulation laboratory. The number of RBCs, their morphological traits, and their

Figure 4–17. Capillary Bed

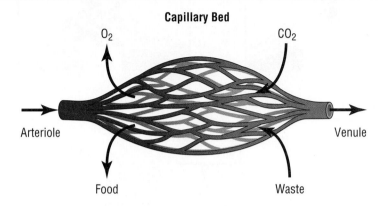

Capillary Bed

O_2 CO_2

Arteriole   Venule

Food   Waste

hemoglobin content can be determined from an anticoagulated blood specimen in the clinical hematology laboratory. Platelets and WBCs can be assessed on the basis of number and morphological features. The results of a WBC differential count enumerate specific cell lines in percentages. Platelet function, as well as each coagulation factor, can be measured from anticoagulated blood specimens in the coagulation section of the clinical hematology laboratory. In addition, bone marrow, which is removed by a physician usually from the iliac crest of the hip, can be stained and studied microscopically in the hematology laboratory for the detection of abnormal numbers and morphological characteristics of blood cells.

Box 4–5	External Bleeding

The nature of the job requires that phlebotomists regularly deal with patients who are bleeding. External bleeding can be described according to the type of blood vessel that is injured and losing blood:

Arterial bleeding is bright red in color (due to high O_2 content), and since the pressure is higher in arteries, bleeding is usually quicker, more abundant, and in spurts (with each heartbeat). Arterial bleeding is the hardest to control and usually requires special attention from the nurse and/or doctor. During a venipuncture procedure, if a phlebotomist accidentally punctures an artery instead of a vein, he or she should follow immediate steps to terminate the procedure and apply pressure to the site. Accidental incidents such as this should be reported to a supervisor immediately.

Venous bleeding is dark red in color (because it lacks O_2), and it occurs in a steady flow. In normal, healthy adults, venous bleeding is easy to stop by simply applying pressure, because venous pressure is lower than arterial pressure.

Capillary bleeding occurs slowly and evenly because of the smaller size of the vessels and the low pressure within the vessels. Capillary bleeding is usually considered minor and is easily controlled with slight pressure or sometimes bleeding stops without intervention. Capillary blood is a color between the bright red of arterial blood and the dark red of venous blood.[2]

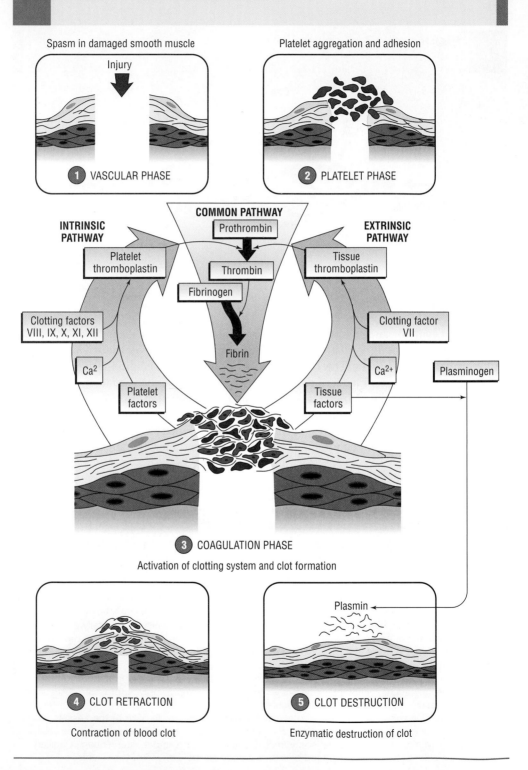

Figure 4–18. Clotting Response

Spasm in damaged smooth muscle

Injury

1 VASCULAR PHASE

Platelet aggregation and adhesion

2 PLATELET PHASE

INTRINSIC PATHWAY

COMMON PATHWAY

Prothrombin

Platelet thromboplastin

Thrombin

Fibrinogen

EXTRINSIC PATHWAY

Tissue thromboplastin

Clotting factors VIII, IX, X, XI, XII

Ca^2

Clotting factor VII

Ca^{2+}

Fibrin

Platelet factors

Tissue factors

Plasminogen

3 COAGULATION PHASE

Activation of clotting system and clot formation

4 CLOT RETRACTION

Contraction of blood clot

Plasmin

5 CLOT DESTRUCTION

Enzymatic destruction of clot

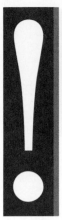

Clinical Alert

When a phlebotomist discovers or anticipates bleeding, it is important to use standard precautions, including gloves, to avoid exposure of the skin and mucous membranes. A mask and protective eyewear or a face shield should also be worn if there is a chance of splattered blood or if the patient is coughing up blood, and a gown should be worn if there is a chance that clothing might become contaminated.

Tests for blood types and cross-matches for donor blood are done in an immunohematology, a transfusion, or a blood-banking laboratory. Serum and plasma constituents, including nutrients, metabolic wastes, respiratory gases, regulatory substances, and protective substances, can all be evaluated from blood specimens in the clinical chemistry laboratory. Refer to Table 4–3 for common chemistry tests. These tests, while conducted on plasma or serum, actually assess the substances that are normally carried in the bloodstream but relate to the functioning of other organ systems besides the cardiovascular system.

Box 4–6	Disorders of the Hemostatic Process

Disorders in the process of hemostasis are serious. Overactive clotting can cause clots within the body, such as an embolus or a thrombus, or disseminated intravascular coagulation (DIC) disease. Drugs such as heparin and Coumadin (warfarin), which suppress clotting factors, can be used to prevent such problems. On the other hand, if clotting factors are not produced by the body, excessive bleeding may occur, as in hemophilia.

TABLE 4–3. Common Blood Chemistries and Examples of Disorders Associated with Abnormal Results

Test	Abbreviation	Normal Range	EXAMPLES OF POSSIBLE DIAGNOSIS	
			Results Increased	Results Decreased
Alkaline phosphate	ALP	30–115 mU/mL	Liver disease, bone disease, mononucleosis	Malnutrition, hypothyroidism, chronic nephritis
Blood urea nitrogen	BUN	8–25 mg/dL	Kidney disease, dehydration, GI bleeding	Liver failure, malnutrition
Calcium	CA	8.5–10.5 mg/dL	Hypercalcemia, bone metastases, Hodgkin's disease	Hypocalcemia, renal failure, pancreatitis
Chloride	Cl	96–10 mEq/L	Dehydration, eclampsia, anemia	Ulcerative colitis, burns, heat exhaustion
Cholesterol	CHOL	120–200 mg/dL	Atherosclerosis, nephrosis, obstructive jaundice	Malabsorption, liver disease, hyperthyroidism
Creatinine	Creat	0.4–1.5 mg/dL	Chronic nephritis, muscle disease, obstruction of urinary tract	Muscular dystrophy
Globulin	Glob	1.0–3.5 g/dL	Brucellosis, rheumatoid arthritis, hepatic carcinoma	Severe burns
Glucose fasting blood sugar	FBS	70–110 mg/100 mL	Diabetes mellitus	Excess insulin
Two-hour postprandial	2-hr PPBS	< 140 mg/dL	Cushing syndrome, brain damage	Addison's disease, CA of pancreas
Lactic acid	LDH	100–225 mU/mL	Acute MI, acute leukemia, hepatic disease	
Potassium	K	3.5–5.5 mEq/L	Renal failure, acidosis, cell damage	Malabsorption, severe burn, diarrhea
Serum glutamicoxaloacetic	SGOT	0–41 mU/mL	MI, liver disease, pancreatitis	Uncontrolled diabetes mellitus with acidosis
Serum glutamicpyruvic transaminase	SGPT	0–45 mU/mL	Active cirrhosis, pancreatitis, obstructive jaundice	
Sodium	NA	135–145 mEq/L	Diabetes insipitus, coma, Cushing syndrome	Severe diarrhea, severe nephritis, vomiting
Free thyroxine	T4	1–2.3 mg/dL	Thyroiditis, hyperthyroidism, Graves disease	Goiter, myeledema, hypothyroidism
Total bilirubin	TB	0.1–1.2 mg/dL	Liver disease, hemolytic anemia, lupus erythemia	
Triglycerides	TRIG	40–170 mg/dL	Liver disease, atherosclerosis, pancreatitis	Malnutrition
Uric acid	UA	2.2–9.0 mg/dL	Renal failure, gout, leukemia, eclampsia	

GI = gastrointestinal; CA = carcinoma, malignant tumor; MI = myocardial infarction

SELF STUDY

KEY TERMS

ABO blood group system
anticoagulant
aorta
arteries
arterioles
atria
basilic vein
basophils
blood
blood pressure
blood vessels
buffy coat
capillaries
cardiovascular system
cell membrane
cephalic vein
cerebrospinal fluid (CSF)
circulatory system
coagulation
cross-match testing
diastolic pressure
differential
eosinophils
erythropoiesis
erythropoietin
extrinsic factors
fibrin
fibrinolysis
granulocytes (basophils, neutrophils, eosinophils)

heart
hematocrit
hematopoietic
hemoglobin
hemostasis
hypoxia
inferior vena cava
intrinsic system
lymphocytes
median cubital vein
megakaryocytes
monocytes
neutrophils
plasma
platelets (thrombocytes)
pulmonary circuit
pulse rate
red blood cells (RBCs or erythrocytes)
Rh factor
serum
superior vena cava
systemic circuit
systolic pressure
vasoconstriction
veins
venae cavae
ventricles
venules
white blood cells (WBCs or leukocytes)

STUDY QUESTIONS

The following questions may have more than one answer.

1. Whole blood consists of which of the following?
   a. water
   b. solutes
   c. cells
   d. tissue

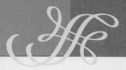

2. Which type of blood cell is most numerous in the circulating blood?
   a. red blood cell
   b. white blood cell
   c. platelet
   d. macrophage

3. Identify the four chambers of the heart.
   a. right atrium, right ventricle
   b. superior vena cava, inferior vena cava
   c. left atrium, left ventricle
   d. ascending aorta, descending aorta

4. The liquid portion of an anticoagulated blood specimen is called
   a. plasma
   b. serum
   c. cellular components
   d. oxygenated blood

5. Which of the following veins are most commonly used for venipuncture procedures?
   a. popliteal
   b. brachial
   c. median cubital
   d. cephalic
   e. basilic

6. Functions of the blood include which of the following?
   a. transportation of gases, enzymes, and hormones
   b. regulation of pH and electrolytes
   c. regulation of body temperature
   d. transportation of waste products

7. Which type of bleeding is easiest to control?
   a. venous bleeding
   b. capillary bleeding
   c. arterial bleeding
   d. systolic bleeding

8. Which of the listed circulating blood cells have no nuclei?
   a. neutrophils
   b. erythrocytes
   c. basophils
   d. eosinophils

9. The most common blood type is
   a. A
   b. B
   c. AB
   d. O

10. The coagulation process occurs in phases that include the
    a. vascular phase
    b. platelet phase
    c. coagulation phase
    d. clot-retraction phase

References

1. Martini, F: *Fundamentals of Anatomy and Physiology,* 3rd ed. Englewood Cliffs, NJ: Prentice Hall, 1995.
2. Limmer, D, O'Keefe, MF, Dickinson, ET, et al: *Emergency Care, Fire Services Edition,* 9th ed., Upper Saddle River, NJ: Prentice Hall, 2003.

Career Pathways: Smooth or Stormy

Derek was a high energy, self motivated type of medical assistant who had worked for the same physician group practice over 10 years. His duties included providing assistance in the laboratory, but his primary job duty was specimen collection, particularly phlebotomy. He was good at what he did and everyone knew it. He was well liked by his coworkers, his supervisors, and the patients. He had been told that the practice was closing their laboratory because several of the physicians were retiring and the others would be sharing laboratory services with another practice. He was devastated at this news and did not know where to turn for a career move.

Questions

1. What types of resources could Derek seek to begin a plan for a job move?
2. Describe the steps he should take in finding a new job.
3. How could professional organizations help him?

Changing Responsibility in Phlebotomy Practice

Ms. Hansen had been working in the hospital clinical laboratory for 4 years as a phlebotomist. She was highly regarded by her laboratory colleagues because of her efficiency in blood collection on three different units of the hospital, her assistance with specimen processing, and overall attention to details. She was recognized by her department as outstanding in her ability to communicate effectively with patients. Outside of work she routinely socialized with her coworkers on weekends. As part of the hospital restructuring plan, she was reassigned to report to a nursing director on a surgical unit of the hospital. Her new work duties included phlebotomy, glucose bedside testing, clerical functions on the unit, and occasional patient transportation from the unit to other parts of the hospital as needed. She was very reluctant to leave her friends and old job duties in the laboratory to be relocated to the surgical unit. Ms. Hansen knew that all the phlebotomists' positions in the hospital were being reassigned, and she did not want to work anywhere else because she felt loyal to the hospital. She was too proud to complain about her unhappiness with the situation.

Questions

1. How could Ms. Hansen become more open to changing her work role?
2. List four character traits that Ms. Hansen should remember about working with health care teams.
3. Describe the positive professional character traits exhibited by Ms. Hansen and how they may be beneficial in her new job assignment.

Collection from the Dorsal Side of the Hand

Mr. Whitefield, a phlebotomist who recently completed his training program at Amber Community College, acquired a position at Oakhaven Hospital on the early morning shift. One morning, he was informed by the nurse on the orthopedic floor that any blood collections from Patient Davis should be taken while Mr. Davis is in the supine position and that all collections should be taken from the left dorsal hand.

Questions

1. Is the dorsal area the same as the proximal area? Explain the similarities or differences.
2. Should Mr. Davis sit up or lie down during the blood collection?
3. Orthopedic refers to what type of specialty?

Communication and Cultural Sensitivity: Keys to Success

Mrs. Rodriguez is pregnant and has come to see her obstetrician for a routine prenatal visit. She is accompanied by her 8-year-old daughter, her mother, and her 2 sisters. None of them speak English very well except the 8-year-old daughter. Mrs. Rodriguez's examination includes laboratory tests and urinalysis. She also needs to be screened for gestational diabetes. Elizabeth, an experienced health care worker who cannot speak Spanish, is assigned to collect the specimens from Mrs. Rodriguez.

Questions

1. Describe possible barriers to the effective communication between Mrs. Rodriguez and Elizabeth.
2. Even though there is limited information presented here, what characteristics seem important to Mrs. Rodriguez?
3. Describe at least five communication strategies that Elizabeth might use during her encounter with Mrs. Rodriquez?
4. What role(s) can the family members play in this situation?
5. Describe career development strategies that Elizabeth might consider to improve her ability to communicate effectively with patients like Mrs. Rodriguez.

Communication and Consent

Ms. Nancy Garcia, a 78-year-old Hispanic woman, was admitted to River Bend Hospital as a result of complications from diabetes mellitus. When the health care worker arrived at her hospital room to collect blood for laboratory tests, he introduced himself and asked her name. She did not respond and looked perplexed.

Questions

1. What should the health care worker do next?
2. What could a health care facility provide to assist in this situation?
3. Has the patient implied her consent to the venipuncture?

An Ethical Dilemma

Ms. Daley was a veteran nurse on a hospital medical floor with mostly cardiac patients. The patient care assistant, Marty, had been performing phlebotomy duties on this floor for about 6 months and had developed a close friendship with Ms. Daley. They had even socialized after work on a few occasions.

One morning two individuals with similar names were admitted to this hospital unit. Their names were Frances L. Johnson and Francis T. Johnston. Ms. Daley was in charge of giving the patients their identification bracelets. Soon after admission, laboratory tests were ordered STAT on both patients so Marty went to collect the specimens. She entered the room expecting to greet Frances L. Johnson. She checked the identification bracelet and noticed that Frances L. Johnson had Francis T. Johnston's identification bracelet, even though the sign on the hospital room was correctly labeled. When Marty mentioned the mistake to Ms. Daley she said, "Oh don't worry, it's just a little mix-up and I'll fix it. Since there was no harm done, I don't see any need to report it. Thanks for letting me know."

Questions

1. What should Marty do next?
2. What corrective actions, if any, should be taken?
3. What ethical situations might arise from this situation?
4. What might the consequences have been if Marty had not noticed the error?

Answers for all case study questions can be found in Appendix 12.

Infection Control

CHAPTER OBJECTIVES

Upon completion of Chapter 5, the learner is responsible for the following:

1. Define the term health-care acquired (nosocomial) infection.
2. Identify the basic programs for infection control.
3. Explain the proper techniques for hand washing, gowning, gloving, masking, double bagging, and entering and exiting the various isolation areas.
4. Identify the potential routes of infection and methods for preventing transmission of microorganisms through these routes.
5. Identify steps to avoid transmission of bloodborne pathogens.
6. Describe the various isolation procedures and reasons for their use.

MediaLINK

Access the accompanying CD-ROM to explore a wide variety of review questions and interactive activities for this chapter, including multiple choice, true/false, and video exercises.

▓▓▓▓ PATHOGENS AND INFECTIONS

The condition in which the body is invaded with pathogenic (causing disease) microorganisms (e.g., bacteria, fungi, viruses, parasites) is called infection. A person normally has microorganisms on the skin, in the respiratory tract, and in the gastrointestinal (GI) tract. Sometimes, these nondisease (nonpathogenic) microorganisms enter parts of the body where they normally do not belong and cause disease (pathogenic). For example, *Escherichia coli,* normally found in the GI tract, can cause a bladder infection from lack of washing hands and other body areas. In health care institutions, the patients are usually very ill because of infection or injury. Health care settings continuously have pathogenic and nonpathogenic microorganisms carried by patients, visitors, and health care providers. The term **bloodborne pathogens (BBPs)** can be used to describe any infectious microorganism present in blood and other body fluids and tissues and include:

- Hepatitis A, B, C, D, and E
- HIV (AIDS)
- Syphilis
- Malaria
- Human T-cell lymphotrophic virus (HTLV) types I and II

Health-care-acquired—**nosocomial**—infections are those that are acquired by a patient after admission to a health care facility, such as a hospital, clinic, nursing home, or psychiatric institution. Approximately 5 percent of all hospitalized patients in the United States get health-care-acquired infections, which account for 87,500 deaths yearly.[1, 2] In an attempt to control them, infection control programs have been developed. Using guidelines established by the Centers for Disease Control and Prevention (CDC), the Joint Commission on Accreditation of Healthcare Organizations (JCAHO), and state regulatory agencies, managers of each health care institution are responsible for developing and implementing an infection control program. These programs address the issues of proper asepsis technique, **isolation procedures,** education, and management of community-acquired infections, as well as health-care-associated infections. An infection control nurse or practitioner usually works closely with or in the clinical microbiology laboratory and communicates with personnel in the health care facility and with home health care providers to make the necessary assessments.

The **Centers for Disease Control and Prevention (CDC),** as part of the U.S. Public Health Service, oversees the investigation and control of various diseases, especially those that are communicable and threaten the U.S. population. CDC provides infection control and safety guidelines to protect health care workers and patients from infection. The cornerstones for infection protection of patients and health care workers, particularly phlebotomists, are **aseptic techniques,** which include the following:

- Frequent hand washing.
- Use of barrier garments and personal protective equipment.
- Waste management of contaminated materials
- Use of proper cleaning solutions
- Following standard precautions
- Using sterile procedures when necessary

These protective procedures must become part of a phlebotomist's routine procedures and standards for practice. These practices are also discussed in Chapters 8 and 9. Because each health care facility has its own infection control program and policy manual, the health care worker should read and be familiar with both.

If the phlebotomist works for a home health care agency, it is imperative to have knowledge of infection control protocols for home health care, because the home is an uncontrolled, unpredictable setting in which to provide care. Infections can be transmitted in a variety of ways, and each health care worker should realize that he or she can be infected and can transmit infectious agents. Tables 5–1 and 5–2 list causative agents for nosocomial infections.

███████ PERSONAL SAFETY FROM INFECTION DURING SPECIMEN HANDLING

Patients' specimens should be handled with caution to prevent the possibility of acquiring an infection, including hepatitis B and C and human immunodeficiency virus (HIV). **Occupational Safety and Health Administration (OSHA),** an agency of the U.S. Department of Labor, requires employers to provide measures that will protect workers exposed to biological hazards. Health care workers who are routinely exposed to blood and body fluids must take the precautions of wearing gloves to protect themselves from infection as well. These requirements have occurred due to the 1991 OSHA standards for occupational exposure to blood-borne pathogens (29 CFR 1930.1030) and the Needlestick Safety and Prevention Act that took effect April 18, 2001, which updated the 1991 OSHA standards.[3,4]

EXPOSURE CONTROL

Any incident of exposure to potentially harmful bloodborne pathogens or other infectious body fluids should be reported immediately to the supervisor and the employer's personnel health department. Each health care worker should know who to contact, where to go, and what to do if possibly exposed to harmful pathogens.[5] The report must include the safety-engineered blood collection device that did not work effectively to protect the health care worker during blood collection. If exposures are not reported, it is difficult to prove retrospectively that an exposure to an infectious agent was work-related. These exposure-control written incidents must also be maintained for legal documentation if lawsuits arise due to an ineffectively safety-engineered blood collection device. (See Clinical Alert on p. 128.)

HEALTH CARE PROVIDERS' HEALTH

Infection control programs also monitor employee health programs. The primary objective is to minimize the risk of infection and hazardous circumstances for employees and patients. Most employees are screened for the following diseases prior to employment: measles, mumps, tuberculosis, hepatitis, diarrheal disease, syphilis, and skin diseases. Immunization for a variety of diseases is often made available initially and throughout employment, free of charge. Often, the hospital stipulates policies for employees with specific infections or employees who have been exposed to certain infections, such as those listed in Table 5–3.

TABLE 5–1.   Microorganisms Causing Health-care Acquired (Nosocomial) Infections in Patients

BODY AREAS	COMMONLY IDENTIFIED PATHOGENIC AGENTS
Blood and cerebrospinal fluid	Any microorganisms
Ear	*Pseudomonas aeruginosa*
	Streptococcus pneumoniae
	Gram-negative bacilli
Eye	*Staphylococcus aureus*
	Neisseria gonorrhoeae
	Gram-negative bacilli
	Moraxella lacunata
	Haemophilus influenzae
	S. pneumoniae
	P. aeruginosa
	Salmonella sp.
Gastrointestinal tract	*Shigella* sp.
	Clostridium difficile
	Enteropathogenic *Escherichia coli*
	Vibrio cholerae
	Campylobacter sp.
	Parasitic protozoans
	Candida albicans
	Some viruses (i.e., Rotavirus)
	N. gonorrhoeae
Genital tract	*Haemophilus vaginalis*
	C. albicans (yeast)
	Streptococcus pyogenes
Respiratory tract	*Corynebacterium diphtheriae*
	Bordatella pertussis
	Staphylococcus epidermidis
	Acinebacter spp.
	S. aureus
	S. pneumoniae
	H. influenzae
	Any Gram-negative bacilli
	Fungi
	Certain viruses (i.e., Influenza A2 and B; Parainfluenza; Rhinovirus)
	S. aureus
	S. pyogenes
Skin	*C. albicans*
	Smallpox
	Herpes virus
	Enterovirus
	Measles
Urinary tract	Any microorganism in sufficient numbers
Wounds and abscesses	Any microorganisms

TABLE 5–2.   Microorganisms Causing Health-care Acquired (Nosocomial) Infections in Hospital Areas

HOSPITAL AREAS	COMMONLY IDENTIFIED PATHOGENIC AGENTS
Burn unit	All Gram-negative bacilli
	Gram-positive rods
	Fungi
Dialysis unit	Hepatitis and other viruses
	Bacteria
	Fungi
Intensive care or postoperative care unit	Any microorganisms
Nursery unit	S. aureus
	Group B Streptococcus
	E. coli
	S. pneumoniae
	Other Gram-negative bacilli
	Viruses (i.e., Rotavirus)

For the employee's protection, many types of warning labels are used. Among these are isolation signs, radiation hazard signs, and biohazard signs (see Figure 5–1 ■). These signs may be posted on or next to the patient's hospital room door or other areas of the health care institution to warn of possible hazards.

■■■■ CHAIN OF INFECTION

Nosocomial infections result when the "chain of infection" is complete (Table 5–4). The three components that make up the chain are the source, mode of transmission, and susceptible host.

SOURCE

In a normal environment, relatively few things are sterile; therefore, potential sources of infection cover a wide range. Inanimate objects, as well as people, have various microorganisms, many of which help carry out normal body functions. Some of these microorganisms, however, are more pathogenic than others. Sources of nosocomial infection are numerous in the health care environment (Table 5–5). For instance, human hands provide a warm, moist environment for microorganisms. Therefore a physician, phlebotomist, or nurse can transmit organisms from themselves or an infected patient to another potential host. Uniforms or other clothing that comes in contact with infectious agents and is then worn around other patients is another potential source of infection. Since tourniquets come in contact with intact skin, a tourniquet should be used on only one patient and discarded.

MODE OF TRANSMISSION

The second link in the chain of infection involves transmission from the source to the next host. Pathogenic agents may be transmitted by five modes:

1. direct contact
2. air

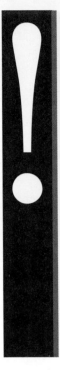

Clinical Alert

OSHA requires managers at health care facilities to provide a confidential medical evaluation, treatment, and follow-up for any employee who has had a blood-borne exposure incident (e.g., needle stick). Immediately after an exposure incident, the employee must

- decontaminate the needle-stick site with an appropriate antiseptic (e.g., iodine) for 30 seconds, or
- flush the exposed mucous membrane site (e.g., eyes) with water for 10 minutes
- then report the incident to his or her supervisor, who will direct the employee to the appropriate clinic for medical evaluation, treatment, and counseling

The medical evaluation involves the following steps:

1. The exposed health care worker (HCW) is identified in a confidential manner and tested for HIV, hepatitis B virus (HBV), and hepatitis C virus (HCV) with permission from the health care worker. Hopefully, the HCW has previously received the HBV vaccine, as required for working in a health care environment.
2. The exposed HCW should receive counseling, medical evaluation, possible antiviral treatment and postexposure testing at 6 weeks, 12 weeks, and 6 months later.
3. The exposed HCW is counseled to be alert for acute viral symptoms within 12 weeks of exposure. This entire medical evaluation must be completely confidential.

<ol start="3">
<li>medical instruments</li>
<li>other objects</li>
<li>other vectors</li>
</ol>

Direct contact involves close or intimate contact with an infected person. For example, some patients acquire staphylococcal infections, chickenpox, hepatitis, or diarrhea after touching other infected individuals. During contact, the infective microorganism rubs off one person onto another. Hand washing is the best means of preventing infections transmitted by this route.

Microscopic airborne droplets may carry infectious agents, such as the causative agent of tuberculosis and Legionnaire's disease. Droplets may become airborne in the following instances: when an individual coughs or sneezes, when linens are shaken, when dust is stirred by sweeping, or when ventilation is inadequate. Preventative measures include wearing a mask, isolating specific patients, and ensuring good ventilation.

As mentioned previously, invasive medical instruments may expose a susceptible patient to pathogenic agents. To prevent instrument-induced infections, health care personnel should discard instruments, such as tourniquets and catheters, after each use. Safety needles and holders should be used only once, then disposed of in appropriate containers. Other inanimate objects, such as toys in the pediatric areas, common toilets and sinks, linens, and water fountains are all potential modes of transmission. Objects that can harbor infectious agents and transmit infection are called **fomites.** Fomites found in health care settings are listed in Table 5–6.

TABLE 5–3.   Employee Infections or Special Circumstances*

DISEASE	WORK STATUS	DURATION OF WORK OR WORK LIMITATIONS
Conjunctivitis, infectious	Off	Until discharge ceases
Diarrheal diseases	Off	Until symptoms resolve
Draining abscess, boils, and so forth	Off	Until drainage stops, if employee has patient contact
Chicken pox (varicella)	Off	For 7 days after eruption first appears in normal host, provided lesions are dry and crusted when he or she returns
Diarrhea Shigella Salmonella	Variable	Individual, depending on extent of symptoms, cultures, and evaluation by Personnel Health Services
Gonorrhea	May Work	
Hepatitis A	Off	Until 7 days after onset of jaundice (must bring note from private physician upon return)
Hepatitis B	Off	Must bring note from private physician upon return
Hepatitis C	May Work	Period of infectivity has not been determined
Herpes simplex	May Work	Evaluation by Personnel Health Services, depending on work area
Herpes zoster (shingles)	No patient contact	If able to work, may do so
Human immunodeficiency virus	May work with restriction	Evaluated by Employee Health Physician
Influenza and upper respiratory infections	Variable	Until acute symptoms resolve
Impetigo	Off	No patient contact until crusts
German measles (rubella)	Off	Until rash clears (minimum of 5 days)
Measles	Off	Until rash clears (minimum of 4 days)
Mononucleosis	Off	At discretion of private physician
Positive PPD Conversion	May Work	Evaluation by chest x-ray and follow-up by Personnel Health Services
Pregnancy (first or second trimester)	May Work	Avoid contact with patients having viral or rickettsial infections, tuberculosis, or those being treated with radioactive material
Pregnancy (third trimester)	May Work	Avoid contact with patients in any type of isolation
Active TB	Off	Until under treatment and smears are negative for 2 weeks
Scabies	Off until treated	
Strep throat (Group A)	Off	May work 24 hours after being placed on appropriate antibiotic therapy and symptom free
Weeping dermatitis	No patient contact	No patient contact until acute symptoms resolve

Abbreviations: PPD, purified protein derivative; TB, tuberculosis.

*Sample guideline for employees with infection; their work status and when they can return to work.

(Sources: Castle M, Ajemian E. *Hospital Infection Control.* New York: John Wiley & Sons; 1987, Bennett J, Brachman P. *Hospital Infections.* 3rd ed. Boston: Little, Brown & Co.; 1992, and Bolyard B, Tablan O, *Am J Infect Control,* 1998; 26(3): 299–301.)

Figure 5–1. Biohazard Sign

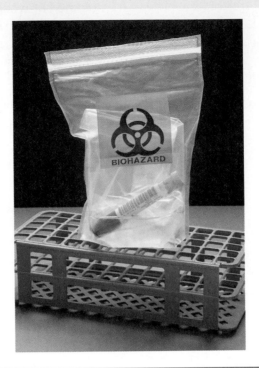

Preventing transmission by fomites can be accomplished by:

- following isolation techniques;
- using sterile technique for injections or venipuncture;
- wearing gloves during equipment handling; and
- restricting the use of common toys or facilities

Many insects (mosquitoes, ticks, fleas, mites) and rodents act as vectors in transmitting infectious diseases, such as plague, rabies, and malaria. Patients may be exposed to these

TABLE 5–4.   Chain of Infection

A **pathogen** must be present

A **source** of disease including patients who have a disease and human carriers of disease (i.e., health care provider, patient's family members) who are unaware they have the disease but can still transmit it to another

A **mode of transmission** for the pathogen to pass directly from the source to the new host (i.e., touching infected individuals, individuals spreading infection through coughing or sneezing, inadequate ventilation, invasive medical instruments)

A **susceptible host** (i.e., hospital patient) that cannot fight off the pathogen (i.e., elderly patient, cancer patient)

TABLE 5–5.   Considerations for Sources of Health-care Acquired (Nosocomial) Infections

Health care personnel (e.g., lack of hand washing between patients)
Visitors
Medical instruments (e.g., contaminated needles, intravenous [IV] catheters, Foley catheters, bronchoscopes, respiratory therapy equipment)
Medical reagents (e.g., IV fluid)
Other patients (e.g., those having severe wound drainage)

vectors in unsanitary conditions in a home setting or in areas where the diseases are prevalent.

SUSCEPTIBLE HOST

The third link in the chain of infection is the susceptible host. Factors that affect a host's susceptibility are age, drug use, the degree and nature of the illness, and the status of the immune system. The patient's progress in the hospital significantly affects his or her chances of acquiring an infection. Underlying diseases, such as diabetes, HIV, acquired immune deficiency syndrome (AIDS), and cancer, as well as therapeutic measures (chemotherapy, radiation therapy, antibiotics), all change the status of the body and make it a potential host for infection.

BREAKING THE CHAIN

Infection control programs aim at breaking the infection chain at one or more links, as shown in Figure 5–2 ■. Hand-washing procedures for sterile technique, proper waste disposal, appropriate laundry services, and housekeeping are ways of controlling the sources. Isolation techniques, control of insects and rodents, and use of disposable equipment and supplies help interrupt the modes of transmission. Host susceptibility is controlled by speeding the patient's recovery. Immunizations, transfusions, proper nutrition, medication, and adequate exercise all help the patient to regain health.

TABLE 5–6.   Fomites Found in Health Care Facilities

Computer keyboards
Door knobs
Telephones
Countertops
Scrub suits
Phlebotomy trays
Eyeglasses
Pens and pencils
Water-faucet handles
Laboratory coats
Manuals and books
Phlebotomy supplies and equipment
IV equipment

Figure 5–2. The Chain of Nosocomial Infection

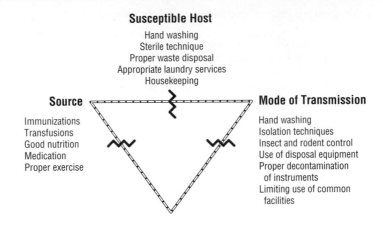

Susceptible Host
Hand washing
Sterile technique
Proper waste disposal
Appropriate laundry services
Housekeeping

Source

Immunizations
Transfusions
Good nutrition
Medication
Proper exercise

Mode of Transmission

Hand washing
Isolation techniques
Insect and rodent control
Use of disposal equipment
Proper decontamination
  of instruments
Limiting use of common
  facilities

■■■■ STANDARD PRECAUTIONS

Isolation procedures, methods of removing diseased individuals from society, date to antiquity. Although the supplies for and methods of isolation have been updated, the fear of being contaminated and the stigma associated with a patient in isolation are still present. The psychological effects of being a patient in isolation are profound. Therefore the health care provider should make an effort to reduce the patient's anxiety by communicating in a calm, professional, and reassuring manner.

Under the CDC's guidelines, the bloodborne pathogen precautions were expanded to assist in the prevention of nosocomial infections. These guidelines are grouped into two levels of protection known as **standard precautions** and **expanded precautions**.[6] Standard precautions are designed to reduce the risk of transmission of microorganisms (see example of isolation signs in Figure 5–3 ■) from both recognized and unrecognized sources of infection in health care facilities. Thus, the precautions provide protection from contact with blood, all body fluids, mucous membranes, and nonintact skin.

The "expanded precautions" cover three sets of precautions based on the routes of transmission. These categories are designed to be used for patients suspected or documented to be infected with pathogens that are highly transmissible. The three types of expanded precautions include:

- **Airborne precautions** reduce the spread of airborne droplet transmission of infectious agents such as rubeola, varicella, and Mycobacterium tuberculosis.
- **Droplet precautions** are used to reduce the transmission of diseases such as pertussis, meningitis, pneumonia, and rubella. These diseases can be transmitted through contact of the mucous membranes of the eye, mouth, or nose with large-particle droplets that occur through sneezing, coughing, or talking.
- **Contact precautions** reduce the risk of transmission of serious diseases such as respiratory syncytial virus (RSV), herpes simplex, wound infections and others through direct or indirect contact.

Figure 5-3. Isolation Signs

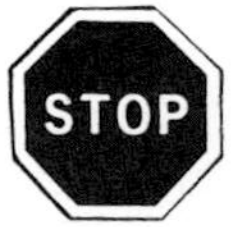

DROPLET PRECAUTIONS

VISITORS: REPORT TO NURSE BEFORE ENTERING

1. Wear surgical mask and eye protection when working within 3 feet of patient.

2. Use surgical mask on patient during transport.

CONTACT PRECAUTIONS

VISITORS: REPORT TO NURSE BEFORE ENTERING

1. Wear personal protective equipment when exposure anticipated (gloves, gowns, mask, and/or eye protection)

2. Use antimicrobial soap for handwashing.

3. After glove removal and handwashing, ensure that hands do not touch potentially contaminated environmental surfaces or items in the patient's room to avoid transfer of microorganisms to other patients or environments.

4. During patient transport drape vehicle with a clean sheet if drainage cannot be contained.

5. Leave routine patient-care equipment in room (examples: BP cuff, stethoscope, thermometer, commode). Clean & disinfect patient-care equipment before use with another patient.

STOP: AIRBORNE ISOLATION

VISITORS: REPORT TO NURSE BEFORE ENTERING.

1. Keep room door closed and patient in room.

2. Respiratory Protection.
   Employees wear respirator when entering the room

3. Use surgical mask on patient during transport.

TABLE 5–7. HICPAC* Recommendations for Transmission-Based Precautions

	CONTACT	DROPLET	AIRBORNE
Purpose	Prevent transmission of known or suspected infected or colonized microorganisms by direct hand or skin-to-skin contact that occurs when providing direct patient care. Conditions in which contact precautions are required: diphtheria, herpes simplex, scabies, staphyloccus infection, hepatitis A, and respiratory syncytial virus wound or skin infection	Prevent transmission of large-particle droplets, larger than 5 microns (μm) (i.e., diphtheria, pertussis, streptococcal pharyngitis, pneumonia, scarlet fever, meningitis, rubella)	Prevent transmission of small-particle residue of 5 microns (μm) or smaller droplets (i.e., measles, varicella, tuberculosis)
Patient Placement	• Private room • Can be placed in room of patient with same microorganism	• Private room • Can be placed in room of client with same diagnosis	• Private room • Can be placed in room of patient with same diagnosis • Monitor negative air pressure • Keep door closed • Keep patient in room
Respiratory Protection	• Mask not necessary	• Use mask when working within 3 feet of patient	• Respiratory protective equipment • Do not enter room of patients with rubeola or varicella if susceptible to these infections
Gloves and Gown	• Wear gloves when entering room • Change gloves after contact with infective material, such as wound drainage or fecal material • Wash hands immediately after removing gloves • Wear gown when working with patients with diarrhea, ostomies, or wound drainage not contained in dressing • Wear gown if contact with patient or environment will occur	• Follow standard precautions	• Follow standard precautions

(continued)

TABLE 5–7.   *Continued*

	CONTACT	DROPLET	AIRBORNE
Patient Transport	• Transport only if essential • Ensure precautions are maintained to minimize risk of transmission	• Transport only if essential • Place mask on patient when outside room	• Transport only if essential • Place mask on patient when outside
Patient Care Items	• Patient care items and environmental surfaces are cleaned daily • Dedicate equipment to single patient use (i.e., stethoscope, thermometer)		

*Hospital Infection Control Practices Advisory Committee.

Adapted from Department of Health and Human Services: CDC, *Federal Register* "Guidelines for Isolation Precautions in Hospitals."

Table 5–7 provides detailed recommendations by the Department of Health and Human Services, CDC, for using these isolation precautions. All three types of precautions may be used at one time when multiple routes of pathogenic transmission are suspected in a patient. These precautions are always used with standard precautions. In Figures 5–4 ■ and 5–5 ■, illustrations are provided of appropriate precautions within a patient's room.

The diseases for which the precautions should be used are shown in Table 5–8.

USE OF STANDARD PRECAUTIONS

Health care providers should follow these guidelines when collecting blood from a patient in order to avoid contracting an infectious microorganism:

1. Use appropriate barrier precautions to prevent skin and mucous membrane exposure when contact with blood or other bloody fluids of any patient is anticipated. Barriers (e.g., gloves, facial masks, respirators, gowns, shields) are also referred to as **personal protective equipment (PPE).**
   • Gloves should be worn
      a. for touching blood and body fluids, mucous membranes, or nonintact skin of all patients;
      b. for handling items or surfaces soiled with blood or body fluids; and
      c. for performing venipunctures and other vascular access procedures.
   • Gloves should be changed after contact with each patient.
   • Masks and protective eyewear or face shields should be worn to prevent exposure of mucous membranes of the mouth, nose, and eyes during procedures that are likely to generate droplets of blood or other body fluids or splashes of blood or other body fluids.
   • A personal respirator should be used if the risk of aerosolized Mycobacterium tuberculosis is present.

Figure 5-4. Transmission-based Precautions

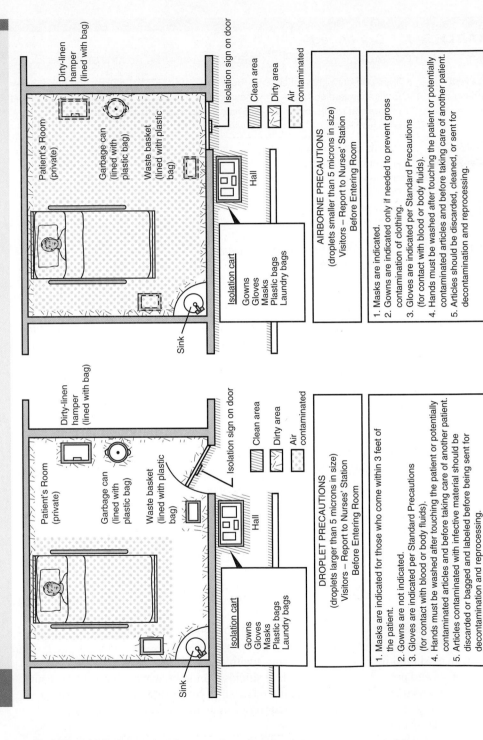

Patient's Room (private)
- Dirty-linen hamper (lined with bag)
- Garbage can (lined with plastic bag)
- Waste basket (lined with plastic bag)
- Sink
- Isolation sign on door

Isolation cart
Gowns
Gloves
Masks
Plastic bags
Laundry bags

Hall

Clean area
Dirty area
Air contaminated

DROPLET PRECAUTIONS
(droplets larger than 5 microns in size)
Visitors – Report to Nurses' Station Before Entering Room

1. Masks are indicated for those who come within 3 feet of the patient.
2. Gowns are not indicated.
3. Gloves are indicated per Standard Precautions (for contact with blood or body fluids).
4. Hands must be washed after touching the patient or potentially contaminated articles and before taking care of another patient.
5. Articles contaminated with infective material should be discarded or bagged and labeled before being sent for decontamination and reprocessing.

AIRBORNE PRECAUTIONS
(droplets smaller than 5 microns in size)
Visitors – Report to Nurses' Station Before Entering Room

1. Masks are indicated.
2. Gowns are indicated only if needed to prevent gross contamination of clothing.
3. Gloves are indicated per Standard Precautions (for contact with blood or body fluids).
4. Hands must be washed after touching the patient or potentially contaminated articles and before taking care of another patient.
5. Articles should be discarded, cleaned, or sent for decontamination and reprocessing.

Figure 5–5. Contact Precautions

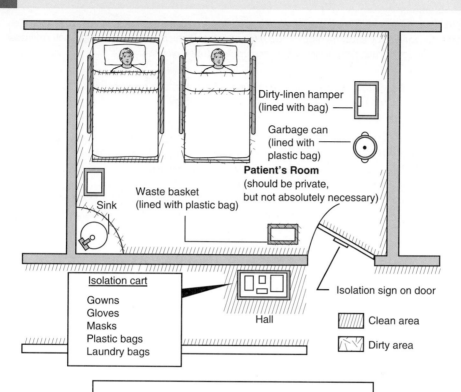

Dirty-linen hamper (lined with bag)

Garbage can (lined with plastic bag)

Patient's Room (should be private, but not absolutely necessary)

Waste basket (lined with plastic bag)

Sink

Isolation sign on door

Isolation cart

Gowns
Gloves
Masks
Plastic bags
Laundry bags

Hall

Clean area

Dirty area

CONTACT PRECAUTIONS
Visitors – Report to Nurses' Station
Before Entering Room

1. **Masks** are not indicated.
2. **Gowns** are indicated if soiling is likely.
3. **Gloves** are indicated for touching infective material.
4. **Hands must be washed after touching the patient or potentially contaminated articles and before taking care of another patient.**
5. **Articles** contaminated with infective material should be discarded or bagged and labeled before being sent for decontamination and reprocessing.

A private room is indicated for Contact Precautions if patient hygiene is poor. A patient with poor hygiene does not wash hands after touching infective material, contaminates the environment with infective material, or shares contaminated articles with other patients. In general, patients infected with the same organism may share a room.

TABLE 5–8. Types of Diseases for Which Precautions Should Be Used

Standard Precautions

Use standard precautions for the care of all patients.

Airborne Precautions

In addition to standard precautions, use airborne precautions for patients known or suspected to have serious illnesses transmitted by airborne droplet nuclei (smaller than 5 microns). Examples of such illnesses include measles, varicella (including disseminated zoster), and tuberculosis.[†]

Droplet Precautions

In addition to standard precautions, use droplet precautions for patients known or suspected to have serious illnesses transmitted by large particle droplets (larger than 5 microns). Examples of such illnesses include:

1. Invasive *Haemophilus influenzae* type b disease, including meningitis, pneumonia, epiglottitis, and sepsis
2. Invasive *Neisseria meningitidis* disease, including meningitis, pneumonia, and sepsis
3. Other serious bacterial respiratory infections spread by droplet transmission:
   - Diphtheria (pharyngeal)
   - Mycoplasma pneumonia
   - Pertussis
   - Pneumonic plague
   - Streptococcal (group A) pharyngitis, pneumonia, or scarlet fever in infants and young children
4. Serious viral infections spread by droplet transmission:
   - Adenovirus*
   - Influenza
   - Mumps
   - Parvovirus B19
   - Rubella

Contact Precautions

In addition to standard precautions, use contact precautions for patients known or suspected to have serious illnesses easily transmitted by direct patient contact or by contact with items in the patient's environment:

1. Gastrointestinal, respiratory, skin, or wound infections or colonization with multidrug-resistant bacteria judged by the infection control program, based on current state, regional, or national recommendations, to be of special clinical and epidemiologic significance.
2. Enteric infections with a low infectious dose or prolonged environmental survival:
   - *Clostridium difficile* infection
   - For diapered or incontinent patients, enterohemorrhagic *Escherichia coli* 0157:H7, *Shigella,* hepatitis A, or rotavirus infection
3. Respiratory syncytial virus, parainfluenza virus, or enteroviral infections in infants and young children
4. Skin infections that are highly contagious or that may occur on dry skin:
   - Diptheria (cutaneous)
   - Herpes simplex virus (neonatal or mucocutaneous)
   - Impetigo
   - Major (noncontained) abscesses, cellulitis, or decubiti
   - Pediculosis
   - Scabies
   - *Staphylococcus furunculosis* in infants and young children
   - Zoster (disseminated or in the immunocompromised host)*
5. Viral hemorrhagic conjunctivitis
6. Viral hemorrhagic infections (Ebola, Lassa, or Marburg)

*Certain infections require more than one type of precaution.

†See the CDC's *Guidelines for Preventing the Transmission of Tuberculosis in Health-Care Facilities,* http://www.cdc.gov/epo/mmwr/preview/rr4313.html

Source: Reprinted with permission from J. S. Garner, Guideline for Isolation Precautions in Hospitals, *Infection Control and Hospital Epidemiology,* Vol. 17, No. 1, pp. 53–80, © 1996, Slack, Inc.

2. Hands and other skin surfaces should be washed immediately and thoroughly if contaminated with blood or other body fluids. Hands should be washed immediately after gloves are removed.

3. Precautions should be taken to prevent injuries caused by needles, scalpels, and other sharp instruments or devices
   - during procedures,
   - during disposal of used needles, and
   - when handling sharp instruments after procedures

4. To prevent infections from **bloodborne pathogens (BBPs)** as a result of needle-stick injuries, health care workers should
   - only use safety engineered needle and sharps devices
   - not recap needles, purposely bend or break them by hand, remove them from disposable syringes, or otherwise manipulate them by hand
   - immediately dispose of the blood tube holder and safety needle as a single unit after blood collection.[7]
   - After they are used, disposable syringes and needles, scalpel blades, and other sharp items should be placed in puncture-resistant containers for transport to the reprocessing center.

5. Health care workers who have exudation lesions or weeping dermatitis should refrain from all direct patient care and from handling patient care equipment until the condition resolves.

6. Pregnant health care workers are not known to be at greater risk of contracting a viral infection (e.g., HIV, hepatitis C, etc.) than health care workers who are not pregnant; however, if a health care worker develops a viral infection during pregnancy, the infant is at risk of infection resulting from perinatal transmission. Because of this risk, pregnant health care workers should be especially familiar with and strictly adhere to precautions to minimize the risk of a viral transmission.

HAND HYGIENE AND GLOVING

Standard Precautions require hand hygiene, including hand washing and antiseptic hand rubbing, as a *major* defense against health-care acquired infections. On October 25, 2002, the Morbidity and Mortality Weekly Report (MMWR) published "Guideline for Hand

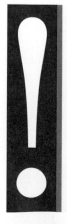

Clinical Alert

- Standard precautions have been designed to be used for patients, health care providers, and visitors in health care facilities.
- Standard precautions reduce the risk of microorganism transmission from health care providers to patients, patients to patients, and health care providers to other health care providers or visitors
- These precautions apply in the following situations:
  - Contact with blood
  - Contact with body fluids
  - Contact with mucous membranes and nonintact skin

1. Wet hands with water. Foot pedals are preferable for controlling the flow of water but they are not available in all health care facilities (Figure 5–6 ■).

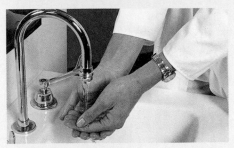

Figure 5–6

2. Dispense a small amount of soap to the hands (1–2 teaspoonfuls or the amount recommended by the manufacturer) (Figure 5–7 ■).

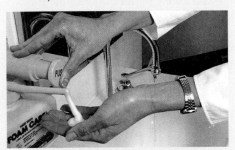

Figure 5–7

3. Rub hands together vigorously for at least 15 seconds, covering all surfaces of the hands and fingers (Figure 5–8 ■).

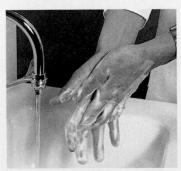

Figure 5–8

4. Rinse hands in a downward motion with water (Figure 5–9 ■) and dry thoroughly with a clean disposable towel. Multiple-use cloth towels of the hanging or roll type are not acceptable for use in health care settings because they can transmit microorganisms.

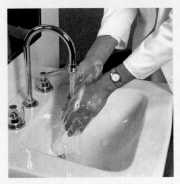

Figure 5–9

5. Turn off the faucet with a dry disposable towel if not using a foot pedal (Figure 5–10 ■).

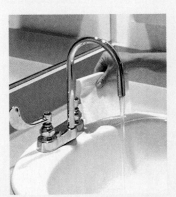

Figure 5–10

Hygiene in Health-Care Settings," which states that while alcohol-based hand antiseptics are not appropriate for use when hands are visibly dirty or contaminated, alcohols are more effective for standard hand washing or hand antisepsis by health care providers than plain or antimicrobial soap (http://www.cdc.gov/mmwr/preview/mmwrhtml/rr5116a1.htm).[8] It is handy to take a plastic bottle of alcohol-based hand antiseptic in the pocket of the laboratory coat just in case the alcohol-based (waterless) antiseptic agent is not available at the patient's bedside.

It is important to wash your hands always after contact with blood, body fluids, or contaminated objects, whether gloves are worn or not. Placing gloves on dirty hands can transfer microorganisms after the gloves are taken off.

ISOLATION FOR HOSPITAL OUTBREAKS

Occasionally, outbreaks of particular infections occur in one or more hospital areas. For example, infection control surveillance may reveal that the nursery unit is having an excessive number of cases of staphylococcal infection. To control the outbreak, the infection control staff may dictate the need for special precautions, isolation procedures, or employee screening for staphylococcal carriers. Any health care worker entering or exiting these areas should be made aware of the special circumstances.

PROTECTIVE, OR REVERSE, ISOLATION

A few hospitals in the United States have large protective isolation facilities for patients with combined immunodeficiencies who must live in an environment that is completely sterile. All food and articles are sterilized before they are taken into the patient's room. Some patients must live in these protected environments when they are recovering from cancer treatments.

INFECTION CONTROL IN SPECIAL HOSPITAL UNITS

Other areas where patients are at a high risk of infection are the nursery, the burn unit, the postoperative care unit, the intensive care unit (ICU), and the dialysis unit. The clinical laboratory plays an important role in infection control in these hospital units and is also subject to specific infection control procedures.

Clinical Alert

- Do not wear artificial fingernails or extenders when collecting blood from patients in high-risk hospital areas (e.g., intensive care unit, premature nursery).
- Keep natural fingernails less than ¼ inch long.
- Wear gloves when there is possible contact with blood or other potentially infectious materials.
- Remove gloves after collecting blood from a patient. DO NOT wear the same pair of gloves for the blood collection of more than one patient.

Infection Control in a Nursery Unit

Newborns are easy targets for infections of all sorts because their immune systems are not fully developed at birth. Neonates may pick up pathogens from their mothers, other babies, or hospital personnel. The best way to minimize infection is to use gloves and an antiseptic for hand washing. Special clothing may be worn by nursery personnel, changed daily, and limited to the unit. Bibs should be used and discarded after contact with only one baby. Often, a baby is assigned a single nurse to limit the possible sources of infection transmission. Babies whose mothers have genital herpes must be isolated from other infants. Mothers with genital herpes must also be isolated. All individuals having contact with either the mothers or the children must be gowned and gloved, and double-bagging procedures must be used for disposal of contaminated articles in the patient's room.

Infection Control in a Burn Unit

Patients with burns are also highly susceptible to infection. In some institutions, infection rates for burn patients are lower because of the availability of a completely isolated environment for each patient. Each bed is surrounded by a plastic curtain with sleeves. Hospital personnel use these sleeves to have contact with the patient. All supplies and equipment are kept outside the curtain. In hospitals lacking these facilities, burn patients are housed in private rooms. Gowning, gloving, double bagging (as described later in this chapter), and strict hand-washing procedures should be used. All articles in the room, as well as the room itself, should be disinfected or sterilized frequently.

Infection Control in an ICU or Postoperative Care Unit

Patients in ICUs are more critically ill and, by nature, more susceptible to infections. In most hospitals, ICUs are open areas, with numerous patients in one large room so as to be more easily monitored. Patients with known infections should be isolated according to the types of infections they have, and strict hand-washing and gloving policies are necessary in all ICUs.

Postoperative patients are susceptible to infection because surgical wounds or drains enable bacteria to gain easy access to deeper tissues. Again, each patient who becomes infected should be isolated and dealt with according to the type of infection acquired.

Infection Control in a Dialysis Unit

Patients needing dialysis are most often immunosuppressed, which makes them a high-risk group for contracting infection, especially hepatitis. Protective gowns and gloves may be worn in the unit, and strict hand-washing and gloving techniques should be adhered to.

INFECTION CONTROL IN THE CLINICAL LABORATORY

The clinical laboratory contributes to infection control programs in the following manner:

1. Maintaining laboratory records for surveillance purposes
2. Reporting on infectious agents, drug-resistant microorganisms, and outbreaks
3. Evaluating the effectiveness of sterilization or decontamination procedures

Laboratory personnel must be cautious because they often handle specimens with infectious agents. Laboratorians have a higher incidence of hepatitis antigen, tuberculosis, tu-

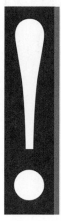

Clinical Alert

Many health care facilities are prohibiting the use of artificial nails or extenders due to the spread of pathogenic infections and fungus to immunosuppressed patients.

laremia, and Rocky Mountain spotted fever than that of other hospital personnel. Many of these infections are acquired by aerosol spray, needle sticks, spills, and eating, drinking, or smoking in the laboratory. Such danger can easily be prevented or minimized by adhering to policies that prohibit eating, drinking, and smoking in the laboratory. Other useful procedures include hand washing; gloving; wearing protective clothing such as laboratory coats, scrubs, and face shields, if appropriate; surface decontamination; and careful disposal of safety needles, holders, and other blood-collection supplies.

The health care worker should remember that the quality of laboratory test results is only as good as the specimen collected. If the specimen is contaminated or improperly collected, laboratory test results reflect this fact and may be misleading. If sloppy techniques are used, the potential for mistakes and infection is greater. Table 5–9 details the infection control policies that health care workers must follow during blood collection.

TABLE 5–9. Infection Control Responsibilities Required in Blood Collection

Frequent handwashing
Use of personal protection equipment
Use of appropriate waste disposal practices
Maintaining good personal hygiene, including wearing clean clothes, keeping hair clean and tied back if necessary, keeping fingernails clean, and washing hands frequently
Maintaining good health by eating balanced meals, getting enough sleep, and getting enough exercise
Reporting personal illnesses to supervisors
Becoming familiar with and observing *all* isolation policies
Learning about the job-related aspects of infection control, and sharing this information with others
Cautioning all personnel working with known hazardous material (this can be done with proper warning labels)
Reporting violations of the policies
Reporting potential candidates for infection control (e.g., patients who are jaundiced)

■■■■ SPECIFIC ISOLATION TECHNIQUES AND PROCEDURAL STEPS

In most hospitals, all supplies required for isolation procedures (see Procesures 5–3 and 5–4) are located in an area or on a cart just outside the patient's room (Figure 5–11 ■). These include:

- Disposable gloves
- Gown
- Mask
- Protective eyewear

ISOLATION ITEM DISPOSAL

The supplies needed for isolation item disposal include:

- Garbage bag
- Linen hamper
- Large red isolation bag
- Specimen container
- Plastic bag with biohazard label
- Laundry bag
- Puncture-resistant disposal container for needle and sharps
- Gloves
- Antiseptic agent or antimicrobial agent

Isolation bags for transporting specimens should be turned halfway inside out and left near the door outside the room; someone may be available to hold the bag outside the door. Only the needed supplies should be taken into the room. Phlebotomy requisitions may be left outside the room on the isolation cart. If collecting a blood specimen, the health care

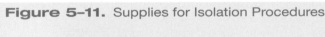

Figure 5–11. Supplies for Isolation Procedures

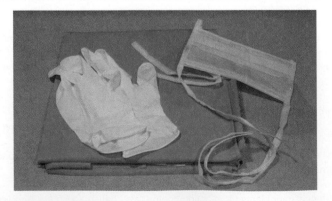

provider may use a tourniquet in the room or leave the one brought in. The specimen should be labeled at the bedside and the pen left in the room. Used needles, swabs, and so forth should be put in appropriate containers inside the room. Any blood on the outside of the specimen container should be removed with a paper towel. While standing in the doorway, and touching only the inside of the isolation bag, the health care worker should place the specimen inside the bag. Gloved hands should be washed in the room. The faucet may be turned off with a paper towel.

PREVENTION OF LABORATORY-ACQUIRED INFECTIONS

As mentioned previously, health care workers must be extremely cautious with biohazardous specimens. Policies and procedures for handling such specimens should be defined in the laboratory policy manual and should be reviewed periodically by health care workers who collect and transport specimens.[9,10] Infections from these specimens may be spread during collection and handling by means of several routes. The actual occurrence of an infection from a biohazardous specimen depends on the virulence of the infecting agent and the host's susceptibility.

STERILE TECHNIQUE FOR HEALTH CARE WORKERS

All health care personnel should realize that bacteria and other microorganisms can be found everywhere. For example, human skin is covered with bacteria. Because of this fact, all health care personnel should be responsible for cleanliness and maintaining sterility when handling instruments, catheters, IV supplies, or other devices that come into contact with patients.

The health care worker is responsible for using sterile supplies for skin punctures and venipunctures and antiseptics for patient preparation. Alcohol pads often are used to cleanse skin sites for venipuncture. Although rubbing with alcohol pads destroys most of the bacteria, it does not destroy all microorganisms. A special decontamination procedure is required to obtain a sterile site. Venipuncture for blood cultures requires this type of preparation, as discussed thoroughly in Chapter 9.

New needles and most blood collection tubes are sterilized by the manufacturers. Once the covering of a needle or a lancet is removed, the needle or lancet should not touch anything until it punctures the skin. If it accidentally touches anything prior to contact with the skin site, it must be discarded appropriately and replaced with a new one. If a needle is used for an unsuccessful venipuncture, it too must be discarded and replaced with a new one before another puncture is attempted.

Sterile technique and isolation procedures may require sterile gloves. If this is the case, the health care worker must make sure that the package of gloves indicates that they are sterile. Some manufacturers produce gloves that are chemically clean but not necessarily sterile. Most sterile gloves are available in various hand sizes. If the gloves do not fit properly, they may interfere with the procedure. Types and use of gloves are also discussed in Chapter 8, "Blood Collection Equipment."

Procedure 5-2   Gowning, Masking and Gloving

To prevent the transmission of microorganisms from health care workers (HCWs) to patients, or from patients to HCWs, the following isolation procedural steps should be followed:

1. Decontaminate hands using an alcohol-based hand rub or soap and water as described in Procedure 5–1 (Figure 5–12 ■).

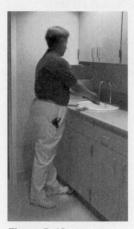

Figure 5–12

2. Gowns should be large enough to cover all clothing (Figure 5–13 ■).

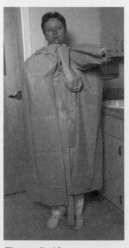

Figure 5–13

3. Touching only its inside surface, place one arm at a time through the gown's sleeves and wrap the gown completely around the body. Gowns are generally made of cloth and paper (Figure 5–14 ■).

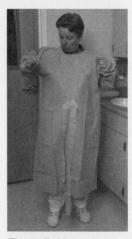

Figure 5–14

4. Sleeves should be pulled down, and then bring waist ties from back to front of gown and tie in back (Figure 5–15 ■).

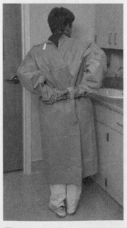

Figure 5–15

continued

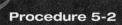

Procedure 5-2   *(continued)*

5. Tie or use Velcro strap to close gown around the neck (Figure 5–16 ■).

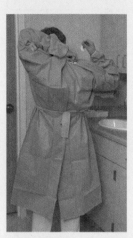

Figure 5–16

6. Don mask (Figure 5–17 ■). Masks protect the health care worker from small-particle droplets that may carry pathogens. Often, a small metal band on the mask can be shaped to fit the nose. Two ties are usually made, the first around the upper portion of the head and the second around the upper portion of the neck. Most masks become ineffective after prolonged use (20 minutes) or if they become wet.[1]

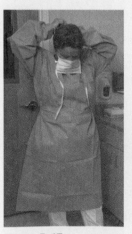

Figure 5–17

7. Face shields or goggles should be worn during procedures that possibly may generate blood or body fluid droplets (i.e., splashes or sprays) such as from severe patient coughing (Figure 5–18 ■).

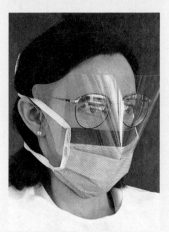

Figure 5–18

8. Gloves should be pulled over the ends of gown sleeves (Figure 5–19 ■). Chemically clean disposable gloves may be used for most isolation procedures. For isolation procedures in which the patient must be protected from any microorganisms, sterile disposable gloves should be used. Rings and other pieces of jewelry should not be worn because they may puncture a glove during patient contact.

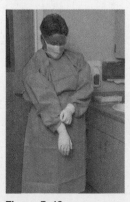

Figure 5–19

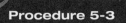

Procedure 5-3   Removal of Isolation Gown, Mask, and Gloves

After completion of blood collection in an isolation room, follow these steps for removing the isolation gown, mask, and gloves:

1. The gown is removed by first breaking the paper tie or untying the sash as shown in Figure 5–20 ■.

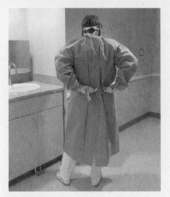

Figure 5–20

2. Next, the gloves are removed as shown in Figure 5–21 ■. The first glove is pulled off in such a manner to turn it inside out. The folled-up glove is placed into palm of the hand that still is gloved. The second glove is removed by slipping the index finger of the ungloved hand between the glove and the hand. Then the glove is pulled down and off as it turns inside out. Dispose of both gloves in a red garbage bag in the isolation room.

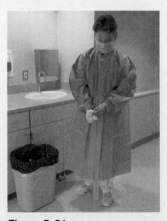

Figure 5–21

3. The gown should be taken off by pulling down from shoulders first and then pulling arms out of gown (Figure 5–22 ■). The gown should be removed and folded with the contaminated side turned inside and with care taken not to touch the uniform.

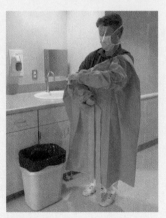

Figure 5–22

4. Gowns are used only once to prevent contamination. The gown should be disposed of in the linen hamper or, if disposable, in a garbage bag in the isolation room (Figure 5–23 ■).

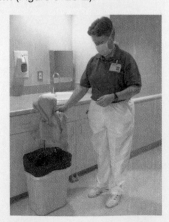

Figure 5–23

continued

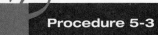

Procedure 5-3   *(continued)*

5. The mask can be removed by carefully untying the lower tie first, then the upper one (Figure 5–24 ■). Only the ends of the ties should be held. The mask should then be properly disposed of inside the room. In some cases, a special container for masks is placed just outside the room to prevent exposure of hospital personnel to airborne pathogens while inside the isolation room.

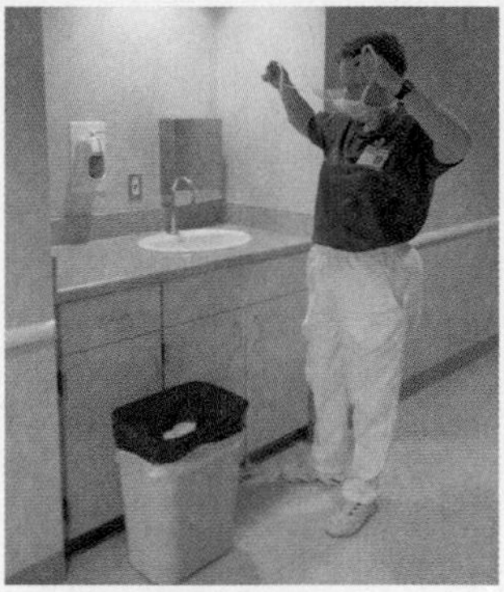

6. Wash hands in the room and again at nearest sink after exiting the room (Figure 5–25 ■). A clean paper towel should be used to open the door. The door shold be held open with one foot and the used paper towels discarded in the wastebasket directly inside the patient's room.

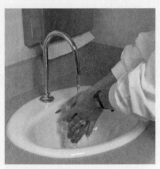

Figure 5–25

Figure 5–24

Procedure 5-4   Disposing of Contaminated Items

Trash, linens, and other articles in an isolation room may be removed by using one sturdy bohazard bag or the double-bagging procedure:

1. Put contaminated material in one bag and seal the bag inside the room as shown in Figure 5–26 ■.

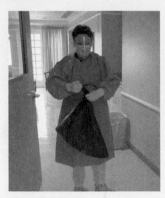

Figure 5–26

2. Another person should stand outside the room with another opened, clean, impermeable bag (Figure 5–27 ■). The person standing outside the room should have the ends of the bag folded over their hands to shield from possible contamination. The sealed bag from the room may then be placed in the clean bag. The person outside the room can then fold over the edges, expel the air, and seal the outer bag. The bag must be labeled with biohazard warnings.

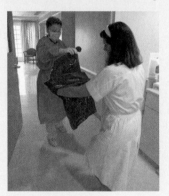

Figure 5–27

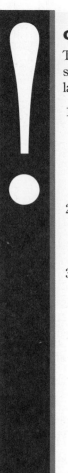

Clinical Alert

The following are possible routes of infection from collected specimens and therefore should be considered when health care personnel must collect or process specimens for laboratory assays:

1. *Skin contact.* Virulent organisms can enter through skin abrasions and cuts or through the conjunctiva of the eye. Thus, scratches from needles and broken glass must be avoided. If the health care worker has a cut or an abrasion, he or she should always wear a laboratory coat, gloves, and protective adhesive tape over the cut or abrasion to prevent possible inoculation from infectious specimens. He or she must also avoid rubbing the eyes.

2. *Ingestion.* Failure to wash contaminated hands and subsequent handling of cigarettes, gum, food, or drinks can result in an infection from a biohazardous specimen. Each employee must comply with the safety rules of the laboratory to prevent transmission of infections.

3. *Airborne.* Aerosol spray created from patient's specimens by careless splashing or centrifugation must be prevented. Dangerous, infectious aerosol spray can be caused from popping tops off blood specimen vacuum tubes. To protect against blood exposure during this hazardous step, cover the tube with a gauze pad while removing the top. Also, manufacturers recently developed different types of items that minimize airborne transmissions (see Chapter 8, Blood Collection Equipment). Prior to centrifugation, vacuum tubes should be inspected for cracks, and tubes with wet rims should be wiped dry. The centrifuge brake should not be applied to save time because braking can cause infectious aerosol formation. Centrifuged infectious specimens must not be poured because of the potential hazards from aerosol formation. Instead, the contents should be transferred by using a disposable pipette with a rubber bulb or its equivalent and gently transferring the contents down the wall of the aliquot tube or tubes.

DISINFECTANTS AND ANTISEPTICS

Disinfectants are chemical compounds used to remove or kill pathogenic microorganisms.[11] Chemical disinfectants are regulated by the Environmental Protection Agency (EPA). A list of EPA-registered products may be obtained by contacting the EPA's Antimicrobial Division. Antiseptics are chemicals used to inhibit the growth and development of microorganisms, but they do not necessarily kill them. Antiseptics may be used on human skin, whereas disinfectants are generally used on surfaces and instruments because they are too corrosive for direct use on skin. A disinfectant with a product label claiming that the disinfectant is HIVcidal or tuberculocidal, or a disinfectant having a chlorine bleach dilution of 1:10, should be used to disinfect tourniquets and items contaminated with blood or other body fluids. A more dilute solution of chlorine bleach (1:100) can be used for routine cleaning of surfaces. Gloves and gowns should be worn when performing decontamination procedures. The minimal contact time for disinfectants to be effective is 10 minutes.

Tables 5–10 and 5–11 lists some of the more common hospital disinfectants and antiseptics.

TABLE 5–10. Common Antiseptics and Disinfectants for the Health Care Setting

COMPOUND	USES AND RESTRICTIONS
Alcohols	
Ethyl (70%)	Antiseptic for skin
Isopropyl (70%)	Antiseptic for skin
Chlorine	
Chloramine	Disinfectant for wounds
Hypochlorite solutions	Disinfectant
Ethylene oxide	Disinfectant (toxic)
Formaldehyde	Disinfectant (noxious fumes)
Glutaraldehyde	Disinfectant (toxic)
Hydrogen peroxide	Antiseptic for skin
Iodine	
Tincture	Antiseptic for skin (can be irritating)
Iodophors	Antiseptic for skin (less stable)
Phenolic compounds	
1–2% phenols	Disinfectant
Chlorophenol	Disinfectant (toxic)
Chlorhexidine	Antiseptic for skin
Hexylresorcinol	Antiseptic for skin
Quaternary ammonium compounds	Antiseptic for skin (ingredient in many soaps)

PREVENTING INFECTIONS FROM GLASS CAPILLARY TUBE USE

Glass capillary tubes have been used for the collection of blood in a variety of health care settings, including hospitals, clinical laboratories, physicians' offices, and blood donation facilities. Accidental breakage of these slender, fragile tubes has been reported when the tubes have been inserted into putty to be sealed, and as a result of centrifugation. To reduce the risk of injury due to breakage of capillary tubes, the Food and Drug Administration (FDA) and OSHA have guidelines indicating that blood collectors use

- Capillary tubes that are not made of glass
- Glass capillary tubes wrapped in puncture-resistant films
- Products that use a method of sealing that does not require manually pushing one end of a tube into putty to form a plug
- Products that allow the blood hematocrit to be measured without centrifugation.

Additional information can be found at the FDA website: www.fda.gov/cdrh/safety.html

TABLE 5–11. Antimicrobial Spectrum and Characteristics of Hand-Hygiene Antiseptic Agents*

GROUP	GRAM-POSITIVE BACTERIA	GRAM-NEGATIVE BACTERIA	MYCOBACTERIA	FUNGI	VIRUSES	SPEED OF ACTION	COMMENTS
Alcohols	+++	+++	+++	+++	+++	Fast	Optimum concentration 60%–95%; no persistent activity
Chlorhexidine (2% and 4% aqueous)	+++	++	+	+	+++	Intermediate	Persistent activity; rare allergic reactions
Iodine compounds	+++	+++	+++	++	+++	Intermediate	Cause skin burns; usually too irritating for hand hygiene
Iodophors	+++	+++	+	++	++	Intermediate	Less irritating than iodine; acceptance varies
Phenol derivatives	+++	+	+	+	+	Intermediate	Activity neutralized by nonionic surfactants
Triclosan	+++	++	+	–	+++	Intermediate	Acceptability on hands varies
Quaternary ammonium compounds	+	++	–	–	+	Slow	Used only in combination with alcohols; ecologic concerns

Note: +++ = excellent; ++ = good, but does not include the entire bacterial spectrum; + = fair; – = no activity or not sufficient.

*Hexachlorophene is not included because it is no longer an accepted ingredient of hand disinfectants.

Source: Guideline for Hand Hygiene in Health-Care Settings. MMWR.10/25/02, Vol. 51, No. RR-16

KEY TERMS

antiseptics

Centers for Disease Control
  and Prevention (CDC)

chain of infection

disinfectants

double bagging

fomites

hand hygiene

infection control programs

isolation procedures

mode of transmission

nosocomial infections

Occupational Safety and Health
  Administration (OSHA)

pathogenic agents

protective (reverse) isolation

source

standard precautions

sterile technique

susceptible host

STUDY QUESTIONS

The following may have one or more answers:

1. Which of the following types of health-care-acquired infections are most prevalent?
   a. dermal infections
   b. wound infections
   c. respiratory tract infections
   d. urinary tract infections

2. Name the links in the chain of infection.
   a. poor isolation technique
   b. susceptible host
   c. source
   d. mode of transmission

3. What is/are the primary function(s) of isolation procedures?
   a. keep the hospital clean
   b. prevent transmission of communicable diseases
   c. protect the general public from disease
   d. provide protective environments

4. Nurses, physicians, and other health care workers are responsible for knowing the procedures of which type(s) of isolation?
   a. strict
   b. drainage/secretion
   c. enteric
   d. droplet
   e. airborne
   f. standard precautions

5. Protective isolation is generally used for
   a. an adult patient with active tuberculosis
   b. a pediatric patient who has an immunodeficiency
   c. an adult patient with meningitis
   d. a pediatric patient who has whooping cough

6. Which of the following laboratory-acquired infections is most prevalent?
   a. HIV infection
   b. Rocky Mountain spotted fever
   c. HBV infection
   d. tuberculosis

7. Airborne precautions may be required for patients with infections such as
   a. tuberculosis
   b. whooping cough
   c. Salmonella
   d. Rocky Mountain spotted fever

8. According to the OSHA standards for occupational exposure to bloodborne pathogens, which of the following is a PPE?
   a. 10 percent household bleach
   b. fluid-resistant gown
   c. goggles
   d. respirator

References

1. Wenzel, RP, and Edmond, MB: The Impact of Hospital-Acquired Bloodstream Infections in CDC's *Emerging Infectious Disease* Mar/Apr 2001; 7(2): 174–177, http://www.cdc.gov/ncidod/eid/vol7no2/pdfs/wenzel.pdf.

2. Jasny, BR, Bloom, FE: It's not rocket science—but it can save lives. *Science,* 1998; 280: 1507.

3. US Department of Labor and Occupational Safety and Health Administration (OSHA): Occupational exposure to bloodborne pathogens; final rule (29 CFR 1910.1030). Federal Register 1991; Dec 6: 64004–64182.

4. OSHA Revised Bloodborne Pathogens Standard 1910.1030. Needlestick Safety and Prevention Bill Act; April 18, 2001.

5. Updated US Public Health Service Guidelines for the Management of Occupational Exposures to HBV, HCV, and HIV Recommendations for Postexposure Prophylaxis. *MMWR,* June 29, 2001; 50(RR11).

6. Updated Guidelines on prevention of agent transmission, Centers for Disease Control (IN PRESS, to be released in 2004)

7. OSHA Disposal of Contaminated Needles and Blood Tube Holders Used in Phlebotomy. Safety and Health Information Bulletin, http://www.osha.gov/dts/shib/shib101503.html, October 15, 2003.

8. Guideline for Hand Hygiene in Health-Care Setting. *MMWR,* 2002; 51(RR16).

9. National Committee for Clinical Laboratory Standards (NCCLS): Protection of Laboratory Workers from Occupationally Acquired Infections, Approved Guideline, 2nd ed. NCCLS Document M29-A. Wayne, PA, 2001.

10. National Committee for Clinical Laboratory Standards (NCCLS): Implementing a Needlestick and Sharps Injury Prevention Program in the Clinical Laboratory, A Report. NCCLS document X3-R (ISBN 1-56238-460-0). (940 West Valley Road, Suite 1400, Wayne, PA): NCCLS, 2002.

11. Luebbert, P: Choosing the appropriate disinfectant. *Lab Med,* 1992; 23(2): 126.

Safety and First Aid

6

CHAPTER OBJECTIVES

Upon completion of Chapter 6, the learner is responsible for the following:

1. Discuss safety awareness for health care workers.
2. Explain the measures that should be taken for fire, electrical, radiation, mechanical, and chemical safety in a health care facility.
3. Describe the essential elements of a disaster emergency plan for a health care facility.
4. Explain the safety policies and procedures that must be followed in specimen collection and transportation.
5. Describe the safe use of equipment in health care facilities.
6. List three precautions that can reduce the risk of injury to patients.

 MediaLINK

Access the accompanying CD-ROM to explore a wide variety of review questions and interactive activities for this chapter, including multiple choice, true/false, and video exercises.

The goal of safety in the health care institution is to recognize and eliminate hazards and provide information on safety education so that employees can work in a healthy environment. Safe working conditions must be ensured by the employer and have been mandated by law under the federal Occupational Safety and Health Administration (OSHA).[1,2] In a health care facility, potential hazards exist, and the health care worker needs to know the proper precautions to take to prevent accidents and injuries. The hazards include:

- Biological infectious agents as discussed in Chapter 5, "Infection Control"
- Fire, bombs, and other explosives such as from oxygen tanks and chemicals
- Laboratory hazards from specimens, equipment, and biological reagents
- Electrical hazards from equipment and high voltage connections
- X-rays and radioactive reagents and equipment
- Chemical spills of toxic reagents or other liquids in the laboratory
- Mechanical hazards from laboratory equipment
- Latex allergies to latex in gloves, blood collection holders, and other health care supplies

Providing protection from hazardous events in the health care environment for the patient and health care worker is part of everyday responsibilities included with the other blood collection responsibilities (Figure 6–1 ■).

▬▬▬ FIRE SAFETY

Fire safety is the responsibility of all employees in the health care institution. Fire or explosive hazards may occur in the laboratory or other areas of the health care facility. Health care workers should be familiar with not only the use and location of the fire extinguishers but also the procedures to follow during a fire. They should also be knowledgeable of the exact locations of fire extinguishers and fire blankets. The blankets should be available to smother burning clothes or to use as a fire shield if fire is blocking the exit. Health care institutions usually conduct periodic safety education programs in which the health care worker can participate to become skillful in and knowledgeable about the use of fire safety equipment (Figure 6–1).

CLASSIFICATION OF FIRES

The components of fire are fuel, oxygen, and heat, plus the necessary chain reaction. Four general classifications of fires have been adopted by the National Fire Protection Association (NFPA).[3] These classifications are as follows:

1. Class A fires occur with ordinary combustible material, such as wood, rubbish, paper, cloth, and many plastics.
2. Class B fires occur in a vapor–air mixture over flammable solvents, such as gasoline, oil, paint, lacquers, grease, and flammable gases.
3. Class C fires occur in or near electrical equipment.
4. Class D fires occur with combustible metals, such as magnesium, sodium, and lithium. These fires are infrequently encountered in health care institutions.

FIRE EXTINGUISHERS

Fire extinguishers are classified to correspond with each class of fire as shown in Figure 6–2 ■.

1. Type A extinguishers contain soda and acid or water and are used to cool the ordinary fire such as of wood, cloth, or paper.

Figure 6–1. Fire Extinguisher and Fire Hose

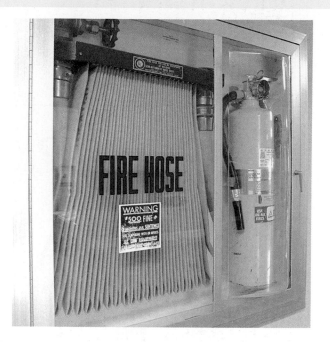

2. Type BC extinguishers contain foam, dry chemicals, or carbon dioxide (CO_2) and are used to combat fires occurring in vapor–air mixtures over solvents such as grease, gasoline, or oil.
3. Type ABC extinguishers contain a dry chemical and are used to to extinguish fires of wood, cloth, paper, oil, grease, and gasoline. These extinguishers are versatile in combating fires and thus are located in fire stations throughout health care institutions.

Class D fires should be fought by fire fighters only.

EMERGENCY RESPONSE TO POSSIBLE FIRE

If a fire or explosion occurs in the workplace, the health care worker should ***not*** do the following:

- Block entrances
- Reenter the building
- Panic
- Run

But instead the health care worker *should:*

- Pull the nearest fire alarm.
- Call 911 or the hospital's fire emergency number, which should be posted on or near the phone.

Figure 6–2. Proper Use of the Extinguisher

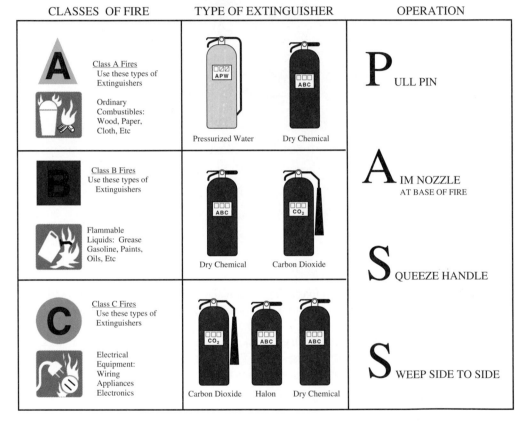

PROPER USE OF FIRE EXTINGUISHERS

*EXTINGUISHER MUST BE RATED FOR TYPE
OF FIRE YOU ARE FIGHTING*

BEFORE YOU BEGIN TO FIGHT A SMALL FIRE

*ACTIVATE FIRE ALARM
CALL UTPD AT 500-4357 (**FROM A SAFE LOCATION**)
BE SURE FIRE IS CONFINED TO SMALL AREA AND IS NOT SPREADING
BE SURE THAT A SAFE AND UNOBSTRUCTED EXIT IS READILY AVAILABLE
BE SURE YOUR EXTINGUISHER IS THE PROPER SIZE AND TYPE FOR THE CLASS OF FIRE*

Courtesy of Environmental Health and Safety, The University of Texas Health Science Center at Houston.

- Remove patients from danger if on patient floor.
- Close windows and doors to prevent spreading of the fire.
- If the fire is small and isolated from other possible fuel sources, use an ABC extinguisher to fight it:
  1. Pull plastic lock off of extinguisher.
  2. Aim extinguisher at the base of fire and squeeze the handle.
  3. Spray the solution toward base of fire, but do not point directly at an individual.
- If the fire threatens to block exits or is not small, leave the area immediately. Take the stairs, not the elevator.
- If clothing is on fire, drop to the ground and roll, preferably in a fire blanket.
- If caught in a fire, crawl to the exit. Because smoke rises, breathing is easier at floor level. Breathing through a wet towel is also helpful.

▆▆▆▆ LABORATORY SAFETY

Laboratory safety includes a variety of policies. All health care workers, however, should remember a few key safety rules at all times:

- Equipment such as centrifuges and quality control biological reagents require the use of PPE.
- Patients' specimens should be covered at all times during transportation and centrifugation.
- Centrifugation of specimens should be performed within a biohazard safety hood.
- All wastes from specimen collections must be disposed of in the correct containers.
- Needles should not be recapped, bent, or broken.
- Phlebotomy collection trays must be disinfected at least once a week with a 1:10 bleach solution.

Specific Environmental Protection Agency (EPA) and OSHA regulations, as well as state and local laws, regulate the disposal of wastes.[4,5] Blood and body fluids should be disposed of through an approved biohazardous waste disposal company in accordance with local, state, and national regulations. Infectious airborne transmission from patients' specimens can occur in the laboratory when:

- Removing top closures from specimen tubes
- Transferring blood or other body fluids between containers, through splashing
- Centrifuging without covering with biological hood
- Not wearing a proper face shield when working with specimens

Needles must not be recapped before disposal.[6] Sharps, such as needles and lancets, should be disposed of in a special container that is spillproof, tamperproof, puncture resistant, and closable (Figure 6–3 ■). The sharps container must be labeled in red or orange, must be maintained upright, and must display the biohazard symbol as shown in Figure 6–3.

CLEANING SPECIMEN COLLECTION AREAS AND BIOLOGICAL SPILLS

In addition, the specimen collection area should be decontaminated with a 1:10 bleach solution. Because a diluted bleach solution becomes unstable when exposed to oxygen, it must be prepared daily. Alternatively, a diluted bleach solution that is stable is available commer-

Figure 6-3. Sharps Container

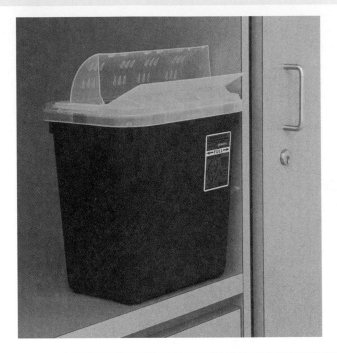

cially. If blood or other body fluids are spilled, encapsulating powder, which is available from manufacturers of safety products (e.g., United Ad Label Direct, Brea, California), should be used to gel the liquid for safe cleanup.

Each laboratory has cleanup procedures, but general recommendations include:

- Wear gloves.
- Use the above described 1:10 bleach solution or commercially prepared solution.
- First clean area with visible blood and then disinfect the entire area of possible contamination.
- Keep the bleach in contact with the contaminated area for at least 20 minutes to ensure complete disinfection.

Colored biohazard labels must be affixed to all containers of regulated waste, refrigerators and freezers containing blood or other body fluids, and other containers used to store, transport, or ship these materials.

If an accident occurs, such as a needle stick, the injured health care worker should immediately cleanse the area with isopropyl alcohol and apply an adhesive bandage. Then he or she should follow the exposure control plan for that facility (e.g. notify the immediate supervisor, fill out the necessary incident and medical forms, and undergo the appropriate laboratory tests). In addition, the health care worker should be counseled and evaluated for HIV and HCV infection at periodic intervals (see "Personal Safety from Infection during Specimen Handling" in Chapter 5).

▰▰▰ ELECTRICAL SAFETY

A major hazard in any area of a health care institution is the possibility of electrical current passing through a person. For example, in the clinical laboratory or physician office laboratory, the health care worker sometimes operates electrical equipment, such as a centrifuge. He or she should be aware of the location of the circuit-breaker boxes in order to assure a fast response in the event of an electrical fire or an electrical shock. In case of power outage, emergency power is delivered to lights by a red toggle switch as shown in Figure 6–4 ■. Power will become available from these switches within 15 to 30 seconds and is supplied from the health care facility's generators.

The health care worker using electrical equipment should consider the following:

- Do not use power cords that are frayed.
- Do not use control switches and thermostats that are not in good working order.
- Always unplug the centrifuge or other electrical equipment before maintenance is performed.
- Any electrical instrument that liquid has been spilled on or in, or whose wiring has come in contact with liquid, should be immediately unplugged and dried prior to further use.
- If equipment has a label with an electrical caution warning, do not open it, since it may contain batteries that store electricity even when the equipment is unplugged.
- Avoid using extension cords.
- While collecting blood, avoid contact with any electrical equipment, since the electricity may pass through you and the needle and shock the patient.
- Use three-prong "hospital-grade" electrical plugs for all equipment (Figure 6–5 ■) since the three-prong has a long prong for grounding of the equipment.

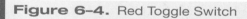

Figure 6–4. Red Toggle Switch

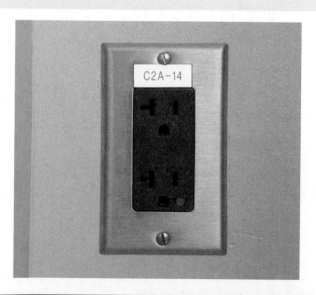

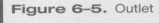

Figure 6–5. Outlet

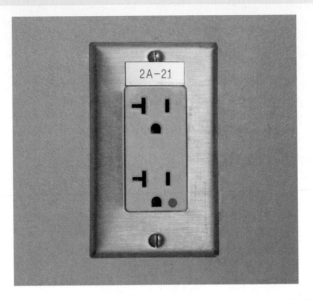

If an electrical accident occurs involving electrical shock to an employee or a patient, the health care worker should be aware of the two points shown in Box 6–1.

Box 6–1   If an Electrial Accident Occurs

1. The electrical power source must be shut off. If this is impossible, carefully remove the electrical contact from the victim, using something that does not conduct electricity, such as placing your hand in a glass beaker and pushing the power supply away from the victim. The rescuer should not attempt to touch the victim without heeding these precautions.

2. Medical assistance should be called and cardiopulmonary resuscitation (CPR) started immediately. The victim should not be moved prior to the arrival of medical assistance. A fire blanket or other warm clothing should be put over the victim to keep him or her warm until medical help arrives.

■■■■■ RADIATION SAFETY

The three cardinal principles of self-protection from radiation exposure are time, shielding, and distance. Radiation exposure is cumulative; thus, limiting the length of exposure at any one time is a major factor in minimizing the hazard.

Areas where radioactive materials are in use and stored must have warning signs (Figure 6–6 ■) posted on the entrance doors. All radioactive specimens and reagents must also be properly labelled with the radioactive sign.

Figure 6-6. Radiation Hazard Sign

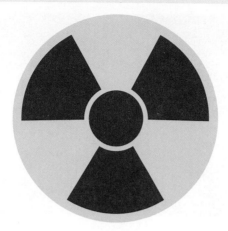

The health care worker will probably encounter potential hazards from radiation exposure only if he or she must collect specimens from patients in the nuclear medicine or x-ray department or must take specimens to the radioimmunoassay section in a research or a clinical chemistry laboratory. Thus the health care worker should be cautious when entering an area posted with the radiation hazard sign and should be knowledgeable of the institution's procedures pertaining to radiation safety. Limit time of exposure to patients who have received radioactive implants. Health care workers who are pregnant should be aware of the potential hazard of radiation to the fetus.

MECHANICAL SAFETY

The centrifuge is a frequently used instrument for blood specimen preparation and testing (Figure 6–7 ■). Thus a health care provider who collects and prepares blood specimens for testing should learn how to maintain this instrument and become familiar with its parts. For example, he or she should know if the carriers are in the correct position prior to use. If the carriers are not in the correct position, they can swing out of the holding disks into the side of the centrifuge. Also, the wrong head, the wrong cups, or imbalanced tubes can lead to the same dangerous problem. If this particular type of accident occurs, tubes containing patients' specimens or spinning chemicals may be propelled onto the side of the centrifuge and broken, and a dangerous, hazardous problem created. Thus it is of utmost importance to abide by the preventive maintenance schedule and procedures for the centrifuge.

CHEMICAL SAFETY

Because a health care worker must sometimes pour preservatives, such as hydrochloric acid (HCl), into containers for 24-hour urine collections and transport these specimens to the patients' floor, he or she should be knowledgeable of chemical safety (Figure 6–8 ■).

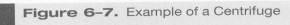

Figure 6–7. Example of a Centrifuge

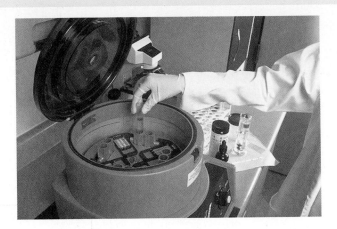

Labeling may be the single most important step in the proper handling of chemicals. Laboratorians should be able to ascertain from appropriate labels not only the contents of the container but also the nature and extent of hazards posed by the chemicals. Carefully read the label before using any reagents.

CHEMICAL IDENTIFICATION

Various chemicals are needed in health care facilities, especially in the clinical laboratory department. Because chemicals may pose health or physical hazards, OSHA amended the Hazard Communication Standard (29 CFR 1910.1200, Right to Know/HCS Standard) to include health care facilities.

In addition to mandating labels, the Right to Know law requires chemical manufacturers to supply **Material Safety Data Sheets (MSDSs)** for their chemicals. The MSDS is re-

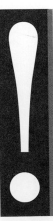

Clinical Alert

ALWAYS add acid to water. NEVER add water to acid!

Figure 6–8. Department of Transportation (DOT) Hazardous Materials Warning Signs

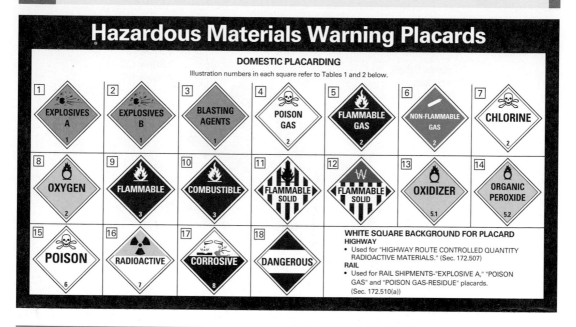

quired for any chemical with a hazard warning label. An MSDS lists general information, precautionary measures, and emergency information.

The NFPA developed a labeling system for hazardous chemicals that is frequently used in health care facilities (Figure 6–9 ■). The system uses a diamond-shaped symbol, four colored quadrants, and a hazard rating scale of 0 to 4. The health hazard is shown in the blue quadrant; the flammability hazard is shown in the red quadrant; the instability hazard is indicated in the yellow quadrant; and the specific hazard is shown in the white quadrant. Common laboratory chemicals such as isopropyl alcohol or diluted bleach (sodium hypochlorite) in squirt bottles require regulatory labels (Figure 6–10 ■).

| Box 6–2 | Chemical Labels |

Labels for hazardous chemicals must:

1. provide a warning (e.g., corrosive) (See Figure 6–8.)

2. explain the nature of the hazard (e.g., flammable, combustible) (See Figure 6–8.)

3. state special precautions to eliminate risks

4. explain first-aid treatment in the event of a chemical leak, a chemical spill, or other exposure to the chemical.

Figure 6-9. NFPA Rating System

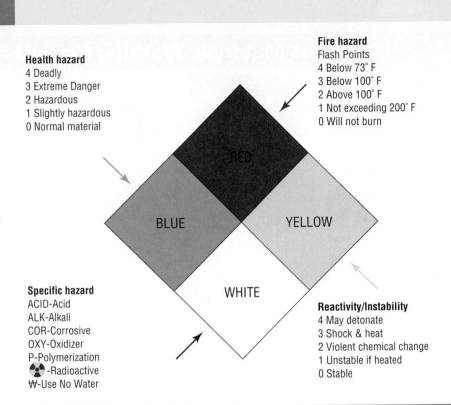

Health hazard
4 Deadly
3 Extreme Danger
2 Hazardous
1 Slightly hazardous
0 Normal material

Fire hazard
Flash Points
4 Below 73° F
3 Below 100° F
2 Above 100° F
1 Not exceeding 200° F
0 Will not burn

Specific hazard
ACID-Acid
ALK-Alkali
COR-Corrosive
OXY-Oxidizer
P-Polymerization
☢-Radioactive
W̶-Use No Water

Reactivity/Instability
4 May detonate
3 Shock & heat
2 Violent chemical change
1 Unstable if heated
0 Stable

SAFETY SHOWERS AND THE EYEWASH STATION

Safety showers should be nearby for use if an accidental chemical spill occurs. Because permanent damage to the skin can result from chemical burns, the victim of a chemical accident must immediately rinse for at least 15 minutes after removing contaminated clothing.

In case of a chemical spill in the eye, the victim should rinse his or her eyes at the eyewash station for a minimum of 15 minutes. Contact lenses must be removed prior to the rinsing in order to thoroughly cleanse the eyes. The victim should not rub the eyes because doing so may cause further injury. If someone is hurt in a chemical spill, it is preferable to take the victim to the emergency department for treatment after his or her eyes have been rinsed for 15 minutes.

CHEMICAL SPILL CLEANUP

If a chemical spill occurs, the health care worker should obtain a spill cleanup kit from the clinical chemistry section. The kit includes absorbents and neutralizers to clean up acid, alkali, mercury, and other spills. The absorbent and neutralizer used depend on the type of chemical spill and have an indicator system that identifies when the spill has been neutralized and can be considered safe for sweep up and disposal. In addition, rubber gloves and other appropriate personal protective equipment (PPE) should be immediately available for

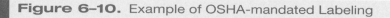
Figure 6–10. Example of OSHA-mandated Labeling

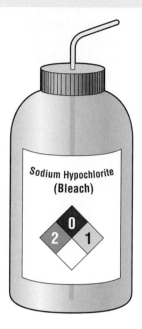

Sodium Hypochlorite
(Bleach)

2 0 1

the cleanup. The health care worker should become familiar with the procedures for cleaning up chemical spills in his or her place of employment.

DISPOSAL OF CHEMICALS

Chemical disposal procedures must comply with all local and state regulations. Certain chemicals can be disposed of in sanitary sewer systems in accordance with the regulations. Thus, the health care worker must be familiar with the laboratory procedures for chemical waste disposal.

Box 6–3   Important Protective Measures for Chemical Use

- The proper personal protective equipment (PPE) and clothing must be worn when a health care worker is working with chemicals.
- A buttoned laboratory coat, safety glasses, face shield, and gloves provide protection and prevent skin contact. The laboratory coat must provide optimal protection against chemicals and infectious agents. Aprons may be used to provide additional protection.
- When transporting acids or alkalis, an acid carrier should be used. It is a specially designed container for carrying large quantities of hazardous solutions.
- The entrance of any room in which hazardous chemicals are in use or in storage must be posted with a caution sign specifying the types of chemicals present.
- No chemicals should be stored above eye level because of the danger of breakage or spillage involved in reaching.
- All explosives should be stored in an explosionproof or a fireproof room that is separate from the flammables.

■■■■■ EQUIPMENT AND SAFETY IN PATIENTS' ROOMS

Each member of the health care team is responsible for the safety of the patient. All health care professionals are responsible for patient safety from the time the patient enters the health care setting until his or her departure. First, when collecting blood from a hospitalized patient, provide privacy for the patient during the procedure (Figure 6–11 ■).

As a matter of general patient safety, the phlebotomist should do the following when in the patient's room:

1. Make certain that all specimen collection supplies, needles, and equipment are either properly disposed of or returned to the specimen collection tray after blood collection.
2. Check to see whether the bed rails are up or down. Always place bed rails up before leaving the patient if they were up when you entered the room.

Figure 6–11. Patient Privacy

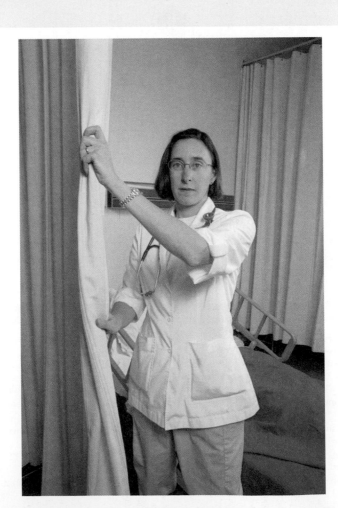

3. Report unusual odors to the nursing station, because a pipe may be broken and leaking gas or liquid.

4. Check for food or liquid spilled on the floor, urine spills, or intravenous (IV) line leakage. Areas on which the patient and health care professionals walk must be dry. They should be free of obstacles and slipping hazards. Thus, in cases of spills, make certain that the area is cleaned and dried for the safety of the patients and hospital personnel.

5. During blood collection, be very cautious not to touch any electrical instrument located adjacent to the patient's bed, because if the instrument malfunctions, the health care worker may ground the patient and, as a result, a microshock could pass through the health care worker and into the patient. A serious problem could result from such a shock if the patient has an electrolyte imbalance or is wet with perspiration or other fluid. Furthermore, the needle inserted in the patient's arm could produce ventricular fibrillation and death if the patient has a pacemaker or an unstable heart ailment.

6. Report the following problem immediately to the nursing station: If the patient has an IV line and the site is swollen and red, the IV needle is probably no longer in the vein and the IV solution is infiltrating into the surrounding tissues. Some chemicals in IV solutions are toxic to body tissue, so gangrene could result from such infiltration. Also, if blood is backing up the IV line from the needle insertion to the IV drip container, the IV solution container is empty. Report this problem immediately.

7. If the patient's alarm for the IV drip is sounding, report this problem to the nursing station immediately.

8. If the patient is in unusual pain or is unresponsive, notify the nursing station immediately.

PATIENT SAFETY OUTSIDE THE ROOM

Health care workers should be aware of possible hazards to patients outside the patients' rooms. As a matter of general safety practice, the following guidelines should be followed:

1. Because trays, carts, and ladders may be placed around a hallway corner, the health care worker should be careful not to travel too quickly from one room to another and around corners.

2. Items lying on the floor, such as flower petals, may cause someone to slip and should be reported for cleanup.

Clinical Alert

Patient identification must be accurate. Thus, use at least TWO patient identifiers—neither of which can be the patient's room number—when collecting blood specimens.

Patient identifiers include: patient's name, identification number, address, telephone number, social security number, or date of birth.[7]

3. Avoid running in a health care facility, because patients and visitors may become alarmed and begin to run as well. Also, someone may be hurt if the health care worker runs into him or her (e.g., a cardiac patient walking in the hall with an inserted-IV stand or another health care worker carrying a specimen collection tray).

PATIENT SAFETY RELATED TO LATEX PRODUCTS

Patients, as well as health care workers, may be allergic to latex products (Figure 6–12 ■). The signs and symptoms of an allergic reaction to latex may include a skin rash, hives, nasal, eye, or sinus irritation, and sometimes, shock. Table 6–1 provides examples of items frequently used in the health care environment that contain latex. Figure 6–13 ■ shows an example of a "Latex-Safe Environment" sign.

Figure 6–12. Latex-Free Cart

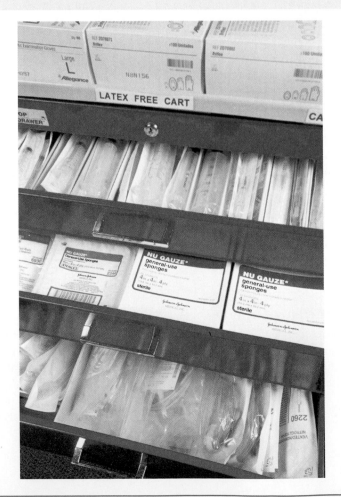

TABLE 6–1. Products Containing Latex

MEDICAL EQUIPMENT	PERSONAL PROTECTIVE EQUIPMENT	OFFICE SUPPLIES	MEDICAL SUPPLIES
Tourniquets	Gloves	Adhesive tape	Condom-style urinary collection device
Syringes	Goggles	Erasers	Enema tubing tips
Stethoscopes	Rubber aprons	Rubber bands	Injection ports
Oral and nasal airways	Surgical masks		Rubber tops of stoppers on multidose vials
IV tubing			
Disposable gloves			Urinary catheter
Breathing circuits			Wound drains
Blood pressure cuffs			

Source: Reprinted from *Preventing Allergic Reactions to Natural Rubber Latex in the Workplace,* The Centers for Disease Control and Prevention, National Institute for Occupational Safety and Health Alert, Atlanta, GA, June 1997.

DISASTER EMERGENCY PLAN

Many health care institutions have developed procedures to be followed in case of a hurricane, flooding, earthquake, bomb threat, and other disasters. The health care worker should become familiar with these procedures because he or she must be prepared to take immediate action whenever conditions warrant such action (Figure 6–14 ■).

Figure 6–13. Latex-Safe Environment Sign

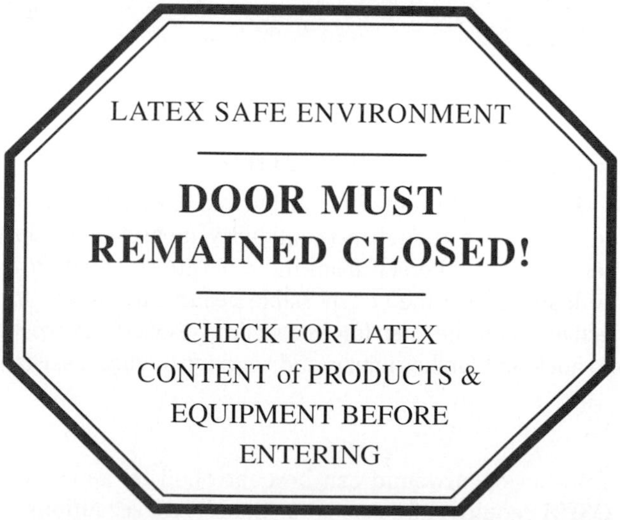

LATEX SAFE ENVIRONMENT

DOOR MUST REMAINED CLOSED!

CHECK FOR LATEX
CONTENT of PRODUCTS &
EQUIPMENT BEFORE
ENTERING

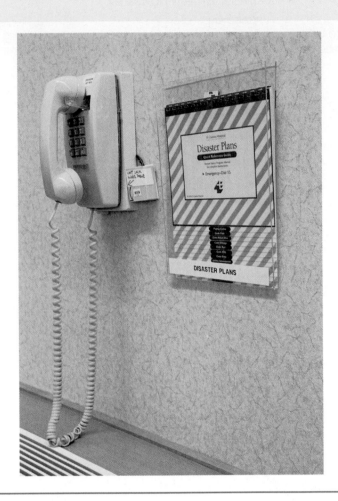

Figure 6–14. Disaster Plans and Phone

EMERGENCY PROCEDURES

The health care worker should become knowledgeable of emergency care procedures because accidents do occur even though precautionary measures are in place. He or she must be able to detach him- or herself from the emergency situation to some degree in order to perform well and deliver the best possible health care. In an emergency situation, the following objectives must be met for the victim: prevent severe bleeding, maintain breathing, prevent shock and further injury, and send for medical assistance.

BLEEDING AID

Severe bleeding from an open wound can be controlled by applying pressure directly over the wound. OSHA requires adherence to "Standard Precautions" when health care

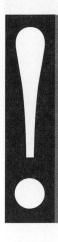

Clinical Alert

If someone telephones and threatens to bomb the health care facility:

- Listen to the person and keep him/her talking
- Listen for background noises for caller's location
- Listen for caller's accent, language, etc.
- Ask the caller where the bomb is located and what time it will go off
- Write down everything the caller states
- Notify the health care facility's security officer

If a bomb threat procedure is in place, it needs to be used by all health care workers

workers respond to emergencies that provide potential exposure to blood and other potentially infectious materials. Health care workers responding to an emergency should be protected from exposure to blood and other potentially infectious materials through the use of PPE (e.g., gloves, mask, etc.). A clean handkerchief or other clean cloth (compress) should be placed over the wound before applying pressure with a gloved hand. In an emergency in which a clean cloth is not available, a gloved hand should be used until a cloth compress can be located. Bleeding of a limb (i.e., an arm or a leg) can be decreased by elevation. The injured portion should be raised above the level of the victim's heart unless the injured portion is broken. Even with elevation, however, pressure should be maintained on the wound until medical assistance arrives. A tourniquet should not be used to control bleeding except in the case of an amputated, mangled, or crushed arm or leg, or for profuse bleeding that cannot be stopped otherwise.

CIRCULATION AID

To maintain circulation in a victim, a health care provider must know the techniques of basic CPR. Thus, he or she should check with the supervisor about the availability of CPR classes at the health care institution, because this emergency technique must be demonstrated so that the employee can learn the proper skills.

SHOCK PREVENTION

Shock usually accompanies severe injury. It may result from bleeding, extensive burns, an insufficient oxygen (O_2) supply, and other traumatic events. Early signs include pale, cold, clammy skin; weakness; a rapid pulse; an increased, shallow breathing rate; and frequently, nausea and vomiting. The main objectives in treating a shock victim are to improve circulation, to provide sufficient O_2, and to maintain normal body temperature.

When a victim's breathing movements stop or his or her lips, tongue, or fingernails become blue, immediate mouth-to-mouth resuscitation is needed. Any delay in using this technique may cost the victim's life. To perform mouth-to-mouth breathing, include the following:

1. See if the victim is conscious by gently shaking the victim and yelling, "ARE YOU OKAY?" However, if any possibility of a neck injury exists, do not shake the victim! If there is no response to the gentle shaking and yelling, call out for help and start aid immediately.

2. Place the victim on his or her back on a firm, flat surface. Caution must be exercised if the person has a spinal or neck injury. No twisting should occur to the victim's body.

3. Open the airway passage by checking for obstructions: tongue, chewing gum, vomitus, and so on.

4. Place one hand on the victim's forehead and, applying firm, backward pressure with the palm, tilt the head back (Figure 6–15 ■). Place the fingers of the other hand under the bony part of the victim's lower jaw, near the chin, and lift to bring the chin forward with the teeth almost to occlusion. The jaw should be supported as the head is tilted back. This position is called the head-tilt/chin-lift.

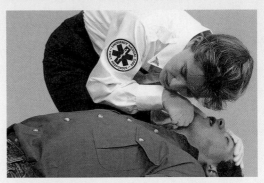

Figure 6–16 *Listen for return of air from victim's mouth and nose.*

6. If there is no breathing, maintain the head-tilt/chin-lift and pinch the victim's nose shut with the hand to prevent air from escaping. Open mouth widely, take a deep breath, and seal mouth over the victim's mouth with a pocket mask (Figure 6–17 ■). Blow into victim's mouth. Watch for the victim's chest to rise. (If it does not, the airway is blocked and must be cleared.)

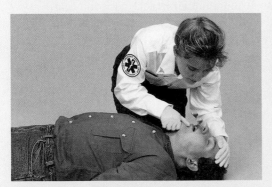

Figure 6–15 *Head-tilt/chin-lift for emergency care.*

5. Listen and feel for return of air from the victim's mouth and nose for approximately 3 to 5 seconds (Figure 6–16 ■). Also, simultaneously, look for the victim's chest to rise and fall.

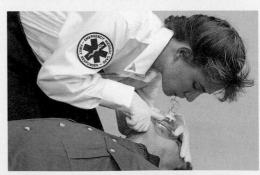

Figure 6–17 *Ventilate with pocket mask.*

7. Give two full ventilations. If this still does not start an air exchange, reposition the head and try again. After two more ventilations, again look, listen, and feel for breathing. Improper chin and head positioning is the most common cause of difficulty with ventilation.

The following six actions are recommended if first aid is given to a shock victim:

1. Correct the cause of shock if possible (e.g., control bleeding).
2. Keep the victim lying down.
3. Keep the victim's airway open. If he or she vomits, turn head to the side so that the neck is arched.
4. In the absence of broken bones, elevate the victim's legs so that the head is lower than the trunk of the body.
5. Keep the victim warm.
6. Call for emergency assistance.

Actions that are *not* recommended include the following:

1. Giving fluids to a victim who has an abdominal injury (The person is likely to require surgery or a general anesthetic.)
2. Giving fluids to an unconscious or semiconscious person

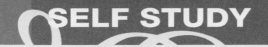
KEY TERMS

cardiopulmonary resuscitation (CPR)
Environmental Protection Agency (EPA)
Material Safety Data Sheets (MSDSs)

Occupational Safety and Health
Administration (OSHA)

STUDY QUESTIONS

The following may have more than one answer:

1. If a fire occurs in or near electrical equipment, which of the following fire extinguishers should be used?
   a. class A extinguisher
   b. class B extinguisher
   c. class C extinguisher
   d. ABC extinguisher

2. What are the major principles of self-protection from radiation exposure?
   a. distance
   b. time
   c. combustibility
   d. shielding

3. Which of the following safety rules should be maintained in patients' rooms?
   a. specimen collection supplies and needles are properly disposed of
   b. unusual odors in the patient's room should be reported to the nursing station
   c. health care providers should not touch electrical instruments located adjacent to the patient's bed
   d. if the patient has an IV line and the site is swollen and reddish, this problem should be reported to the nursing station

4. The main objectives of treating a shock victim are to:
   a. improve circulation
   b. provide sufficient drinking water
   c. provide sufficient oxygen
   d. maintain normal body temperature

5. In an emergency situation, which of the following is/are objective(s) that must be met for the victim?
   a. prevent severe bleeding
   b. maintain breathing
   c. prevent shock
   d. send for medical assistance

6. Which of the following should occur first if a fire breaks out in the health care facility?
   a. run from the floor where the fire is located
   b. call the assigned fire number
   c. use the fastest elevator to escape from the floor where the fire is located
   d. close all windows before leaving the area of the fire

7. The Right to Know law originated with:
   a. CDC
   b. CAP
   c. OSHA
   d. NFPA

8. The hazard labeling system developed by the NFPA has the blue quadrant of the diamond to indicate:
   a. flammability hazard
   b. health hazard
   c. instability hazard
   d. specific hazard

9. If an electrical accident occurs involving electrical shock to an employee or a patient, the first thing that the health care worker should do is:
   a. move the victim
   b. shut off electrical power
   c. start CPR
   d. place a blanket over the victim

References

1. US Department of Labor, Occupational Safety and Health Administration (OSHA): *Occupational exposure to bloodborne pathogens, final rule* (29 CFR 1910.1030). Federal Register, December 6, 1991: 64004–64182.

2. US Department of Labor, Occupational Safety and Health Administration (OSHA): *Occupational exposure to bloodborne pathogens: final rule* (29 CFR 1910.1030). Amendment: Needlestick Safety and Prevention (January 18, 2001).

3. National Fire Protection Association (NFPA): *National Fire Codes.* Quincy, MA: http://www.NFPA.org.

4. Occupational Safety and Health Administration (OSHA): *Hazard Communication Standard.* 29 CFR 1910.1200. Washington, DC: OSHA, 1986.

5. Occupational Safety and Health Administration (OSHA): *Toxic and Hazardous Substances.* 29 CFR 1910.1001–1047. Washington, DC: OSHA, 1989.

6. National Committee for Clinical Laboratory Standards: *Protection of Laboratory Workers from Occupationally Acquired Infections, Approved Guideline,* 2nd ed. NCCLS Document M29-A. Wayne, PA: National Committee for Clinical Laboratory Standards, 2001.

7. Auxter, S: How JCAHO's New Patient Safety Goals will affect labs. *Clin Lab News,* October 2002; 28 (10): 1, 3, 6.

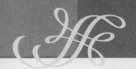

Additional Sources for Safety Information

Centers for Disease Control
  and Prevention (CDC)
Division of Biosafety
1600 Clifton Road, NE
Atlanta, GA 30333
(404) 639-3883
http://www.cdc.gov

College of American Pathologists (CAP)
325 Waukegan Road
Northfield, IL 60093-2750
(800) 323-4040 or (847) 832-7000
http://www.cap.org

Department of Transportation (DOT)
Materials, Transportation Bureau,
  Information Services Division
Washington, DC 20402
(202) 366-4000

Joint Commission on Accreditation
  of Healthcare Organizations (JCAHO)
One Renaissance Blvd
Oakbrook Terrace, IL 60181
(630) 792-5000
http://www.jcaho.org

National Committee for Clinical Laboratory
  Standards (NCCLS)
940 West Valley Road S-1400
Wayne, PA 19087-1898
(610) 525-2435
http://www.nccls.org

National Fire Protection Association (NFPA)
One Batterymarch Park
Quincy, MA 02269-9101
(617) 770-3000
http://www.nfpa.org

Occupational Safety and Health
  Administration (OSHA)
U.S. Department of Labor
200 Constitution Avenue, NW
Washington, DC 20210
(202) 523-8148
http://www.cdc.gov/niosh

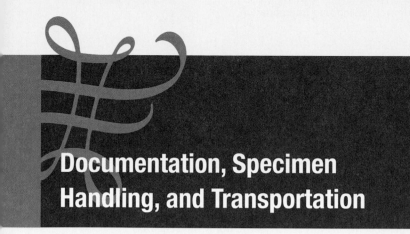

Documentation, Specimen Handling, and Transportation

7

CHAPTER OBJECTIVES

Upon completion of Chapter 7, the learner is responsible for the following:

1. Describe the basic components and uses of a medical record.
2. Describe acceptable guidelines for maintaining privacy and confidentiality.
3. Describe essential elements of requisition and report forms.
4. Name three methods commonly used to transport specimens.

 MediaLINK

Access the accompanying CD-ROM to explore a wide variety of review questions and interactive activities for this chapter, including multiple choice, true/false, and video exercises.

▆▆▆▆ FUNDAMENTALS OF DOCUMENTATION

Documentation in all health care organizations provides a record of the patient's visit and progress. Health care workers document progress in a clinical (or medical) record for each patient. As mentioned in Chapter 2, it is an important legal document and is admissible in a court of law. Any clinically significant information should be included in the medical record, including laboratory results. The format of the medical record varies by setting— for example, a hospital versus a doctor's office—or by the amount of documentation that is required—open-ended forms versus checklists, for instance. Some or all of the medical records may be kept and/or maintained via computer with restricted access, e.g., computerized patient records (CPRs).

Documentation of all clinical events is important for the following reasons:[1,2]

- **Monitoring the quality of care.** Documentation is used to describe what has been done and how the patient responds. State and JCAHO regulations mandate quality assessment activities including the following: nosocomial infection rate, use of unnecessary procedures and tests, discharge planning, and the occurrence of avoidable

| Box 7–1 | Components of a Medical Record |

The following components are commonly used in medical/clinical records. In some cases, these components are combined into one section.

Personal Information: Patient's name, date of birth (DOB), social security number (SSN) or other identification number, address, marital status, closest relative, known allergies, and physician's name and diagnosis.

Personal and Family Medical History: Initial assessment completed by the physician (MD or DO) and the nurse (RN).

Ordering Documentation: Includes MD's and/or other qualified provider's (nurse practitioner's [NP], clinical nurse specialist's [CNS], physician assistant's [PA]) orders for laboratory, radiology, pharmacy, etc.

Consent and Release Forms: Consent forms, authorization forms for release of medical information, and other forms for patient's preferences (e.g., do-not-resuscitate orders, etc.).

Patient's Plan of Care: MD and nursing care diagnoses, interventions, and patient outcomes. Can include flowcharts or checklists indicating recordings of the patient's temperature, pulse rate, respiratory rate, blood pressure, glucose screening levels, weight, and other assessments.

Diagnostic Test Results: Results from all tests performed on the patient: laboratory, radiology, etc.

Medication Administration Record: Medication dosage and timing, route of administration, site, and date.

Progress Notes: Notes from qualified health providers (MD, NP, CNS, PA) about the patient's progress, interventions used, and treatment effectiveness.

Consultations: Evaluation summaries by clinical specialists: infectious disease specialists, endocrinologists, etc.

Health Care Team Notes: Progress notes from other departments such as Nutrition, Physical Therapy, Occupational Therapy, Counseling, etc.

Discharge Plan or Summary: Plans for after discharge from a hospital, including special diets, medications, home health visits, and follow-up appointments.

discomfort or death. The College of American Pathologists (CAP) Laboratory Accreditation Program (LAP) also requires quality monitoring including the following: turnaround times for laboratory results, measures to reduce the volume of blood needed for testing, etc.

- **Coordination of care.** Collaboration among health care providers to plan interventions, evaluate progress, and assist the health care team in making effective decisions. It provides for communication among all health care providers involved with the patient.
- **Accrediting and licensing.** JCAHO and other such agencies require standards for documentation in each patient's clinical, or medical, record. They usually include some guidelines for containing an assessment, a plan of care, medical orders (e.g., laboratory, radiology), progress notes, and a discharge summary.
- **Legal protection.** Documentation in the clinical records provides "proof" that the action was performed. Documentation can serve as supporting evidence in disability, personal injury, malpractice, and mental competency cases. Appropriate documentation is the key to winning or losing a case for individuals or employees of the health care facility. (If a health care worker does not write down what he or she did to a patient, it is assumed that it was not done.)
- **Research.** In teaching institutions, documentation provides important data for research on new therapies, procedures, or drugs.

THE LABORATORY COMMUNICATION NETWORK

The major purpose of a clinical laboratory is to acquire and analyze appropriate patient specimens and to communicate timely results to the physician. Specimen collection procedures are the first and most critical steps in this process. The number of persons and steps involved varies greatly depending on the size of the institution and the type of laboratory involved. Clinical laboratories may be centralized or decentralized, with satellite laboratories in various locations. With each additional location or person involved, another potential source of error or delay is introduced into the system.

As mentioned in Chapter 1, there are many ways to conceptualize the cycle of performing laboratory tests, flowing from preanalytical phases of the initial test request, to

Box 7–2	Important Tips for Documenting Clinical Information

- **Be accurate, objective, short, and legible.** Record only the facts in short phrases, not opinions or assumptions; write in ink and if handwriting is difficult to read, print the words. Documented comments should not assign blame (e.g., "Blood was not collected from Mr. Jones because nurse Daly did not complete the proper requisition"). Likewise, comments about staffing shortages or working overtime are discouraged because they may not have a direct influence on the patient's medical condition.
- **Errors should not be erased.** Records should never be changed or falsified to cover a mistake. Errors should be noted by marking a single line through it and writing the word "Error" next to it with one's initials next to the correction.
- **Include all relevant information in a timely manner.** Notes should be made about each event, procedure, or problem that occurs as soon as possible with the exact time and date. For example, if a phlebotomist is unable to identify a patient because of a missing armband, the notation should include the time, the date, the name of the nurse who positively identified the patient, and the phlebotomist's name. Computerized notations should be done by authorized personnel and according to the organization's policies.

Figure 7–1. Laboratory Testing Cycle: Preanalytical and Analytical Phases

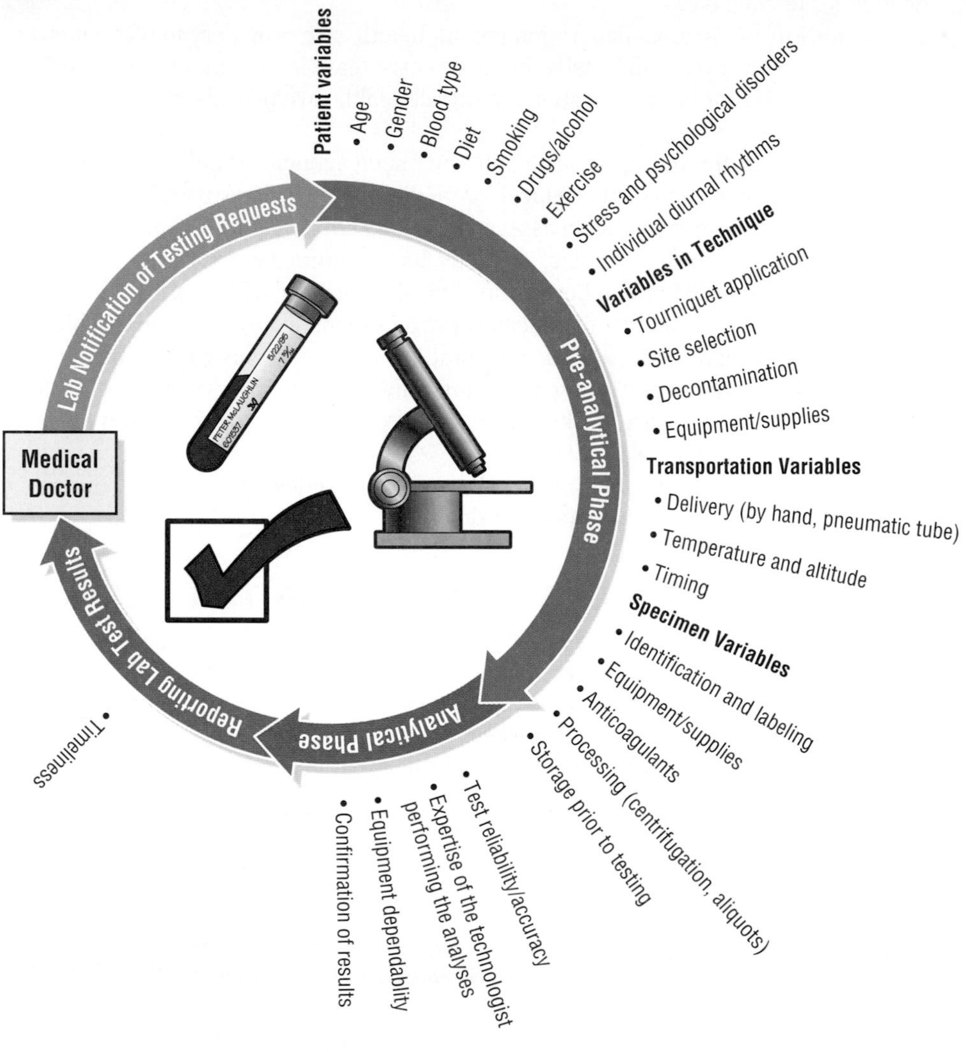

The laboratory testing cycle begins with a physician's (medical doctor, MD) request for specific tests. Once the laboratory is notified, the phlebotomist begins the preanalytical process by obtaining a specimen. It is then transported, processed, and prepared for the analytic phase. The analytic process entails performing clinical analyses on the specimen and reporting the results back to the physician. Note the many variables that affect the entire process.

the specimen collection, to the analytic phase, to the final reporting of results, as shown in Figure 7–1 ■. The phlebotomist is the vital link in the preanalytical phase of laboratory testing.

POLICIES AND PROCEDURES

All health care facilities have policy and procedure manuals that document and guide practices within the organization. Employees usually spend time during their orientation/training period to learn the policies. Phlebotomists commonly utilize the manuals that are summarized in Table 7–1 in a variety of settings. In particular the College of American Pathologists (CAP), an accrediting agency for clinical laboratories, requires that a specimen collection manual (electronic or hard copy) be available to phlebotomists at all sites where specimens are collected. According to the CAP, phlebotomists should be appropriately instructed and evaluated on competencies for all procedures.

CONTINUING EDUCATION

Certain types of continuing education (CE), such as training in universal standard precautions, fire safety, and radiation safety, are required periodically and are offered by larger organizations. Many of the professional organizations listed in Chapter 1 also provide continuing educational courses that are required for employment and/or state licensure. Thus phlebotomists should maintain documentation of all CE coursework related to their careers.

COMMUNICATION OUTSIDE THE LABORATORY

Communication with other health care workers working outside the laboratory is enhanced by using a paper-based or computerized information bulletin, or "floor book," of laboratory services. It should contain a directory of the laboratory departments, staff members, the location of the laboratory, telephone numbers, operating hours, reference ranges, instructions, and pertinent standard procedures of the laboratory. The methods used for collection of all specimens, as well as the proper identification, storage, preservation, and transportation mechanisms to be used, are clearly specified. In addition, an alphabetical listing of all laboratory determinations, specimen requirements, special instructions, and tables with reference ranges for each measurement are often included. This is particularly helpful to phlebotomists, medical students, residents, fellows, and trainees.

Box 7–3   Preanalytic Variables

Preanalytic variables that are inherent in phlebotomy duties include the following:

- **Patient variables.** Identification, fasting versus nonfasting, diurnal variations, refusal to cooperate, patient unavailable, stress or anxiety, etc.
- **Transportation variables.** Specimen leakage, tube breakage, excessive shaking, etc.
- **Specimen processing variables.** Adequacy of centrifugation, sample registration and distribution, delays in processing, contamination of the specimen, exposure to heat or light, etc.
- **Specimen variables.** Hemolysis, inadequate volume in the tube, inadequate mixing of anticoagulant, etc.

TABLE 7–1.   Manuals and Procedures Important to Phlebotomists

The following topics are generally covered in procedure manuals and are particularly important for phlebotomists.

Specimen Collection Manual
- Patient preparation
- Type of collection container and amount of specimen required
- Timing requirements (e.g., creatinine clearance, therapeutic drug monitoring, etc.)
- Type and amount of preservative or anticoagulant needed
- Special handling or transportation needs (e.g., refrigeration, immediate delivery, etc.)
- Proper labeling requirements
- Need for additional clinical data when indicated (e.g., fasting vs. nonfasting, etc.)[3]

Administrative Procedures
- Performance evaluation procedures and job descriptions
- Disciplinary policies and confidentiality/nondisclosure policies
- Compensatory time, annual leave, and overtime policies
- Attendance and punctuality policies
- Holiday schedules
- Handling of employee accidents
- In-service requirements
- Vaccination policies (e.g., hepatitis)
- Telephone etiquette policies
- Translation procedures for non-English-speaking patients
- Release of information policies
- Sexual harassment policies
- Quality improvement plan
- Patient billing methods
- Dress code

Safety Manuals
- Fire safety
- Internal and external disaster plan
- Radiation safety
- Exposure control plan
- Hazard communication manual

Infection Control Procedures
- Handling specimens
- Precautions
- Isolation procedures
- Disposal policies
- Decontamination procedures
- Hand-washing procedures
- Accidental percutaneous needle sticks
- Postexposure procedures

Quality Control (QC) Procedures
- Maintaining appropriate supplies
- Monitoring reagents and equipment
- Proper use, storage, and handling of supplies
- Stability of reagents and expiration dates
- Measuring precision and accuracy

(continued)

TABLE 7–1.   Continued

Other Procedures Important to Phlebotomists	<ul><li>Reporting of critical values</li><li>Maintaining confidentiality</li><li>Laboratory test or billing codes</li><li>Inventory procedures for equipment and supplies</li><li>Acceptable symbols, abbreviations, and units of measure (Refer to the Appendices for examples)</li><li>Interdepartmental loans of supplies and equipment</li><li>Use of library resources</li><li>Handling specimens going to or coming from outside organizations</li><li>Instrument and maintenance manuals</li></ul>

USE OF THE TELEPHONE

The telephone is the most frequently used method of two-way communication in any setting. Health care workers must be aware of the procedures for operation, documentation, and for releasing information. These procedures usually include the following:

- Using effective customer service manners
- Transferring calls
- Placing the caller "on hold"
- Using the intercom system
- Modifying and using voice mail messages
- Organizing conference calls
- Using the speaker phone
- Writing legible, complete messages

Box 7–4   Telephone Tips

- Always speak in a polite and professional tone.
- State the department, clinic, or unit name.
- Be mindful of the patient's privacy and confidentiality when speaking.
- To establish a cooperative relationship, always use phrases such as the following:

    May I help you?

    Pardon me, could you please repeat that?

    Please spell your name.

    I am sorry that I cannot assist you with that, may I refer you to someone who can?

    Thank you.
- If speaking to patients and family members, try to use words that are easy to pronounce, concise, direct, and uncomplicated.
- Articulate words clearly; do not use slang.
- Spelling a term may help you or the receiver understand or recognize what is being said.
- Restate sentences to make sure that you understand the message or instructions.
- Remain neutral in a controversy.
- Reflecting on a response before answering will help clarify your answer; however, pauses that are too long may indicate a lack of interest.
- Ask pertinent questions and have the ability to say that you do not know the answer.

Clinical Alert

Occasionally a phlebotomist may overhear communication between a physician and the patient. This communication is considered privileged and must not be shared with others without the prior consent of the patient. This assures compliance with the Health Insurance Portability and Accountability Act of 1996 (Public Law 104-191), HIPAA, which details specific rights for patients regarding protection of their health information. HIPAA prohibits disclosure of any health information unless a written consent has been obtained from a patient.

CONFIDENTIALITY AND PRIVACY

Clinical documents such as laboratory and radiology test results must be kept confidential and private. Health care workers, including phlebotomists who have access to this information, must be careful not to disclose patient information in a casual, unnecessary fashion. Discussion that does not directly relate to the health care worker's role in caring for the patient should be avoided.

Health care providers are required to create "privacy-conscious" practices, which include informing patients about the use and disclosure of their health information and require that only the minimum amount of health information necessary be disclosed. Furthermore, providers and insurance companies must ensure internal protection of medical records, employee privacy training and education, proper handling of privacy complaints, and designation of a privacy officer.[4]

FAX TRANSMISSION OF LABORATORY INFORMATION

HIPAA laws also affect policies related to electronic transmission of laboratory information. Fax machines are widely used because they are efficient, timely, and cost effective, especially when off-site services are offered. However, since the patient's permission is needed to disclose information, each health care facility or laboratory should have clear policies related to the use of test requisitions or results that are sent or received by facsimile or via computer.

COMPUTERIZED COMMUNICATIONS

Personal, handheld, and mainframe computers and networks have become essential instruments in the clinical laboratory and health care setting; thus, the health care worker needs to become acquainted with computer systems. For example, computer systems carry out functions such as:

- Entering lists of test requisitions for a patient
- Generating patients' labels, specimen collection lists, and schedules

- Updating the laboratory specimen accession records
- Printing lists that identify which test procedures need to be performed on patient's specimens
- Reporting test results
- Storing test results
- Sending laboratory test results to the nursing stations either as individual test reports or cumulative summaries of the patient's laboratory records
- Sending patient charges to the accounting office

▆▆▆▆ LABORATORY TEST REQUISITION FORMS

Laboratory tests are requested by means of the laboratory requisition form or a computer-generated order. Multiple-part requisition forms that serve as both laboratory request and report forms are considered a more traditional manual system. These forms may also be used when computer failures occur. The forms are usually of a convenient size to be easily attached to 8½-by-11-inch paper, as is customarily used for patients' medical records. Also, these forms are easy to transport, handle, sort, and store, and they are cost effective. The forms are manufactured to provide clear copies and easy detachment (perforated edges). Color coding can be used for different request forms for ease of identification, both in the ordering of tests and in the charting of results. The name of the institution is usually included on each request form.

▆▆▆▆ BARCODES

The use of barcoded labels (Figure 7–3 ■) for patients' samples, to reduce transcription errors and speed up sample processing, is commonplace. Barcodes represent a series of light and dark bands that relate to specific alphanumeric symbols (i.e., numbers and letters). In other words, each letter of the alphabet and each number has a specific code. When these bands are placed together in a series, they can correspond to a name (of a patient, plebotomist, or test) or a number (identification or test code). This technology is very accurate and fast, and it keeps personnel from entering or typing information, which reduces errors substantially.

Radio frequency identification (RFID) is another form of identification tag that is rapidly emerging in health care for identifying and tracking records, equipment and supplies, specimens, and patients. RFID tags are tiny silicon chips that transmit data to a wireless receiver. In contrast to a barcode, RFID does not require line-of-sight reading with a scanner. It is possible to identify and/or track many items simultaneously. The frequency (and cost) varies depending on the application being used and the distance that the RFID tag needs to be from the wireless receiver. Lower frequencies can be used in situations where the range of distance is relatively short. While technology is very promising, there are still issues that are being addressed for the health care market, including cost, standardization, and privacy protection measures.

Figure 7–2. Multiple-part Sample Requisition Forms

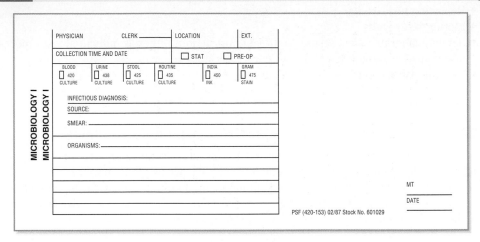

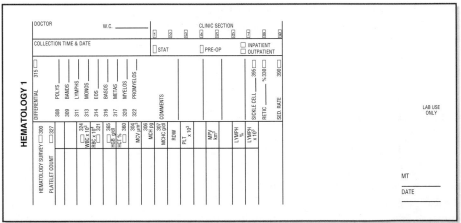

Use of multiple-part requisition forms is helpful in a manual system or as a temporary request until the formal request can be entered into a computer system.

 TRANSMITTAL OF THE TEST REQUEST TO THE LABORATORY

A test request initiates the cyclic procedure of the laboratory communication network. Two systems are commonly used for this activity:

- an online interactive computer system; or
- a manual request system

Sometimes barcodes are used; other times a totally manual system is used in which the request form also serves as the final report.

Figure 7-3. Barcode Labels

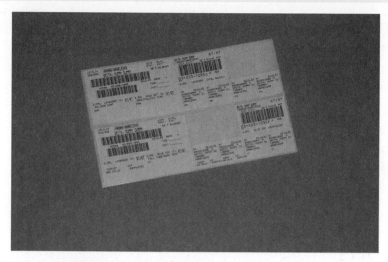

Note that various sizes of labels are printed on one sheet and can be peeled off as needed for each collection tube or microscopic slide.

Online computer input of information is the most error-free means of making requests. Because a computer system can perform automatic checks on the input, it may not accept a request for any test that is not in its test-information database or that is from an unauthorized person. Likewise, it may not accept a sample of plasma or urine for a test restricted to serum. It also allows the person entering the test request to obtain accurate and up-to-date information about specific determinations, such as revised specimen collection requirements, delivery instructions, assay techniques, reference ranges, and fees. Even with handheld computers that are used for barcode scanning, special comments may be added regarding the patient or sample (e.g., "nonfasting" or "drawn from a CVC line").

Box 7-5　Use of Barcodes

Information that can be converted to barcoded symbology for laboratory uses include the following:[5]

- Name and identification number (of patient and/or phlebotomist)
- Date of birth (DOB)
- Test codes
- Specimen accession or log numbers
- Expiration dates for inventory of supplies and equipment
- Product codes for needles, syringes, specimen collection tubes, etc.
- Billing codes to facilitate accounting
- Identification numbers for a group of samples tested on one analyzer at one time, i.e., a "batch-run."

Figure 7–4. Sample Documentation Form for Emergency (STAT) Verbal Test Requests

> **EMERGENCY REQUEST FOR LABORATORY TESTS**
>
> Requesting Nurse:
>
> Requesting Physician:
>
> Patient name: Patient ID (if available):
>
> Location:
>
>   Room #: _____   ICU: _____   ER: _____   Other location: _____
>
> Laboratory requisitions to follow: _____   Pick up on unit _____   Computer entry
>
> List tests ordered:
>
>
>
> Requested by:
>
> Order taken by:
>
> Date: _____   Time: _____ am / pm

Verbal emergency, or STAT, laboratory requests can be accepted only from authorized personnel and must later be followed by an appropriately completed laboratory requisition (manual or computerized).

In a manual system, the multipart request forms are more subject to human error (e.g., transcription mistakes, lost requisitions, duplicate orders, etc.). These problems can be minimized by instituting a centralized location for all requisition forms, using a sorting system once the requisition slips reach the laboratory, and using a blood collection log. Regardless of the method for submitting a laboratory test request, the information submitted must include the following:[3]

- patient identification (name, registration or identification number, location)
- name of physician or legally authorized person ordering the test
- tests requested
- time and date of specimen collection
- other pertinent clinical information when appropriate

A verbal test request is occasionally used in cases of emergency, called a "STAT request." The request should be documented on a standardized form in the laboratory prior to the specimen collection, as shown in Figure 7–4 ■. After the blood is collected, the official laboratory request slip must be completed and accompany the specimen to the laboratory in the routine manner; alternatively, a computerized request can be entered.

◼◼◼ SPECIMEN LABELS AND BLOOD COLLECTION LISTS

Clear and accurate specimen identification is essential and must begin immediately upon collection, and it must continue through disposal of the specimen. Identification methods vary from manually copying all patient identification information onto the container to using prenumbered, barcoded labels. Manually labeling specimens can be time-consuming and prone to transcription errors. These problems can be prevented by using preprinted labels, which are available from many commercial sources. Labeling systems include those that can imprint a patient identification card or electronically print patient identification information onto the specimen label.

Among the most accurate and efficient labels are those generated by a hospital computer system. On the basis of the laboratory orders, the computer can generate the correct number of labels containing the following information:

- patient identification for each tube required to be drawn
- specific tests requested
- types of specimen collection tubes required for the requested tests
- unique accession numbers or sample numbers to be used for that particular collection time
- smaller transfer labels may be used to label aliquot tubes, collection tubes, cuvettes, and microscope slides
- blood drawing lists by floor or unit

This type of system eliminates the manually written entry log used at smaller facilities for recording the tests and accession number requested for each patient. Additional test requests ordered later in the day are entered into the computer, which assigns a specific time to the tests so that they can be easily separated from those requested in the morning. Labels for later collection can be computer printed or made with an Addressograph machine. For even greater accuracy, speed, and convenience, handheld scanners and/or printers can be used at or near the patient's bedside.

Box 7-6   Use of a Blood Drawing List

A blood drawing list (usually generated each morning) is useful in a hospital setting for each floor or nursing unit. The phlebotomist should initial the blood drawing list after the patient's blood has been drawn, and a copy should be left at the nursing unit so that caregivers attending the patient can see which specimens have already been collected. Any additional specimens collected later in the day are documented also. In this way, the personnel on the health care team have a complete list of the specimen collections taken from each patient throughout the day.

◼◼◼ SPECIMEN HANDLING

Both the communication network and the quality of laboratory test results depend on the time that specimens are received for processing. Blood and other specimens must always be delivered expeditiously. The National Committee for Clinical Laboratory Standards (NCCLS) defines standards for handling and processing after consideration of numerous variables that might affect laboratory testing during precentrifugation (after the specimen

TABLE 7–2.   Recommendations for Handling and Processing Blood Specimens

This table provides an overview summary of essential recommendations adapted from the NCCLS Approved Guideline entitled *Procedures for Handling and Processing of Blood Specimens.*[6] The Guideline is much more detailed and provides numerous references and resources for further information. Since every laboratory is under pressure to balance transportation, time, test accuracy, and specimen rejection issues, each laboratory should undergo it's own assessment of processing/handling specimens by reviewing published clinical studies in the literature, following the manufacturer's recommendations, and/or evaluating their own practices. Conclusive evidence from these sources may warrant adjustments for specimen handling when testing for specific analytes.

Precentrifugation Refers to specimen handling/processing after collection and prior to centrifugation

Serum or plasma should be removed from cells as soon as possible and not exceed 2 hours from the time of collection

Other considerations:

- For potassium, ACTH, cortisol, catecholamines, and lactic acid, a shorter time is recommended.
- Many studies have been conducted on the effects of time on analytes' stability. Some show that analytes such as albumin, alkaline phosphatase, ALT, bilirubin, calcium, cholesterol, CK, creatinine, magnesium, phosphorus, sodium, total protein, triglycerides, T3, T4, urea nitrogen, and uric acid may *not* be affected even if the serum is not removed for 48 hours; others demonstrate stability for longer periods.
- Some analytes *are affected* significantly after 2 hours if the serum/plasma is not removed; glucose level decreases, potassium increases, and LD increases.
- Analyte stability is also affected by temperature.

Tubes with additives should be gently inverted 5–10 times to mix the specimen with the additive.

- Tubes with sodium citrate should be inverted 3–4 times.

Specimens without anticoagulant additives (serum specimens) should be clotted prior to centrifugation, which usually takes 30–60 minutes at room temperature (22–25°C).

- Clotting time is affected (often delayed) by anticoagulant therapy that the patient may be taking.
- Chilling the specimen will delay clotting.
- Clotting may be accelerated by activators such as glass or silica particles, thrombin, snake venom/thrombin. They may reduce clotting times to 15–30 minutes.

Anticoagulated specimens (plasma specimens) can be centrifuged immediately after collection.

Some constituents are thermolabile and need to be chilled immediately.

- Chilling a specimen inhibits blood cell metabolism and stabilizes most constituents.
- If potassium (K) is being tested, the specimen cannot be chilled more than 2 hours because it causes K to leak out of the cells causing a false elevation.
- Specimens for electrolytes should not be chilled.
- Specimens that require chilling are blood gases, gastrin, ammonia, lactic acid renin, catecholamine, pyruvate, and parathyroid hormone.

Excessive agitation causes hemolysis.

- Hemolysis causes chemical interference with the laboratory assays listed: elevated for LD, AST, K, plasma hemoglobin, iron, ALT, phosphorus, total protein, albumin, magnesium, acid phosphatase; decreased for T_4

TABLE 7–2.   Continued

Some analytes are light sensitive and should be wrapped with aluminum foil or placed in an amber specimen container to shield the specimen from light.

- Photosensitive analytes include bilirubin, Vitamins A & B6, beta-carotene, and porphyrins
  Tubes should be kept closed at all times. If it is necessary to remove the closure, it is often done behind a shielded plastic box or within a biological safety cabinet to protect the worker from aerosols created when the top is removed.
- Some laboratories still use the practice of removing the tube closure to "rim the tube" with a wooden applicator stick. This releases a blood clot attached to the tube closure or to the sides of the tube. However, this practice is not recommended because of the aerosol dangers and it may cause hemolysis. It is not necessary either since there have been many manufacturer improvements in the tube/closure systems in recent years.

Centrifugation Refers to specimen handling/processing during centrifugation

Manufacturer's specifications generally indicate the speeds and times of centrifugation.

Blood specimens should be allowed to clot before centrifugation.

Tubes should be centrifuged with closures in place.

The centrifuge should have a top that secures appropriately.

Since centrifuges generate internal heat, they should be temperature-controlled so that heat-sensitive analytes are protected.

Specimens should not be centrifuged more than once; and specimens that contain separation devices should never be re-centrifuged.

Many types of gel and non-gel devices are available to enable a barrier to form between the serum/plasma and the blood clot/cells during centrifugation. They all have a particular viscosity and specific gravity that is between the clot/cells and the serum/plasma. They may be incorporated into the tube as an additive or they may be added just prior to centrifugation. Whatever the case, the manufacturer's directions should be followed.

Postcentrifugation Refers to specimen handling/processing after centrifugation and prior to removal of serum or plasma.

Serum or plasma should be physically separated from cells as soon as possible and no longer than 2 hours from the time of collection (unless there is conclusive evidence that longer times do not affect specific test results.)

Many studies have been done to test stability of specimens at varying temperatures for varying time durations. Evidence suggests that separated serum/plasma should remain at 22 degrees C for no longer than eight hours. If testing cannot be completed within 8 hours, it should be refrigerated (2–8 degrees C).

Unless manufacturers' directions instruct otherwise, if testing is not completed within 48 hours, the separated serum/plasma should be frozen at or below −20 degrees C.

- Serum/plasma should not be repeatedly frozen and thawed due to destruction or deterioration of some analytes.
- Frost-free freezers are not suitable for storage.

(continued)

TABLE 7–2.   Continued

Serum/plasma may be left in contact with a gel barrier or separator device as recommended by their respective manufacturers.

- The tube should be inspected after centrifugation to check for a complete barrier between the serum/plasma and the cells.
- The tube should be stored in an upright position with a secure closure.

Serum/plasma and whole blood should be kept covered at all times to avoid contamination, evaporation, changes in concentration, accidental spills, and/or creation of aerosols.

Plunger-type filters are sometimes used to separate serum/plasma from the clot/cells after centrifugation. The device (a plastic tube with a filter on the end) is inserted into the centrifuged blood tube and slowly moved into the specimen. The serum/plasma flows into the tube while the filter acts as a barrier to keep the clot/cells out. It is recommended that filters be used only if they can fully prevent backflow (particulate matter passing into the filtered serum/plasma).

is collected but before centrifugation), centrifugation (while the specimen is in the centrifuge), and postcentrifugation (after centrifugation of the specimen but before removal of an aliquot of serum or plasma for testing).[6] There are currently hundreds of laboratory assays, chemical reagents, and manufacturers' instructions for testing specimens. With all the data, it is not surprising that some evidence on specimen variables may be conflicting. However, Table 7–2 summarizes basic NCCLS recommendations for handling and processing blood specimens.

BASIC HANDLING GUIDELINES

Every health care facility has a specific protocol for specimen transportation and processing. Most laboratories require the use of a leakproof plastic bag for enclosing and transporting the primary specimen tube, i.e., the blood samples taken directly from the patient.

Figure 7–5. Transportation Bag for Blood Specimens

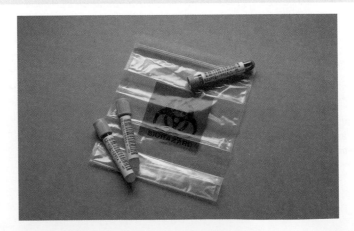

Clinical Alert

Glycolytic action (the breakdown of glucose) from the blood cells interferes in the analysis of various chemicals (e.g., glucose, calcitonin, aldosterone, phosphorus, enzymes). Also, rough handling and agitation of the specimen can have an effect on coagulation tests (e.g., platelet activation and shortened clotting times).[7] Because of these interfering factors, the blood samples should be transported to the clinical laboratory *as soon as possible* from the time of collection so that the sample can be processed appropriately, that is, so serum or plasma can be separated from the blood cells. The serum or plasma that is separated from the cells must be handled according to specified testing procedures, but in general, sera can remain at room temperature for testing, be refrigerated, be stored in a dark place, or be frozen, depending on the prescribed laboratory method.

This bag protects the health care worker from pathogenic (disease-producing) microorganisms during specimen transportation.

The transport bag may have a pouch on the outside for the laboratory request slip, thus eliminating the potential for contamination. If possible, the blood specimens in evacuated tubes and microcollection tubes should be maintained in a vertical position with the tube cap or closure on top to promote complete clot formation and to reduce the possibility of agitating the sample which may cause hemolysis. Handling blood specimens in a gentle manner also reduces the chances of hemolyzing the specimens.

For transportation of specimens from remote ambulatory sites, including home health collections, the phlebotomist must still follow the handling guidelines according to Standard Precautions. The phlebotomist should use the same safety equipment he or she would use in a hospital environment (e.g., closed venipuncture system, gloves, disposable laboratory coat, plastic blood collection tubes, and a biohazardous disposal container). In addition, all blood collection equipment and specimens should be transported in an enclosed or lockable container to avoid spills should the automobile be in a collision. The container should have a biohazard warning label on it and notification procedures in case of an accident. Cold packs should be used in the container for transport during hot weather, or the reverse, the vehicle should be heated in freezing weather. For home collection, the phlebotomist must be extra careful to dispose of waste properly and to place blood specimens in leakproof plastic bags in an upright position inside a labeled transport container.

CHILLED SPECIMENS

For special types of specimens, chilling is required. If a health care worker is requested to transport an arterial specimen for blood gas analysis, he or she should be aware that the specimen must be transported in an airtight heparinized syringe and placed in a mixture of ice and water. The airtight container and the ice water decrease the loss of gases from the specimen. It is important to use ice water rather than solid chunks of ice; otherwise, parts of the specimen may freeze and hemolysis will result.

Speed in specimen transportation is essential to prevent the loss of blood gases. Thus specimens that may require chilling are:[6]

- Blood gases
- Gastrin

Figure 7–6. Chilled Specimen Ready for Transportation to the Laboratory

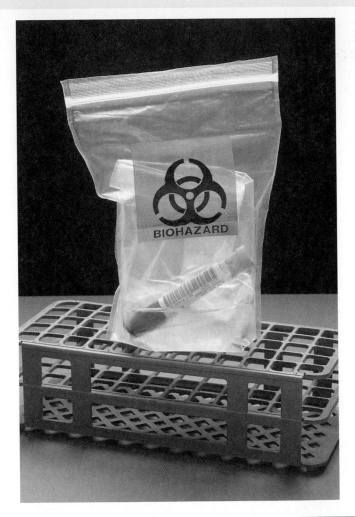

- Ammonia
- Lactic acid
- Renin
- Catecholamine
- Parathyroid hormone
- Pyruvate

PROTECTION OF SPECIMENS FROM LIGHT

Some chemical constituents in blood, such as bilirubin, are light sensitive and decompose if exposed to light. Thus, blood collected for light-sensitive chemical analysis should be protected from bright light with an aluminum foil wrapping around the tube. Light-sensitive constituents include the following:

- Bilirubin
- Vitamin B_{12}
- Carotene
- Folate

MICROBIOLOGICAL SPECIMENS

Blood and urine specimens for microbiological culture need to be transported to the laboratory as quickly as possible so that the blood can be transferred to culture media and the urine analyzed. This enhances the likelihood of detecting pathogenic bacteria. Specimens for blood cultures can also be collected directly into culture media, which minimizes possible contamination and speeds the contact with the culture media.

WARMED SPECIMENS

Specimens that require warming (to body temperature, 37°C) include those for testing cold agglutinins and cryofibrinogen. These special cases require a heat block for transportation and handling purposes.

■■■■■ SPECIMEN DELIVERY METHODS

In larger facilities the laboratory is most often the department responsible for the delivery of blood specimens to the location where they will be analyzed. However, other types of specimens, such as urine, sputum, etc., are commonly delivered by transportation or nursing staff members. Whatever the site, guidelines should be available for safe and efficient delivery of specimens; these may include a schedule of pick-ups, how to deliver STAT specimens, where to place specimens, how to "log in" specimens, etc. Appropriate documentation procedures and open communication among all departments are the keys to successful and efficient specimen delivery.

Courier services are also used to transport specimens to or from off-site areas such as reference laboratories, blood drawing stations, or remote clinics. Again, considerations prior to and during transportation should include adequate packaging and handling. This is especially true in hot or cold temperatures.

HAND DELIVERY

Many specimens are hand-carried and require guidelines for timeliness of delivery to the laboratory. A log sheet for specimens that are hand-delivered to the laboratory is commonly used and is depicted in Figure 7–7 ■. For health care workers in a hospital setting, the blood collection trays or carts are typically arranged to hold specimens awaiting delivery to the laboratory using test tube racks, a holder for microscopic slides, plastic holders, cups, and/or a leakproof container for ice water.

PNEUMATIC TUBE SYSTEMS

These systems are commonly used to transport patient records, messages, letters, bills, medications, x-rays, and laboratory test results. Considerations in the use of pneumatic tubes for transporting specimens are mechanical reliability, distance of transport, speed of carrier, control mechanisms, landing mechanism, radius of loops and bends, shock ab-

Figure 7–7. Sample Log Sheet to Document Delivery of Patient Specimens to the Laboratory

SPECIMEN DELIVERY LOG

Patient name & ID	Location (Rm #)	Specimen(s) (CSF, blood, urine, sputum)	Test(s) ordered	Date	Time specimen collected	Time specimen was delivered to laboratory	Escort name

sorbency, sizes of carriers, cleaning methodology, and laboratory assessment of chemical and cellular components in transported specimens versus hand-carried specimens. If specific documentation does not already exist, the pneumatic tube system should be evaluated for these effects on laboratory results. However, the NCCLS reports that many studies have documented the validity of laboratory results after this type of transport and suggest that tests most affected (lactate dehydrogenase, potassium, plasma hemoglobin, and acid phosphatase) are due to the disruption of the red cells. Also, if heparin is monitored by the activated partial thromboplastin time (APTT), the sample should not be sent through the pneumatic tube system.[6] However, the majority of analytes are not usually affected so this is an efficient means of specimen transport. It is recommended that blood collection tubes be placed in the pneumatic tube with shock-absorbent inserts padding the sides and with the tubes separated from one another to prevent spillage or breakage. Plastic clear liners are also commercially available so that if leaks do occur, they are visible and are contained to prevent contamination of the tube system, the carrier, and the personnel handling the specimens.

TRANSPORTATION BY AUTOMATED VEHICLES

Some manufacturers provide transport systems that are motorized and/or computerized. Delivery of specimens can be by means of a small container car attached to a network of track that is routed to appropriate sites in the laboratory, nursing stations, or other specimen collection areas. Again, a thorough evaluation of such automated delivery systems needs to include the same factors mentioned for pneumatic tube systems. When plans are made to renovate a laboratory area so that it includes this type of transport system, extra space above the ceiling tiles should be considered because the transport vehicles require a sizable right-of-way.

■■■■■■ SHIPPING INFECTIOUS SUBSTANCES

With the expanded worldwide transport of specimens and the increased attention to security, many air carriers, couriers, customs agents, and federal and state agencies have become more cautious about monitoring transport of hazardous agents. The United Nations

Box 7-7	Shipping Biohazardous Specimens

It is the organization's and/or employee's responsibility to comply with the following requirements:

- Provide information and training to all employees who are involved in preparation of specimens for transport
- Properly identify, classify, pack, mark, label and document accordingly
- Make advance arrangements with all carriers of the specimens
- Receive confirmation of prompt delivery
- Notify all carriers of all shipping details

General packing requirements for infectious substances being shipped by passenger or cargo aircraft involve the following:

- Packaging must include an inner, or primary, package, a secondary container, an outer package, and the name and telephone number of the person responsible for the shipping in durable, legible ink.
- The inner primary packaging must have a watertight primary receptacle (e.g., specimen tubes), a watertight secondary packaging container, and an absorbent material between the primary and secondary containers that must be capable of absorbing all contents of the primary receptacle.
- Multiple primary specimen tubes must be individually wrapped, separated, and supported to avoid contact among them.
- The secondary packaging must be sufficiently strong, have an overall dimension of at least 100 mm (4 inches), and have an itemized list of contents enclosed between it and outer packaging.
- All outer packages must be marked with "Infectious Substances" labels, the net weight of dry ice (if applicable), the name/address/phone number of the shipper, and a Shipper's Declaration indicating "Inner Packaging Complies with Prescribed Specifications" and "Prior arrangements as required by the IATO Dangerous Goods Regulations 1.3.3.1 have been made."
- Up to 500 mL of blood can be shipped in a primary receptacle and in outer packaging not exceeding 4 liters.
- Substances shipped at ambient or higher temperatures need to be in leakproof primary containers of glass, metal, or plastic.
- When specimens are refrigerated or frozen, the refrigerant must be placed outside the secondary packaging with internal support to secure the secondary packaging after the refrigerant has evaporated/dissipated. If dry ice is used, the pack and outer packaging must allow for the release of CO_2 gas.
- After receiving a specimen from an outside source, it should be immediately identified, logged in, and checked for sample integrity.

The packing instructions for diagnostic specimens are slightly less restrictive but differ only in requirements for the strength of the outer packaging material. For infectious substances, the outer packaging must comply with stringent pressure, puncture, vibration, and temperature tests. For diagnostic specimens, the outer packaging should be of sufficient strength for its capacity, weight, and designated use to pass a stacking test and a drop test from a height of not less than 1.2 meters. There are serious fines and legal ramifications for failure to comply with these requirements.[8,910]

Committee of Experts has defined nine hazard classes of dangerous goods as "articles or substances that are capable of posing a significant risk to health, safety, or to property when transported by air." Infectious substances, defined as substances known to contain, or reasonably expected to contain, pathogens (including bacteria, viruses, rickettsia, parasites, fungi, or recombinant microorganisms), are in Class 6 and require specific packaging and handling. Infectious substances include diagnostic specimens, that is "any human or animal material such as excreta, secreta, blood and blood components, tissue, and tissue fluids being shipped for diagnostic or investigative purposes."[8]

■■■■■ REPORTING LABORATORY RESULTS

WRITTEN REPORTS

Both the JCAHO and the CAP state that laboratory results should be confirmed, dated, and accompanied by permanent reports that are available in the laboratory, as well as on the patient's medical record via an electronic transmission or a hard copy. The CAP also states that each report should contain adequate patient identification, contain the date and hour when the procedures were completed, and be signed and initialed by the laboratory personnel performing the procedure. When electronic reports are used, laboratory documentation on instrument-generated worksheets by personnel performing the procedures is sufficient. The CAP has suggested that health care personnel consider the following when designing a report form:

1. Identification of patient, patient location, and physician
2. Date and time of specimen collection
3. Description, source of specimen, and labeled precautions
4. Compactness and ease of preparing the package for shipment
5. Consistency in format
6. Clear understandability of instructions or orders
7. Logical location in patient's chart for reference laboratory reports
8. Sequential order of multiple results on single specimens
9. Listing of reference ranges or normal and abnormal/critical values
10. Assurance of accuracy of request transcription
11. Administrative and record-keeping value

Any unique institutional requirements for an acceptable report should be stated in the laboratory procedure manual and may include criteria such as quality control (QC) limits and/or delta checks (QC that allows for detection of clinically significant changes in laboratory results). Results can be documented in one of the following three ways: manual recording of test results, laboratory-instrument-printed reports, and electronically generated reports.

VERBAL REPORTS

The use of verbal and telephone reports has declined because of easier, more reliable computer access and the concern for privacy. Verbal reports, although useful for reporting STAT results and panic (or critical) values are more prone to error. Verbal reports should be accompanied by documentation with the following information: patient name and hospital number, name of person receiving the report, date and time, information given, and name of person issuing the report, as shown in Figure 7–8 ■.

COMPUTERIZED REPORTS

Various computer-transmission devices can provide a rapid online report system and are more reliable than verbal reports. Hospitals may have terminals located in each patient unit. After the tests have been completed and verified in the laboratory, the results can be

Figure 7–8. Sample Form Used for Reporting Verbal Laboratory Results

PATIENT NAME: PATIENT ID #:
PHYSICIAN:
PERSON REQUESTING INFORMATION:
DATE OF TEST RESULTS:

INFORMATION GIVEN:

DATE & TIME OF INQUIRY:

REPORTED BY:

Reporting of laboratory results is a serious responsibility, and each health care facility has policies for who is authorized to do so and under which conditions. Compliance with HIPAA regulations assures that patients' privacy and confidentiality wishes are maintained. Only employees who are authorized to do so should complete the required documentation when the situation is appropriate.

immediately displayed in each patient unit. A printer can be attached to each terminal to generate a temporary hard-copy report. However, steps must be taken to ensure privacy and confidentiality of patient results after they are printed.

A health care facility's computer system can easily provide daily laboratory reports and cumulative reports for the patient's computerized medical record. All reports should be available at times convenient for making clinical decisions by the medical staff.

The business office of the health care facility also receives data online regarding laboratory procedures. This office must be notified of all laboratory charges, according to data requested and procedural code for patient billing. It is financially advantageous to send reports promptly.

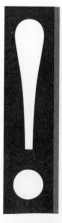

Clinical Alert

A critical laboratory value, sometimes referred to as a "panic value," is a test result that "represents a pathophysiologic state at such variance with normal as to be life-threatening" unless action is taken by the patient's physician. According to the Clinical Laboratory Improvement Act (CLIA), health care workers are required to report critical values to physicians in a timely manner. This often means paging or telephoning a physician at home and/or during off-hours. While this can be an unwelcomed task, it is important for the patient's welfare and to avoid liability risks. All laboratories should have policies about what should be done when results are within a critical range.[11]

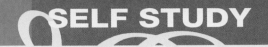

SELF STUDY

KEY TERMS

analytic phase
barcodes
clinical (or medical) record
confidentiality
critical value
diagnostic specimens
e-mail
fax machines
Health Insurance Portability and
 Accountability Act (HIPAA)

infectious substances
light sensitive
"panic value"
pneumatic tube systems
preanalytical phases
privacy
radio frequency identification
reference ranges
requisition form
specimen collection manual

STUDY QUESTIONS

The following may have more than one answer:

1. The key elements common to most medical records are which of the following:
   a. name, DOB, SSN
   b. personal and family medical history
   c. plan of care
   d. discharge summary

2. Medical records serve what purpose?
   a. coordination of care
   b. meet accrediting and licensing
   c. provide legal protection
   d. provide research data requirements

3. Guidelines for documentation in health care include which of the following:
   a. accuracy
   b. personal opinions of the situation
   c. completion for each event or proce-
      dure
   d. objectivity and timeliness

4. Which of the following data should be considered confidential?
   a. laboratory test results
   b. radiology reports
   c. patient's diagnosis
   d. universal precautions

5. Barcodes can be used for which type(s) of information?
   a. identification of patient names
   b. identification of patient numbers
   c. designation of test to be performed
   d. inventory of supplies

6. What is the most error-free method for requesting a laboratory test?
   a. handwritten requisition
   b. computerized method
   c. verbal method
   d. verbal STAT method

7. Sources of preanalytic error can be categorized as follows:
   a. processing variables
   b. specimen variables
   c. physician's attitude
   d. patient variables

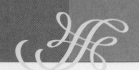

8. Telephone responsibilities for health care workers usually include:
   a. using effective customer service manners
   b. using an intercom system
   c. transferring calls
   d. placing people on hold

9. A specimen should be protected from light for which of the following determinations?
   a. bilirubin concentration
   b. hemoglobin level
   c. glucose level
   d. blood cultures

10. A specimen should be chilled for which of the following analyses?
    a. complete blood count (CBC)
    b. bilirubin level
    c. blood gas
    d. glucose level

References

1. Clinical Skillbuilders: *Better Documentation*. Springhouse, PA: Springhouse Corporation, 1992.

2. Fiesta, J: *20 Legal Pitfalls for Nurses to Avoid*. Allentown, PA: Delmar Publishers, 1994.

3. College of American Pathologists (CAP): Laboratory Accreditation Program (LAP), Checklist: Laboratory General, www.cap.org, March 2003 (325 Waukegan Road, Northfield, IL 60093, 800-323-4040 or 847-832-7000 in IL).

4. QuadraMed: Internet Forum on HIPAA Preparedness, Executive Summary, www.hipaa-iq.com/summary.htm, last updated January 30, 2001.

5. Garza, D: Phlebotomy and bar coding: Improving accuracy in specimen handling. *Adv Med Lab Professionals,* March 22, 1999: 22–27.

6. National Committee for Clinical Laboratory Standards (NCCLS): Procedures for the Handling and Processing of Blood Specimens; Approved Guideline, 2nd edition, volume 19, Number 21, H18-A2, October, 1999.

7. Lawrence, JB: Preanalytical variables in the coagulation laboratory. *Laboratory Medicine,* January 2003; 1: 34, 49–57.

8. Roane, PA: Transporting infectious substances, Packaging is everything! *Adv Med Lab Professionals,* October 18, 1999: 7–10.

9. Occupational Safety and Health Administration (OSHA), U.S. Department of Labor, OSHA 3128: Bloodborne Pathogens and Acute Care Facilities, 1992, www.osha.gov/Publications/OSHA3128/osha3128.html, last viewed on June 17, 2003.

10. James, E.: Guarding Specimen Integrity, Protecting Samples Requires Proper Pachaging. *Adv Med Lab Professionals,* April 5, 2004: 24–26.

11. Dalton-Beninato, K: Critical value notifications are never welcome news. *Lab Med,* 2000; 31(6): 319–323.

Blood Collection Equipment

8

CHAPTER OBJECTIVES

Upon completion of Chapter 8, the learner is responsible for the following:

1. List the various types of anticoagulants used in blood collection, their mechanisms for preventing blood from clotting, and the vacuum-collection-tube color codes for these anticoagulants.

2. Describe the latest phlebotomy safety supplies and equipment and evaluate their effectiveness in blood collection.

3. Identify the various supplies that should be carried on a specimen collection tray when a skin puncture specimen must be collected.

4. Identify the types of safety equipment needed to collect blood by venipuncture.

5. Describe the special precautions that should be taken and the techniques that should be used when various types of specimens must be transported to the clinical laboratory.

MediaLINK

Access the accompanying CD-ROM to explore a wide variety of review questions and interactive activities for this chapter, including multiple choice, true/false, and video exercises.

■■■■ INTRODUCTION TO BLOOD COLLECTION EQUIPMENT

Phlebotomists use several types of supplies and safety equipment in the collection of blood and its transportation to the specimen processing center. The collection equipment is used for venipuncture (blood collection from a vein), skin puncture (blood collection from a finger and/or an infant's heel), and arterial puncture. Venipuncture equipment includes vacuum tubes and safety-needle collection devices that allow the blood collector to collect a patient's blood, plus a tourniquet to assist in locating a vein, supplies to cleanse the puncture site, labeling supplies, gloves, and special trays for transportation of the blood specimens. Box 8–1 lists equipment used in routine venipuncture procedures.

■■■■ VENIPUNCTURE EQUIPMENT

Venipuncture with a vacuum (evacuated) tube (VACUTAINER), as shown in Figure 8–1 ■, is the most direct and efficient method for obtaining a blood specimen. The evacuated tube system requires evacuated sample tube, the double-pointed needle, and a special safety plastic holder (adapter) (Figure 8–2 ■) that covers the needle after blood collection. One end of the double-pointed needle enters the vein, the other end pierces the top of the tube, and the vacuum aspirates the blood. Due to state and federal laws for the requirement to have safety-engineered devices, manufacturers have designed different types of safety devices on the needle and/or plastic holder that covers the needle after venipuncture to protect the phlebotomist from a needlestick injury.

■■■■ BLOOD COLLECTION TUBES AND ADDITIVES

The tubes are available in different sizes, in safety-engineered plastic to reduce risk of tube breakage and blood spill. Glass collection tubes are not desirable since risk of exposure to bloodborne pathogens is increased due to possible breakage. The external tube diameter

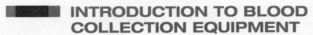

Box 8–1	Equipment for Routine Venipuncture

Antimicrobial hand gel or foam to wash hands

Safety needle collection device

Needles

Vacuum (evacuated) collection tubes

Safety syringes

Safety winged infusion sets (safety butterfly sets)

Needle disposal container

Tourniquet

70 percent isopropyl alcohol, iodine pads, or swab sticks

Disposable gloves

Gauze pads

Bandages

Marking pens and labels

Specimen collection tray

Vacuum (evacuated) tube systems

Figure 8–1. Vacuum Tubes

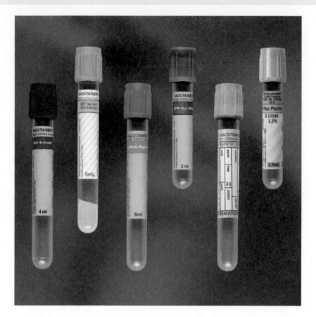

Courtesy of BD VACUTAINER Systems, *Preanalytical Solutions,* Franklin Lakes, NJ

and length plus the maximum amount of specimen to be drawn into the vacuum tube are the two criteria used to describe vacuum tube size (Table 8–1). The smaller sizes (e.g., 2 mL) are useful for pediatric and geriatric collections and can be purchased with different types of anticoagulants, as well as in chemically clean or sterile glassware. Each vacuum tube is color coded according to the additive contained within the tube (see Table 8–2).

Many tubes are specifically designed to be used directly with chemistry, hematology, or microbiology instrumentation. In these cases, the tube of blood is identified by its barcode and is pierced by the instrument probe, and some sample is aspirated into the instrument for analyses. Use of these closed systems minimizes laboratory personnel's risk of exposure to blood. In addition, some tubes have plastic tops or screw-on enclosures around the rubber stopper to minimize exposure to blood left on the top of the cap or blood splatters that can occur during cap removal.

The expiration dates of tubes should be monitored continuously. Such monitoring is most easily accomplished with a computer.

Traditionally in most clinical laboratories, serum, plasma, or whole blood has been used to perform various assays. More recently, though, heparinized whole blood has become the specimen of choice for the latest clinical laboratory instruments used in STAT (immediate) situations. Using whole blood as a specimen decreases the time involved in acquiring the test result, because centrifugation is not required prior to laboratory testing.

Many coagulation factors are involved in blood clotting, and coagulation can be prevented by the addition of different types of anticoagulants. These anticoagulants often

Figure 8-2. Vacuum (Evacuated) Tube Holder System and Parts

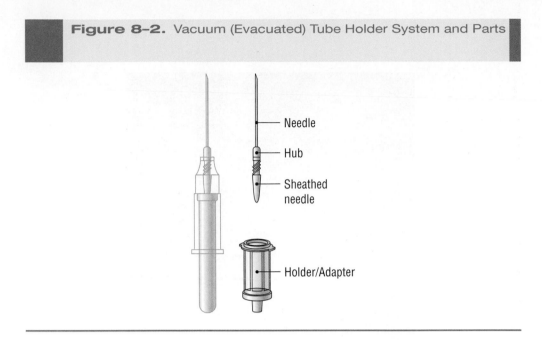

contain preservatives that can extend the metabolism and life span of the red blood cells (RBCs) after blood collection. Anticoagulants and preservatives are used extensively in blood donations to ensure the biochemical balance of certain components of RBCs, such as hemoglobin, pH, adenosine triphosphate (ATP), and glucose. Once transferred, anticoagulants, such as acid citrate dextrose (ACD), ensure that the RBCs provide the recipient with the means of delivering oxygen (O_2) to the tissues.

Another major use of anticoagulants and preservatives is in the collection of plasma for laboratory analysis. Specific anticoagulants or preservatives must be used depending on

TABLE 8–1.   Typical Sizes of Blood Collection Vacuum Tubes for Full, Partial or Pediatric Draws

EXTERNAL DIAMETER × LENGTH (MM)	DRAW VOLUMES (ML)
10.25 × 64	2.0
13 × 75	2.0
13 × 75	2.0 and 3.0
13 × 75	4.0
13 × 100	4.5
13 × 100	6.0
16 × 75	7.0
16 × 100	8.5
16 × 125	12.5

TABLE 8–2.　Specimen Type and Collection Vacuum Tubes

SPECIMEN TYPE	COLLECTION TUBES (STOPPER COLOR/TYPE)	ADDITIVE
Clotted blood/serum	Gray and red	Polymer barrier
	Yellow and red	Polymer barrier
	Gold	Polymer barrier
	Red	None
	Orange	Thrombin
	Yellow and gray	Thrombin
	Brown	Polymergel
Whole blood/plasma	Green and gray	Polymer barrier and lithium heparin
	Green (yellow top)	Polymer barrier and lithium heparin
	Light green	Polymer barrier and lithium heparin
	Light blue	Trisodium citrate
	Lavender (purple)	EDTA (K_3) or EDTA (K_2) or EDTA (Na_2)
	Gray	Sodium fluoride and potassium oxalate
	Green	Lithium heparin
	Green	Sodium heparin or ammonium heparin
	Royal blue	Sodium heparin or EDTA (Na_2)-sterile tube for toxicology and nutritional studies
	Pink	Blood Bank (EDTA)
	Tan	EDTA (K_2) tube for lead testing
Clotted blood/serum	Royal blue	No additive; but sterile tube for trace elements, toxicology, and nutritional studies
	Brown	No additive or sodium heparin, but lead-free glass and sterile for lead determinations
Whole blood	Lavender (purple)	EDTA (K_3) or EDTA (K_2) or EDTA (Na_2)
	Green	Lithium heparin, sodium heparin, or ammonium heparin
	Black	Sodium citrate
	Yellow	Sodium polyanetholesulfonate (SPS) or acid citrate dextrose (ACD)

the test procedure ordered. Anticoagulants cannot be substituted for one another. Appendix 4 lists the various laboratory assays along with the types of anticoagulants required and the approximate amount (in milliliters) of blood that must be collected for each assay.

Coagulation of blood can be prevented by the addition of oxalates, citrates, ethylenediamine tetra-acetic acid (EDTA), or heparin. Oxalates, citrates, and EDTA prevent the coagulation of blood by removing calcium and forming insoluble calcium salts. These three anticoagulants cannot be used in calcium determinations; however, citrates are frequently used in coagulation blood studies. EDTA prevents platelet aggregation and is therefore used for platelet counts and platelet function tests. Fresh EDTA-anticoagulated blood allows preparation of blood films with minimal distortion of white blood cells (WBCs). Heparin, a mucopolysaccharide used in assays, such as ammonia and plasma hemoglobin, prevents blood clotting by inactivating the blood-clotting chemicals—thrombin and Factor X. "Partial collection" tubes are available through manufacturers for patient blood collec-

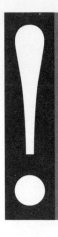

Clinical Alert

Two important things to remember for using vacuum blood collection tubes:

1. These tubes have been designed for a certain amount of blood to be collected into the tube by vacuum as related to the amount of prefilled anticoagulant in the tube.
2. If an insufficient amount of blood is collected in the anticoagulated tube, the laboratory test results may be erroneous because of the incorrect blood-to-anticoagulant ratio.

tions in which it is anticipated that a "short draw" will be collected. These partial collection tubes will provide accurate laboratory results even though a short draw is collected.

GRAY-TOPPED TUBES

Gray-topped vacuum tubes usually contain (1) potassium oxalate and sodium fluoride or (2) lithium iodoacetate and heparin. This type of collection tube is primarily used for glycolytic inhibition tests. Thus, sometimes "antiglycolytic agent" or "glycolytic inhibitor" are the terms for this tube's additive.

Box 8-2

Because sodium fluoride destroys many enzymes, the gray-topped tube should not be used in blood collections for enzyme determinations that include:

- creatine kinase [CK]
- alanine aminotransferase [ALT]
- aspartate aminotransferase [AST]; or
- alkaline phosphatase [ALP]

Likewise, oxalate distorts cellular morphologic features. Thus, gray-topped tubes should not be used for hematology studies.

GREEN-TOPPED TUBES

The anticoagulants sodium heparin, ammonium heparin, and lithium heparin are found in green-topped vacuum tubes. These tubes are used in various laboratory assays requiring plasma or whole blood, which are mainly chemistry tests. For potassium measurement, heparinized plasma or whole blood, rather than serum, is preferred because sporadic increased potassium levels can occur in serum as a result of potassium released from platelets during blood clotting.[1]

Lithium heparin tubes are used for many assays that include:

- Glucose
- Blood urea nitrogen (BUN)
- Ionized calcium
- Creatinine
- Electrolyte studies

However, this anticoagulant is not suitable for tests involving the measurement of lithium or folate levels.[2] Similarly, sodium heparin tubes should not be used for assays that measure the sodium concentration. In other cases, a particular procedure will require sodium heparin without lithium, or vice versa.

Green-topped vacuum tubes should not be used for collections for blood smears that are to be stained with Wright's stain, because the heparin causes the Wright's stain to have a blue background. When used for cytogenetic studies, these tubes must be sterile.

PURPLE-TOPPED AND LIGHT-BLUE-TOPPED TUBES

The purple-topped vacuum tubes (containing EDTA) are used for most hematology procedures. Also, this tube is used for molecular diagnostic testing.

Box 8-3

If a purple-topped tube is underfilled, the patient will have

- falsely low blood cell counts,
- falsely low hematocrits,
- staining alterations on blood smears, and
- erroneous morphologic changes to RBCs.

Many coagulation procedures, such as PT and APTT, are done on blood collected in light-blue-topped vacuum tubes, which contain sodium citrate at a concentration of 3.2 or 3.8 percent. It is becoming preferred to use 3.2 percent since this concentration reduces falsely negative or falsely positive results.[3] If a light-blue-topped tube is underfilled, coagulation results will be erroneously prolonged.

RED-TOPPED, ROYAL-BLUE-TOPPED, BROWN-TOPPED, AND TAN-TOPPED TUBES

The red-topped tubes indicate a tube without anticoagulant for the collection of serum. Thus, the collected blood will clot in this tube. The royal-blue-topped tubes are used to collect samples for nutritional studies, therapeutic drug monitoring, and toxicology. The royal-blue-topped tube is the trace element tube. The brown-topped tube contains heparin or no additive and is used for blood lead values. The tan-topped tube is also used for lead testing and contains EDTA.

BLACK-TOPPED TUBES

From certain manufacturers, a black-topped tube with buffered sodium citrate is available for blood collections used to determine the erythrocyte sedimentation rate (ESR).

YELLOW-TOPPED TUBES

Sterile blood specimens are also ordered for blood cultures when the patient is suspected of having septicemia (symptoms of sepsis). A major problem with collecting blood for culture is that the patient's sample can become contaminated with microorganisms from the skin. Thus the blood must be collected in a sterile container (vacuum tube, vial, or syringe) under aseptic conditions. (See Chapter 13 for blood culture collections.) The additive, sodium polyanethol sulfonate (SPS) is in the yellow-topped tubes for blood culture specimen collections in microbiology. Also, as shown in Figure 8–3 , blood can be collected directly into vacuum vials that contain culture media.

This type of collection minimizes the risk of specimen contamination. The vacuum vials can be purchased with different types of culture media, an unplugged venting unit for aerobic incubation, or a plugged venting unit for anaerobic incubation.

It should be noted that tubes containing ACD (acid citrate dextrose) also use the yellow color code. These tubes are used for specialty blood banking, such as HLA typing.

Figure 8–3. BD BACTEC Culture Vials in Blood Culture Procedural Tray

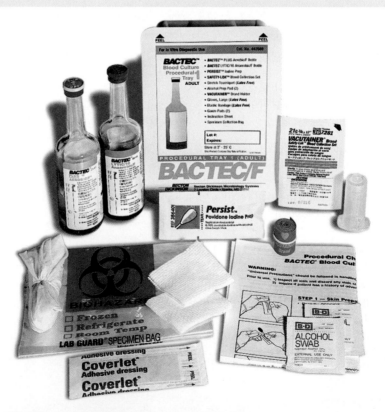

Courtesy of BD (Becton-Dickinson and Company), Sparks, MD.

SERUM SEPARATION TUBES (MOTTLED-TOPPED, SPECKLED-TOPPED, AND GOLD-TOPPED TUBES)

Another collection method is to collect blood in a serum separation tube, such as the VACUETTE® serum tube (Figure 8–4 ■) or BD VACUTAINER Plus SST tube. These tubes contain a polymer barrier that is present in the bottom of the tube. The specific gravity of this material lies between the blood clot and the serum. During centrifugation, the polymer barrier moves upward to the serum-clot interface, where it forms a stable barrier separating the serum from fibrin and cells. Serum may be aspirated directly from the collection tube, eliminating the need for transfer to another container.

PINK-TOPPED TUBES

These tubes contain EDTA and are used for blood bank collections.

MOLECULAR DIAGNOSTICS TUBES

Special sterile vacuum tubes for molecular diagnostic studies are available containing different additives (e.g., sodium citrate, sodium heparin) as required for the different testing procedures. Manufacturers have different color tops for these tubes.

▇▇▇ SAFETY SYRINGES

Some patients' veins are too fragile for blood collection with vacuum tubes. Thus safety syringes are generally used for the collection process. Syringes are hazardous and pose an increased risk of accidental needlesticks.

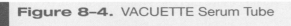

Figure 8–4. VACUETTE Serum Tube

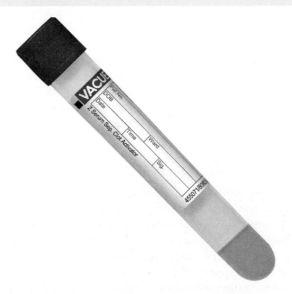

Courtesy of Grenier Bio-One, Monroe, NC.

Figure 8–5. Example of a Syringe

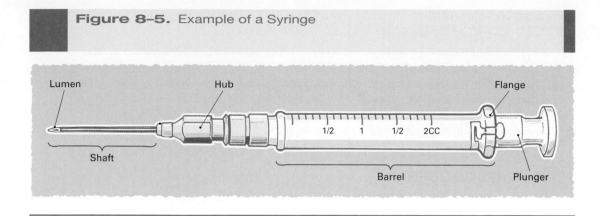

Syringes are sometimes used for collecting blood from central venous catheter (CVC) lines. This procedure is discussed in detail in Chapter 13. Major parts of the syringe consist of the needle, hub, barrel, and the plunger (Figure 8–5 ■). The barrel and the plunger are made to fit together tightly so that when the plunger is in the barrel and drawn back, a vacuum is created. To fit properly, the needle and syringe must be compatible and are attached together by the hub. This vacuum allows blood or other fluids to be aspirated, or sucked, into the barrel as the plunger is pulled back. The barrel of the syringe has graduated measurements in milliliter increments. Sizes range from approximately 0.2 to 50.0 mL; however, for specimen collection purposes, 5- to 20-mL syringes are most often used. In addition, the health care worker should ensure that the syringe is the correct size for the amount of blood to be collected.

A safety syringe shielded transfer device (Figure 8–6 ■) needs to be used to avoid possible exposure to the patient's blood. The plunger must not be pushed down if the tubes are being filled from the syringe because it is extremely hazardous. Also, pushing the plunger may damage cellular components and cause hemolysis because of the forceful expulsion of blood. The syringe needle should be shielded after blood collection, removed, and discarded in a sharps disposal container.[4] The BD Blood Transfer Device is attached to the syringe, and a vacuum tube is inserted into the transfer device. The blood is transferred from the syringe to the tube using the tube's vacuum. Specialized tubes and bottles that may fit the adapter are also available for blood culture collection.

■■■■■ SAFETY NEEDLES/HOLDERS

The gauge and length of a needle used on a syringe or a vacuum tube is selected according to the specific task. The gauge number indicates the diameter of the needle; the smaller the gauge number, the larger the needle diameter and higher the flow rate.

When blood is collected from a child, a 21- to 23-gauge needle is usually used with a tuberculin, or 3-mL, syringe or with a winged infusion set. The length of the needle depends on the depth of the vein to be punctured. Needles are usually available at either 1- or 1.5-inch. The needle attaches to the safety holder/adapter, or syringe, at its hub.

Needles are sterilized and packaged by vendors in sealed shields that maintain sterility. These sealed shields are packaged individually. For example, the BD Eclipse safety-shielding

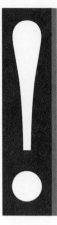

Clinical Alert

- Safety engineering controls (engineered sharps injury protection) and safe work practices must be used if collecting blood with a syringe.
- Needleless safety blood transfer devices must be used to place the blood from the syringe to the vacuum tube.

Figure 8–6. BD SafetyGlide Needle and BD Blood Transfer Device

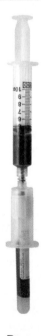

Courtesy of BD VACUTAINER Systems, *Preanalytical Solutions,* Franklin Lakes, NJ.

Box 8-4   Needle Sizes Used for Blood Collection

- Larger (16- to 18-gauge) needles are used for collecting donor units of blood (e.g., 450 ml)
- Smaller (21- and 22-gauge) needles are used for collecting specimens for laboratory assays.

Figure 8–7. BD Eclipse Blood Collection Needle Attached to a Holder

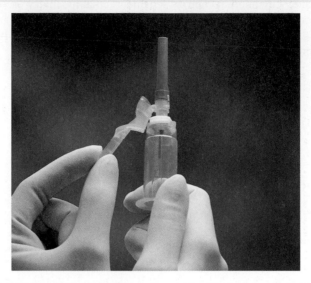

Courtesy of BD VACUTAINER Systems, *Preanalytical Solutions,* Franklin Lakes, NJ.

blood needle attaches to a holder (Figure 8–7 ■). After the blood collection tubes are filled, the BD Eclipse shield is activated immediately after the needle is removed from the vein. When the thumb pushes forward on the shield as shown in this figure, an audible click indicates that the safety shield is locked in place. This single-use adapter provides immediate containment of a used needle.

Another protective holder that provides effective, immediate containment of a used needle is the Venipuncture Needle-Pro (Figure 8–8 ■). After removing the needle from the patient's vein, the phlebotomist activates the needle guard by holding the tube holder and pressing the needle guard against a hard surface so that the guard swings over the needle. Once engaged, both ends of the needle are covered, protecting the blood collector from an accidental needlestick. It reduces the risk of reusing a contaminated holder since it is a onetime-use-only safety-engineered device.

The Vanishpoint blood collection tube holder offers engineered sharps injury protection and features patented technology, which automatically retracts the needle directly from the patient upon activation:

- Automated retraction virtually eliminates exposure to contaminated sharps by protecting the user from both ends of the blood collection needle.
- The tube holder accommodates conventional multisample blood collection needles up to 1½ inches in length and is nonreusable.
- A small-diameter-tube adapter is available for use with 10.25 mm tubes.
- The Vanishpoint blood collection tube holder and small-diameter-tube adapter contain no natural rubber latex (Figure 8–9 ■).

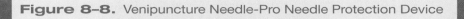

Figure 8-8. Venipuncture Needle-Pro Needle Protection Device

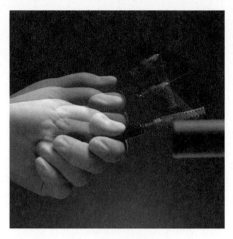

Courtesy of Portex, Inc., Keene, NH

Another vacuum tube assembly developed to prevent needlestick injuries is the PUNCTUR-GUARD Blood Collection Needle (www.bio-plexus.com). PUNCTUR-GUARD is actually two needles, one inside of the other. The internal "needle" is hollow and has a flat, or blunt end. This blunt needle is recessed inside of the outer sharp needle. When blood collection is performed, the sharp needle accesses the vein. Blood is collected into vacuum tubes. Once the last tube is filled, the health care worker activates the safety feature, while the needle is still in the patient. Activation of the safety feature advances the inner blunt needle forward, past the sharp tip of the outer needle.

The VACUETTE QuickShield Safety Tube Holder is used to prevent accidental needlestick injuries during venous blood collection. It can be used in conjunction with VACUETTE blood collection needles. The device is used by pressing the protective cover over the needle with the aid of a stable surface and then disposing of the needle and holder into a sharps disposal container.

Sarstedt, Inc., has the S-Monovette Blood Collection System (Figure 8–10 ■), which is an enclosed multiple-sampling blood collection system that collects blood using either an aspiration or vacuum principle of collection. Using the aspiration procedure replaces syringe draws for patients with difficult veins and can prevent uncomfortable resticks. All tubes are plastic with screw caps, which minimizes the risk of breakage and aerosol formation when caps are removed. Each needle has an integral holder that does not require assembly before use and cannot be disassembled. Thus, it prevents reuse of the holder.

For any of these blood collection needle and tube holder devices, disposing of the tube holder while it is still attached to the needle ensures that the tube-puncturing needle re-

Figure 8–9. Vanishpoint Blood Collection Tube Holder

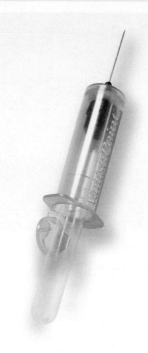

Courtesy of Retractable Technologies, Little Elm, Texas

mains protected during and after disposal. Thus, it significantly reduces the risks of needle-stick injuries and blood exposure from the tube-puncturing needle to automatically retract into it after blood collection.

NEEDLES

The gauge and length of a needle used with a vacuum tube holder system is selected according to the specific task. For example, larger (18-gauge) needles are used for collecting donor units of blood (450 mL or less), whereas smaller (21- and 22-gauge) needles are used for collecting specimens for laboratory assays. When blood is collected from children, a 21- to 23-gauge needle is usually used with a tuberculin, of 3-mL, syringe or with a winged infusion set. The gauge number indicates the diameter of the needle; the smaller the gauge number, the larger the needle diameter and higher flow rate. The length of the needle depends on the depth of the vein to be punctured. Needles are usually available as either 1 or 1.5 inch.

Needles are sterilized and packaged by vendors in sealed shields that maintain sterility. These sealed shields are packaged in individual containers that are color coded according to the gauge size of the needles and must be twisted apart before the needles are used in blood collection.[5]

Figure 8–10. Sarstedt S-Monovette Venous Blood
Collection System

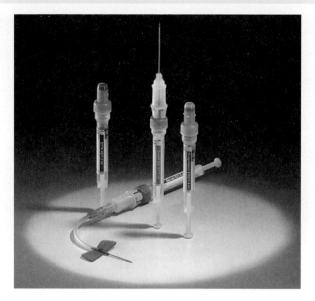

Courtesy of Sarstedt Inc., Newton, NC

The tip of each needle should be checked for damage. A blunt or bent tip can be harmful to the patient's vein and may result in failure to collect blood.

Multiple-sample needles are used with vacuum collection tubes and the holder to allow for multiple tube changes without blood leakage within the plastic holder. The multiple-sample needle has a plastic cover over the tube-top puncturing portion of the needle; this cover creates a leakage barrier.

It is important to use needles with holders or syringes that are compatible with the needle to avoid the possiblity of leaking blood and blood exposure.

THE BUTTERFLY NEEDLE (BLOOD COLLECTION SET)

The butterfly needle, also referred to as a blood collection set or winged infusion set, is the most commonly used intravenous device. It is a stainless steel beveled needle and tube with attached plastic wings on one end and a Luer fitting attached to the other. The most common butterfly needle sizes are 21-, 23-, and 25-gauge, and the length of these needles range from ½ to ¾ inches long. The smaller angle of insertion can occur with the shorter needle. The butterfly needle is sometimes used in the collection of blood from patients who are difficult to stick by conventional methods (e.g., geriatric patients, cancer patients, pediatric patients).

Numerous types of safety butterfly needles are available and must be used according to OSHA regulations. These safety needles each have a shield that automatically covers the contaminated needle point upon withdrawal from the patient's vein. One example is the Kendall Monoject Angel Wing blood collection set (Figure 8–11 a & b ■). It has a stainless

Figure 8–11A. Angel Wing Blood Collection Set with Female Luer

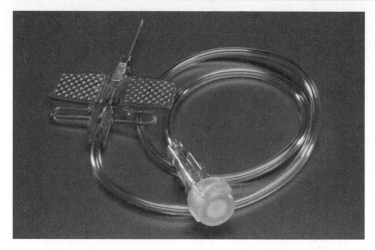

Courtesy of Tyco Healthcare/Kendall Co., LP, Mansfield, MA

steel safety shield that automatically resheaths the needle during withdrawal from the patient. The system includes multisample needle-shielded tube holders and sets for use in drawing blood specimens directly into blood collection tubes and blood culture bottles, as well as multisample needle-shielded transfer tube holders and sets for transferring blood from syringes into collection tubes and blood culture bottles.

BD VACUTAINER Systems *Preanalytical Solutions* has the BD VACUTAINER Push Button Blood Collection Set (see Figure 8–12 ■), which provides immediate protection against needle stick injury when properly activated within the vein and in accordance with the BD directions.

Greiner Bio-One manufactures the VACUETTE® safety blood collection set (Figure 8–13 ■). It is a winged needle device with a safety shield. Bio-Plexus produces the PUNCTUR-

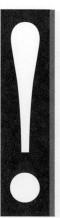

Clinical Alert

Winged infusion sets (butterfly needles) have accounted for the HIGHEST percentage of needlestick injuries.

Figure 8–11B. Angel Wing Blood Collection Set with Male Luer

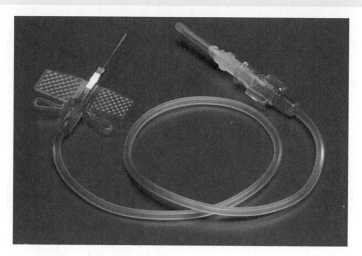

Courtesy of Tyco Healthcare Kendall Co. LP, Mansfield, MA.

GUARD winged set for blood collection. The safety device uses an internal hollow blunt built within the sharp outer needle. When the blood samples have been withdrawn, the "internal blunt" is activated prior to removing the needle from the vein, thus reducing exposure to a sharp contaminated needle. Terumo Medical Corp. manufactures the Surshield Safety Winged Blood Collection Set (Figure 8–14 ■) that is a safety-engineered butterfly device for blood collection or IV insertion. No matter what type of safety blood collection set is used, it is imperative to use a Luer adapter from the same manufacturer to avoid possible blood leakage and exposure.

NEEDLE AND OTHER SHARPS DISPOSAL

Needles, syringes, and lancets (sterile, disposable sharp devices used in skin puncture) must be discarded in rigid, leakproof, plastic containers, reducing the possibility of needle sticks for the phlebotomist. Each unit is usually orange or red and is disposable as biohazardous waste (Figure 8–15 ■). Several sizes of sharps disposal containers are available for use at the bedside, on the cart, in isolation, and on home health care trays. Before beginning a blood collection procedure, the phlebotomist should note the location of the nearest sharps container.

■■■■■ TOURNIQUETS

The tourniquet is a key to successful venipuncture: it provides a barrier to slow down venous flow. Tourniquets are used in specimen collection to apply enough pressure to the arm to slow the return of venous blood to the heart. This slowing of venous return causes pooling of blood in the veins, which makes the veins more visible and easier to feel and find. A tourniquet should not restrict arterial blood flowing into the arm. Blood should

Figure 8–12. BD VACUTAINER Push Button Blood Collection Set

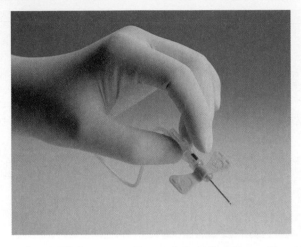

Courtesy of BD VACUTAINER Systems, *Preanalytical Solutions,* Franklin Lakes, NJ.

 Figure 8–13. VACUETTE Safety Blood Collection Set

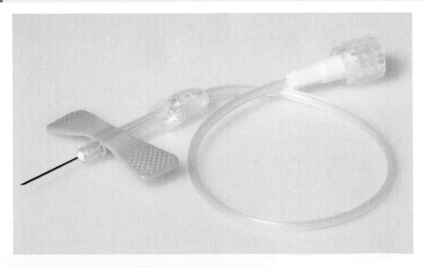

Courtesy of Greiner Bio-One, Monroe, NC.

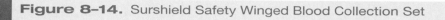

Figure 8–14. Surshield Safety Winged Blood Collection Set

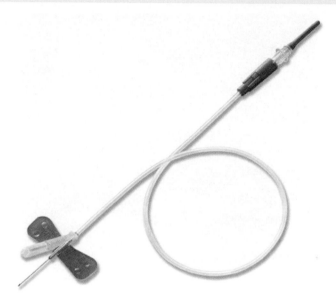

Courtesy of Terumo Medical Corp., Somerset, NJ.

enter the arm at a normal rate and, with the use of a tourniquet, return to the heart at a slower rate.

Tourniquets that are usually used include the pliable strap, the Velcro type, and the blood pressure cuff. The blood pressure cuff can be used successfully when veins are difficult to find. The most efficient blood barrier provides a resistance that is less than systolic blood pressure but greater than diastolic, or stated another way, so that blood flows in but not out. The blood pressure cuff can determine these pressures; consequently, it is a perfect tourniquet.[6]

Another type of tourniquet is the Seraket, which uses a seat-belt design. It allows the phlebotomist to release the venous pressure partially by using a lever that releases some pressure, but not all. Thus, if the phlebotomist needs to tighten the tourniquet again, the lever can be used to adjust the tourniquet. Because errors in laboratory test results can occur from prolonged tourniquet pressure, the Seraket provides a solution to this problem. One drawback of this type of tourniquet, however, is the difficulty in cleaning and decontaminating it if it is soiled with blood.

Velcro-type tourniquets are popular because they are easy to apply and comfortable for the patient. Alternatively, because of major concern for infection control in health care institutions, many facilities now use a disposable natural latex tourniquet strap to help prevent cross-contamination. Many patients are allergic to latex, and thus other types of tourniquets must be available to use to avoid an allergic reaction. Nonlatex disposable tourniquets are now available as a good option for the blood collector and patient. If the tourniquets used in the health care facility are not disposable, they must be wiped fre-

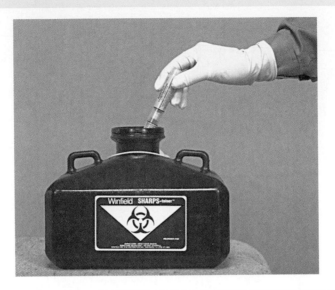

Figure 8–15. Sharps Disposal Container with the Required Biohazard Sign

quently with 70 percent isopropyl alcohol and disinfected with a chlorine bleach dilution of 1:10 if contaminated with blood or other body fluids.

 BLEEDING-TIME EQUIPMENT

Bleeding time is an assay used to assess the contributions of platelet function and blood vessel integrity to primary blood-clotting abilities.[7] The test is performed by making a minor standardized incision in the forearm or earlobe and recording the length of time required for bleeding to stop. Many procedures have been used to measure bleeding time. Mechanical devices are used to create uniform and reliable skin incisions for bleeding-time determination. One such device is the Surgicutt which provides a uniform surgical incision. The procedure for determining bleeding time is provided in Chapter 13.

 GLOVES FOR BLOOD COLLECTION

Safety guidelines have been established for health care workers to help them prevent the possibility of acquiring infections, such as hepatitis or those associated with AIDS. These guidelines include the use of gloves during collection of blood from patients (Figure 8–16 ■). It is recommended that phlebotomists not use gloves with talc powder containing calcium, because tubes of patients' blood may become contaminated with this powder, and such contamination can result in falsely elevated calcium values.

Latex gloves have proved effective in preventing the transmission of infectious diseases to health care workers. However, exposures to latex may result in an allergic reaction in some individuals. A latex allergy is a reaction to certain proteins in latex rubber.

Increasing exposure to latex gloves or the lubricant powder in some gloves also increases the risk of developing allergy symptoms. NIOSH has valuable information on their

Figure 8–16. Use of Gloves

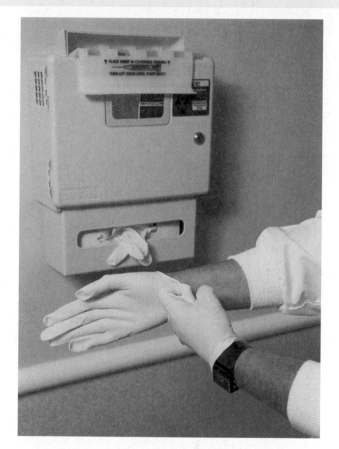

Gloves should be changed after each patient's blood collection.

website (www.cdc.gov/niosh/98-113.html) regarding latex allergy prevention, and suggests the following steps to protect oneself from latex exposure:

- Use nonlatex gloves for activities that are not likely to involve contact with infectious materials: housekeeping, maintenance, etc.
- Use powder-free gloves with reduced protein content
- "Hypoallergenic" latex gloves do not reduce the risk of latex allergy, but may reduce reactions to chemical additives in the latex
- When wearing latex gloves, do not use oil-based hand creams, which can cause glove deterioration
- Wash hands with mild soap after using latex gloves
- Clean areas frequently that have been contaminated with latex-containing dust
- Learn the symptoms of latex allergy
- Attend latex allergy educational programs

Clinical Alert

- Change gloves between patients' blood collections.
- Do not wash, disinfect, or reuse the gloves.

ANTISEPTICS, STERILE GAUZE PADS, AND BANDAGES

The health care worker needs antiseptics, sterile gauze pads, and bandages for blood collection by either venipuncture or microcollection. Therefore, 70 percent isopropyl alcohol preparation and iodine swab sticks or pads (for blood cultures) are essential items for blood collection. In home health care and other ambulatory health care environments where soap and water may not be available, a waterless antiseptic agent (Figure 8–17 ■) should be carried with other blood collection items and used before and after blood collection.

MICROCOLLECTION EQUIPMENT

Usually, skin puncture blood-collecting techniques are used on infants because venipuncture is excessively hazardous. These techniques are also useful for adults and older children in the circumstances listed in Box 8–5.

Clinical Alert

A latex allergy can begin within minutes of exposure. Mild reactions to latex include skin redness, rash, hives, or itching. Severe reactions may involve respiratory symptoms including sneezing, itchy eyes, scratchy throat, asthma, and sometimes, shock.

The allergy can occur in patients and/or health care workers. In these instances, ALL latex products should be avoided, including latex gloves, bandages, and tourniquets. (See "Patient Safety Related to Latex Products" in Chapter 6, "Safety and First Aid.")

Figure 8–17. Waterless Antiseptic Agent

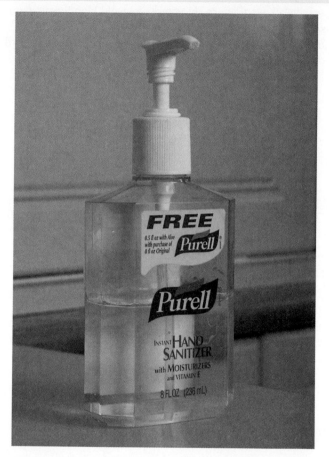

Waterless antiseptic agents should be carried with other blood collection supplies.

Box 8-5   Skin Puncture Blood Collection

Skin puncture collection is indicated for adults and older children when they:

- are severely burned or scarred in venipuncture areas
- have veins that are difficult to stick because of their small size or location
- must undergo bedside clinical testing
- are receiving IV therapy
- require frequent blood tests
- are geriatric patients
- are extremely obese
- must perform home glucose testing

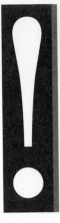

Clinical Alert

- Disposable, sterile lancets that are retractable to avoid bloodborne pathogen exposure should be used to puncture the skin for skin puncture collections.
- Surgical blades should not be used for skin puncture due to the hazard to the patient and phlebotomist.

The volume of plasma or serum that generally can be collected from a premature infant is approximately 100 to 150 uL, and about two times that amount can be taken from a full-term newborn. Larger volumes are obtained from older children and adults.[8]

LANCETS AND TUBES

For infants, the National Committee for Clinical Laboratory Standards (NCCLS) recommends a penetration depth of less than 2.0 mm on heel sticks to avoid penetrating bone.[8] The BD Quikheel lancet (Figure 8–18 ■) is available for two different incision depths, dependent upon the needs of the infant. The teal-colored Quikheel Infant lancet has a preset incision depth of 1.0 mm and width of 2.5 mm, and the purple-colored Quikheel Preemie lancet has a preset incision depth of 0.85 mm and width of 1.75 mm. This lancet blade retracts permanently after activation to assure safety to the health care worker.

Figure 8–18. BD Quikheel Lancet

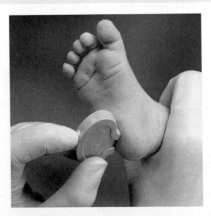

Courtesy of BD VACUTAINER Systems, *Preanalytical Solutions,* Franklin Lakes, NJ.

Figure 8–19. BD Genie Lancet

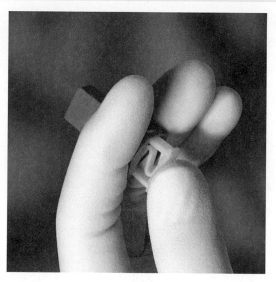

Courtesy of BD VACUTAINER Systems, *Preanalytical Solutions,* Franklin Lakes, NJ.

Also, the BD Genie lancet (Figure 8–19 ■) is a safety-engineered device for skin puncture blood collection. The Genie lancet is available in an assortment of puncture widths and depths, as well as in a needle lancet for glucose testing.

LifeScan, Inc., produces the Unistik 2 Neonatal, a single-use disposable lancing device that has a penetration depth of only 1.8 mm. It provides protection for infants and for health care workers who have to obtain patient blood samples.

ITC has produced fully automated, single-use, automatically retracting, disposable devices that provide safety both for the neonate and for the health care worker (Figure 8–20 ■). Tenderlett Jr. for children, Tenderlett for adults, and Tenderlett Toddler for infants and toddlers are engineered to incise to the least invasive but most effective depth for optimal blood flow. The Tenderlett incises 1.75 mm deep, Tenderlett Jr. incises 1.25 mm deep, and Tenderlett Toddler incises only 0.85 mm deep. The retracting blade of each of these devices eliminates potential injury from an exposed blade contaminated with blood.

Another safety device for microcollection is the Monoject Monoletter Safety Lancet (Figure 8–21 ■) for finger stick collections. The Greiner Bio-One lancet (Figure 8–22 ■) is a safety microcollection device available for various puncture depths.

A laser-based device that is FDA-approved for blood collection is the Lasette. The laser penetrates to a depth of 1 to 2 mm and width of 250 mm. This is a smaller puncture hole than other devices make. Up to 100 mL of blood can be collected.[9]

To collect a reliable small-volume blood sample, it is important to use properly designed blood microcollection tubes that are made of plastic for safety. See "Preventing Infections from Glass Capillary Tubes Use" in Chapter 5, "Infection Control." The microcontainers recommended for use for skin puncture collections are listed in Box 8–6.

Figure 8–20. Tenderlett Automated Skin Incision Device

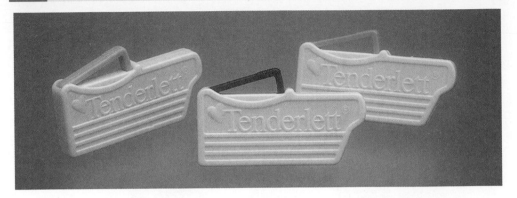

Courtesy of ITC, Edison, NJ.

Microhematocrit capillary tubes are disposable narrow-bore pipettes that are used for packed red cell volume in microcentrifugation. These plastic tubes also have colored bands; a red band indicates a heparin-coated tube, and a blue band indicates no anticoagulant. Plastic microcollection devices for general laboratory collections (e.g., chemistry, immunology) are usually color coded according to the established protocol for blood collection vacuum tube tops. Thus, purple- or lavender-topped tubes contain EDTA, green-topped tubes contain heparin, red- or pink-topped tubes have no additive, and gray-topped tubes have sodium fluoride to inhibit blood enzymes that destroy glucose.

Figure 8–21. Monoject Monoletter Safety Lancet

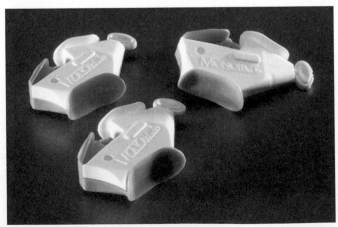

Courtesy of Tyco/Healthcare/Kendall, Mansfield, MA.

Figure 8–22. Greiner Bio-One Lancets for Microcollection

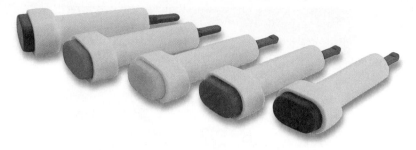

Courtesy of Greiner Bio-One, Monroe, NC.

Tyco/Healthcare/Kendall Co. manufactures the Samplette micro blood collector, which is offered with a full range of anticoagulants and serum and plasma separation gels. One of their collectors is an amber capillary blood separator that provides protection for light-sensitive analytes (e.g., bilirubin).

Electrolytes and general chemistry microspecimens can be collected in the BD Microtainer tube, which has its own capillary blood collector, self-contained serum separator, and Microgard closure, which is safety engineered to reduce the risk of tube leakage and specimen splatter. Each tube is imprinted with two markings, a minimum 250 mL line and a maximum 500 mL, to assist in collecting appropriate volumes (Figure 8–23 ■).

Alternatively, two or more capillary tubes can be used for electrolyte and general chemistry collection. One advantage of these tubes is that if blood hemolyzes in one capillary tube, another capillary tube containing the patient's sample can be used for the chemical analyses.

The Microvette capillary blood collection system is another microcollection system that is offered with a full range of anticoagulants and serum separation gel. This system can be used to collect, store, and separate samples in the same unbreakable, disposable container.

RAM Scientific, Inc., has developed an unbreakable plastic capillary-receptacle system called the SAFE-T-FILL capillary blood collection system. The device consists of a plastic capillary inserted into a microtube receptacle (Figure 8–24 ■). With the attached receptacle, blood flows directly to the bottom of the tube. This system makes the blood drawing safe and clean. The capillary can then be removed, and the tube is closed with the appropriate color-coded cap.

For most chemical assays using the various types of microcollection devices, lithium and ammonium salts of heparin are the anticoagulants of choice for microcollections. They have rarely been reported to interfere with the determination of electrolytes and most other chemical assays.

Another type of microcollection device is the Unopette, shown in Figure 8–25 ■. This device serves as a collection and dilution unit for blood samples and, thus, increases the speed and simplicity of laboratory procedures. These devices are prefilled with specific amounts of diluents or reagents, or both, for different types of laboratory assays. Some of

Figure 8–23. BD Microtainer Tube

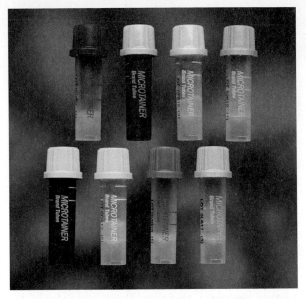

Courtesy of BD VACUTAINER Systems, *Preanalytical Solutions,* Franklin Lakes, NJ.

the more prevalent procedures in which Unopette devices are used include the WBC count, RBC count, platelet count, and RBC fragility.

The standard Unopette test comprises:

1. a disposable, self-filling diluting pipette consisting of a straight, thin-walled, uniform-bore, glass capillary tube fitted into a plastic holder, and
2. a plastic reservoir containing a premeasured volume of reagent for diluting

TRANSPORTING MICROSPECIMENS

Glycolysis in RBCs and WBCs causes a decrease in blood pH that can be detected after a blood gas sample has been stored at room temperature for approximately 20 minutes. Therefore, blood gas microsamples should be immersed in a slurry of ice water from the time of collection until they are delivered to the clinical laboratory. Plastic containers that

Box 8-6	Plastic Microcollection Devices—Various Types Needed

- Serum or plasma separator devices in different color codes (same colors as for vacuum color-topped tubes described earlier according to additives, e.g., purple—EDTA, etc.)
- Disposable plastic calibrated microcollection tubes
- Plastic microhematocrit tubes
- Microdilution systems (e.g. BD Unopette)

Figure 8–24. Safe-T-Fill Capillary Blood Collection Device

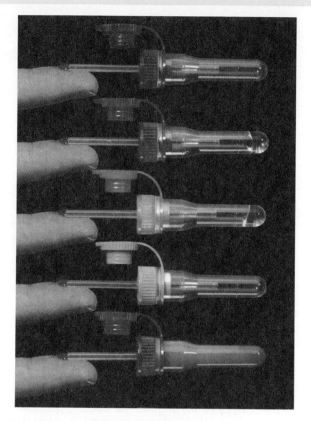

Courtesy of Ram Scientific, Inc., Needham, MA.

are small enough to hold these specimens with ice and water should be carried on the specimen collection tray. Ice is usually available on the patient ward. Other items to be carried on a microcollection tray include the following:

1. Seventy percent isopropyl alcohol and iodine or Betadine pads
2. Marking pens for labels
3. Microcollection blood serum separator tubes
4. Capillary whole blood cell collectors with 0.23 mg of EDTA (200 mL)
5. Safety lancets for skin puncture
6. Sterile gauze pads or bandages
7. Unheparinized plastic microcollection tubes
8. Heparinized plastic microcollection tubes (250, 400, and 500 mL)
9. Heparinized Natelson tubes (75 mL)
10. Unopette devices for collection and dilution procedures
11. Disposable gloves
12. Appropriate warming device

Figure 8–25. Unopette, a Collection and Dilution Unit for Blood Samples

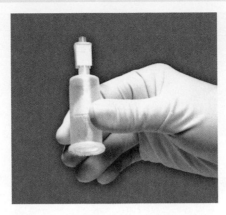

Courtesy of BD VACUTAINER Systems, *Preanalytical Solutions,* Franklin Lakes, NJ.

13. Thermometer
14. Biohazardous waste containers for sharps
15. Glass microscope slides
16. Capillary safety tube sealer
17. Antimicrobial hand gel or foam to wash hands without water and soap

BLOOD-DRAWING CHAIR

There are many chair styles and options available for making phlebotomy procedures easier and safer. Options include adjustable armrests, leg extensions, neck pillows or supports, scale mounts, storage cabinets, hydraulic lifts, and foot covers. An option for outpatient health care facilities to have in case the blood-drawing chairs are not available is the use of the exam table. The patient can lie on the exam table as the blood is collected. Thus, if

Clinical Alert

In an outpatient clinic that requires blood collections, a blood-drawing chair should be available for patients. The blood-drawing chair:

- Is needed for maximum safety and comfort of the patient plus easy accessibility to either arm of the patient.
- Should have an armrest for the patient's use during blood collection.
- Should have an armrest that locks in place so that the patient cannot fall from the chair if he/she becomes faint.
- Should have an armrest that adjusts in an up-and-down position so that the best venipuncture position for each patient can be achieved.

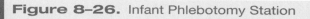

Figure 8–26. Infant Phlebotomy Station

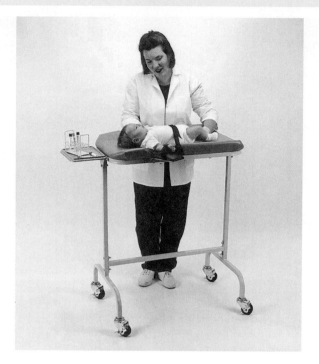

Courtesy of www.customcomfort.com

he/she feels faint during the blood collection, the patient will not fall since he/she is already in a safe, reclined position.

INFANT PHLEBOTOMY STATION

As health care services are increasingly being provided at ambulatory sites, including home visits, a safe site is frequently needed for infant blood collections. An infant phlebotomy station provides safety for infant blood collections at off site locations (Figure 8–26 ■).

SPECIMEN COLLECTION TRAYS

The health care worker needs a specimen tray (Figure 8–27 ■) to take on blood-collecting rounds. The tray is usually made of plastic (preferably latex-free) and must be amenable to sterilization. The tray should include all necessary collection equipment, and its contents usually differ from one hospital or clinic to another, depending on the patient population. For example, if the phlebotomist works in a children's hospital, he or she needs trays containing microcollection equipment, such as that described earlier. For home health care providers and reference laboratory couriers, the necessary collection supplies, equipment, and collected blood must be carried in an enclosed container with the biohazard symbol shown on the outside. It should be lockable to protect the contents from tampering or acci-

Figure 8-27. Specimen Collection Tray

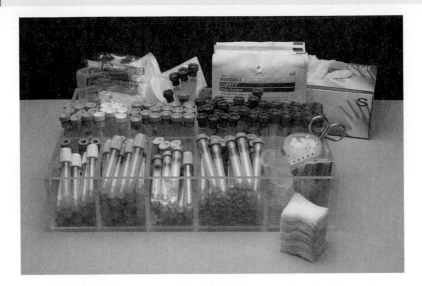

dental contamination. It also should have a tight seal to reduce the risk of infection from bloodborne pathogens due to spills or accidents.

Health care workers who collect blood from adults usually have the following equipment on their trays or in their safety container:

1. Marking pens or pencils
2. Vacuum tubes containing the anticoagulants designated in the clinical laboratory blood collection manual
3. Safety holders for vacuum tubes
4. Safety needles for vacuum tubes and syringes
5. Safety syringes
6. Tourniquet (nonlatex)
7. Safety blood collection sets (butterfly needle assembly)
8. Seventy percent isopropyl alcohol, iodine pads, or swab sticks
9. Sterile gauze pads
10. Bandages
11. Biohazardous waste containers for used needles, holders, and lancets
12. Safety lancets for skin puncture
13. Unopette devices for finger-stick blood collection
14. Microcollection blood serum and plasma separator tubes
15. Microcollection capillary whole blood collectors with 0.23 mg of EDTA (200 mL)
16. Disposable gloves
17. Cloth towel or washcloth
18. Thermometer
19. Antimicrobial hand gel or foam to wash hands without water and soap

▬▬ WEB ADDRESSES FOR SUPPLIERS OF SAFETY BLOOD COLLECTION EQUIPMENT

Baxter Healthcare Corp.
http://www.baxter.com

Becton Dickinson and Co.
http://www.bd.com

Bio-Plexus, Inc.
http://www.bio-plexus.com

Greiner Labortechnik
http://www.vacuette.com

Healthmark Industries Co.
http://www.hmark.com

Helena Products
http://www.helena.com

International Technidyne Corp.
http://www.itcmed.com

The Kendall Co. LP
http://www.kendallhq.com

Lab Safety Supply
http://www.labsafety.com

Lifescan, Inc.
http://www.lifescan.com

Owen Mumford, Inc.
http://www.owenmumford.com

RAM Scientific
http://www.ramscientific.com

Retractable Technologies, Inc.
http://www.vanishpoint.com

Sarstedt, Inc.
http://www.sarstedt.com

Portex, Inc.
http://www.portexusa.com

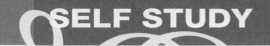

SELF STUDY

KEY TERMS

acid citrate dextrose (ACD)
anticoagulants
antiseptics
arterial blood gas
blood-drawing chair
capillary tubes
citrates
disposable sterile lancet
ethylenediamine tetra-acetic acid (EDTA)
gauge number
heparin

holder (adapter)
latex allergy
lithium iodoacetate
microcontainers
multiple-sample needles
oxalates
single-sample needle
sodium fluoride
sterile gauze pads
vacuum (evacuated) tube

STUDY QUESTIONS

The following may have more than one answer.

1. Which of the following anticoagulants prevent coagulation of blood by removing calcium through the formation of insoluble calcium salts?
   a. EDTA
   b. ammonium oxalate
   c. sodium citrate
   d. sodium heparin

2. Which of the following anticoagulants is found in a green-topped blood-collection vacuum tube?
   a. EDTA
   b. ammonium oxalate
   c. sodium citrate
   d. sodium heparin

3. For capillary collection from newborns, a lancet of which of the following lengths should be used to avoid penetrating bone?
   a. 1.75 mm
   b. 2.75 mm
   c. 3.00 mm
   d. 3.25 mm

4. Which of the following blood chemical constituents is light sensitive?
   a. glucose
   b. bilirubin
   c. phosphorus
   d. blood gases

5. When blood is collected from a patient, the serum should be separated from the blood cells as quickly as possible to avoid:
   a. hemoconcentration
   b. hemolysis
   c. glycolysis
   d. hemostasis

6. The color coding for needles indicates the:
   a. length
   b. gauge
   c. manufacturer
   d. anticoagulant

7. From the listed needle gauges, which one has the largest diameter?
   a. 19
   b. 20
   c. 21
   d. 23

8. Which of the following is/are skin puncture equipment?
   a. Tenderlett
   b. Lasette
   c. Samplette
   d. winged infusion set

9. Which of the following laboratory tests requires that the blood be transported in a slurry of ice water to the laboratory?
   a. bilirubin
   b. CK
   c. blood gas analysis
   d. complete blood cell (CBC) count

References

1. Hyman, D, Kaplan, N: The difference between serum and plasma potassium (letter). *N Engl J Med,* 1985; 313: 642.

2. National Committee for Clinical Laboratory Standards (NCCLS): Tubes and Additives for Venous Blood Specimen Collection, Approved Standard, 5th ed. NCCLS Document H1-A5. Wayne, PA: NCCLS, 2003.

3. Adcock, DM, Kressin, DC, Marlar, RA: Effect of 3.2% versus 3.8% sodium citrate concentration on routine coagulation testing. *Am J Clin Pathol,* 1997; 107: 105–110.

4. Occupational Safety and Health Administration (OSHA), US Dept. of Labor: OSHA Safety and Health Information Bulletin (SHIB): Re-Use of Blood Tube Holders. October 15, 2003.

5. National Committee for Clinical Laboratory Standards (NCCLS): Procedures for the Collection of Diagnostic Blood Specimens by Venipuncture, Approved Standard, 5th ed. NCCLS Document H3-A5. Wayne, PA: NCCLS, 2003.

6. Scranton, PE: *Practical Techniques in Venipuncture.* Baltimore: Williams & Wilkins, 1977, p. 66.

7. Harker, LA, Slichter, SI: The bleeding time as a screening test for evaluation of platelet function. *N Engl J Med,* 1972; 287: 155.

8. National Committee for Clinical Laboratory Standards (NCCLS): Procedures and Devices for the Collection of Diagnostic Capillary Blood Specimens. NCCLS Document H4-A5. Wayne, PA: NCCLS, 2004.

9. News & Views: Lasers to replace lancets? *Lab Med,* 1997; 28(11): 689.

Running Late on the Day Shift

A phlebotomist named John was running behind schedule for his early-AM hospital blood collections. As he entered the room of the last patient on the nursing unit, he left his supplies on the table by the window and picked up only the tubes and needle assembly that he needed. He proceeded with patient identification and the venipuncture which was successful. As he was finishing and about to pull out the needle, he realized he had left the gauze on his supply tray. As he reached over toward the supplies to try to get some gauze, he inadvertently pushed the needle into the nerve below the vein. The patient yelled and John withdrew the needle immediately, however, the damage had been done.

Questions

1. What were the fundamental problems in this case?
2. How could problems have been prevented?

A Supervisor's Folly

Helen is a phlebotomy supervisor who has worked in a small community hospital for 27 years. She relies on her early training experience in her daily work practices. These habits include not always wearing gloves during venipuncture procedures, washing hands after the procedure but not before, and using syringe/needles to routinely collect blood specimens. Her co-workers and a few of her subordinates occasionally express concern about the safety of her patients and herself. She laughs and says that she "has never had any problems and you can't teach an old dog new tricks."

Questions

1. Describe the issues that might pose some legal risk for Helen and her employer.
2. What measures can her coworkers or subordinates take to protect Helen and the patients?
3. In what ways should Helen modify her practices?

Stocking Supplies in Phlebotomy Practice

The phlebotomists were having an in-service with supervisory technologists to discuss options for improving productivity, accuracy, and for minimizing the number of preanalytical errors occurring in the laboratory. In the previous two years, the specimen collection workload had increased threefold, including the hospital and in-house clinics. Preanalytical errors had also increased and on several occasions they had run out of certain evacuated tubes, used expired tubes, or used capillary tubes that broke easily during processing. It was mentioned that they were behind on the inventory counts, restocking, and ordering. One phlebotomist named Billy Bob suggested that barcodes be used as a method to improve productivity and accuracy. He had worked at a hospital where they had been in use for several years and thought it could have a positive impact. He began to highlight the benefits of bar code technology and explain how they might be used.

Questions

1. What could Billy Bob say about the benefits and drawbacks of barcode technology?
2. In what ways could inventory/control management of supplies help reduce pre-analytical errors?

Traumatic Transport

A specimen tube for chemistry analysis was sent to the laboratory via a pneumatic tube system. Upon arrival it was noted that the specimen appeared to be grossly hemolyzed. There were no initials on the specimen label to indicate who performed the collection.

Questions:

1. What are the likely causes of the hemolysis?
2. What other factors are of concern in this brief scenario?

Accidental Injury

Sally Landers had been on the job for only 8 months. She was a phlebotomist at a rural hospital in the Southwest where she had been hired to do early morning blood collections and deliver specimens to the centralized laboratory. She was tired when she went to work one Friday morning. She drew blood from a frail middle-aged man, Mr. Johnson. She had trouble with the collection procedure in that she had to stick him twice before she acquired the blood specimen. She was relieved when she finally finished the procedure. As she began to clean up and discard the used equipment, she noticed that the biohazard container was full. She decided, however, that it could probably hold the needles she had used on Mr. Johnson. She used her fingers to push the used needles and needle holders into the container and she felt a sharp puncture. She realized that she had stuck herself with a contaminated sharp object. She gathered the specimens she had drawn and quickly left. She immediately reported the injury to her supervisor.

Questions

1. Describe what Sally did correctly and incorrectly.
2. What procedures would need to be reviewed with Sally?
3. What additional education would you recommend for Sally?

Transporting Specimens from Homebound Patients to the Laboratory

The medical assistant, Larry Smith, works for Mackin Home Health Agency. His job is multifaceted because he performs history and physical assessments, and when required to, he draws blood for laboratory testing. One day he went to collect blood and urine samples on Mr. Gonzales, an 80-year-old man who spoke very little English. He greeted Mr. Gonzales and found the bathroom and a suitable spot to draw blood from him. He felt confident that Mr. Gonzales had understood his communication. He was successful on the first attempt to collect the blood sample, and he helped Mr. Gonzales to the bathroom to collect the urine. Mr. Gonzales followed directions except he did not close the urine bottle tightly because he lacked the strength. Larry did not notice that the lid was not on tightly. He placed all the specimens in the container he had brought. He decided to leave the lid open because he knew his next stop was just 1 block away. On the way to the next house, a car ran a stop sign so Larry had to jam on his brakes, and the container with specimens fell off the seat of the car. The urine specimen spilled all over the floor of his vehicle.

Questions

1. What could Larry have done to avoid the situation?
2. What should Larry do now?

Answers for all case study questions can be found in Appendix 12.

Venipuncture Procedures

CHAPTER OBJECTIVES

Upon completion of Chapter 9, the learner is responsible for the following:

1. Describe the patient identification process.
2. List supplies used in a typical venipuncture procedure.
3. Describe methods for hand hygiene.
4. Identify the most appropriate sites for venipuncture and situations when these sites might not be acceptable. Identify alternative sites for the venipuncture procedure.
5. Describe the process and time limits for applying a tourniquet to a patient's arm.
6. Describe the decontamination process and the agents used to decontaminate skin for routine blood tests and blood cultures.
7. Describe the steps of a venipuncture procedure.
8. Describe the "order of draw" for collection tubes.
9. Explain the importance of collecting "timed specimens" at the requested times.
10. Define the terms "fasting" and "STAT" when referring to blood tests.

 MediaLINK

Access the accompanying CD-ROM to explore a wide variety of review questions and interactive activities for this chapter, including multiple choice, true/false, and video exercises.

◼◼◼◼ BLOOD COLLECTION

Several essential steps are part of every successful blood collection procedure. This chapter discusses the blood collection process in the same order as these steps. However, each phlebotomist generally establishes a routine that is comfortable for him or her even though some facilities vary the sequence of steps based on the characteristics of their patient populations. In some cases, steps may occur simultaneously (e.g., assessing the patient's physical disposition while confirming his or her identity). In other cases, a problem may arise that precludes the phlebotomist from going further in the procedure (e.g., the verbal identity of the individual does not match the written documentation; the supplies needed for the venipuncture have expired, etc). Each step of the patient encounter must be evaluated carefully by the phlebotomist in a detailed manner, being careful not to omit any of the essential components. Thus, the basic steps involve the following:[1,2]

1. Preparation of the health care worker, including hand hygiene and reviewing laboratory test orders
2. Approaching, identifying, and positioning the patient
3. Assessing the patient's physical disposition, including diet and/or if the patient is sensitive to latex
4. Selecting and preparing equipment and supplies
5. Finding a puncture site
6. Preparing the puncture site
7. Choosing a venipuncture method
8. Collecting the samples in the appropriate tubes and in the correct order
9. Discarding contaminated supplies
10. Labeling the samples
11. Assessing the patient to ensure bleeding has stopped
12. Maintaining hand hygiene
13. Considering any special circumstances that occurred during the phlebotomy procedure
14. Assessing criteria for sample recollection or rejection
15. Prioritizing patients and sample tubes

◼◼◼◼ HEALTH CARE WORKER PREPARATION

Prior to performing any type of specimen collection, the health care worker should have all protective equipment, phlebotomy supplies, test requisitions, writing pen, and appropriate patient information. If patient information is incomplete on test requisitions, the health care worker may not be able to identify the patient correctly, or he or she may not know in which tubes to collect the blood. In such cases, assistance from a laboratory supervisor or a nurse is required prior to collecting the sample.

In addition, the health care worker needs a positive, professional disposition prior to beginning the patient encounter. A clean and neat appearance instills confidence. Refer to Chapter 1 to review an example of a dress code policy. A clear and open mind aids the phlebotomist in successful dialogue, listening skills, the venipuncture, and exiting graciously.

Clinical Alert

Phlebotomists must be familiar with policies regarding precautions for handling blood and body fluids. *All specimens should be treated as if they are hazardous and infectious,* according to the universal precautions described in detail in Chapter 5. Hands should be decontaminated before and immediately after specimen collection procedures. Refer to Appendix 3, "CDC Recommendations for Hand-Hygiene in Health Care Settings;" and Box 9–1, "Issues in Hand Hygiene." A clean pair of gloves should be put on in the presence of the patient as a safety-conscious gesture for both the patient and the health care worker. Refer to Procedure 9–1, "Gloving Technique." A clean, pressed uniform with a laboratory coat also instills a sense of professionalism and cleanliness, which is gratifying to patients and promotes a safer work environment for health care workers.

EXERCISING UNIVERSAL PRECAUTIONS

Normal human skin is colonized with microorganisms; thus, transmission of pathogens by health care workers from one patient to another can occur easily. Based on studies reported by the CDC, health care workers vary widely in the number of times they actually wash their hands (from 5 times per shift to over 100 times per shift). There is also great variability in the both the duration that workers perform the hand-washing process (5 seconds to 24 seconds), and the coverage of surface area on the hands, wrist, and fingers. Adherence to hand-hygiene techniques (hand washing or use of alcohol-based hand rubs) has been shown to significantly reduce outbreaks of infections, including antimicrobial-resistant infections (e.g., methicillin-resistant Staphylococcus aureus).[3]

NEEDLESTICK PREVENTION STRATEGIES

As covered in previous chapters, the Needlestick Safety and Prevention Act has mandated changes in the workplace to protect phlebotomists. It is a fact that those who use needles are at increased risk of a needlestick injury. These injuries may lead to serious or fatal infections with bloodborne pathogens such as hepatitis B virus (HBV), hepatitis C virus (HCV), or human immunodeficiency virus (HIV). However, needlestick injuries are preventable with the use of safety devices, precautionary practices, and safe handling/disposal of needles and specimens. In addition, the diseases may be prevented by preexposure vaccination and/or postexposure prophylaxis. Phlebotomists must report all needlestick injuries as soon as possible so that disease detection and prevention measures can be quickly initiated.[4]

Box 9–1   Issues in Hand Hygiene

The CDC Recommendations for Hand-Hygiene that apply to phlebotomists are listed in Appendix 3. Phlebotomists must be knowledgeable of the recommendations and have appropriate training for performing and maintaining hand hygiene. Refer to Chapter 5 for procedures to maintain hand hygiene. Key issues are summarized below.[3]

INDICATIONS FOR HAND WASHING AND HAND ANTISEPSIS

- If hands are visibly dirty, contaminated, or soiled, they should be washed with either an antimicrobial soap and water or a non-antimicrobial soap and water.
- If hands are not visibly soiled, an alcohol-based hand rub can be used routinely for decontaminating hands. Washing hands with antimicrobial soap and water is also acceptable.
- Hands should be decontaminated before and after contact with a patient, blood, or body fluids.
- Hands should be decontaminated before and after wearing gloves.
- Hands should be decontaminated before eating and after using a restroom.
- Antimicrobial-impregnated wipes are not as effective as alcohol-based hand rubs or antimicrobial soap and water.

HAND-HYGIENE TECHNIQUE

- Alcohol-based hand rubs—Apply to palm on one hand and rub hands together, covering all surfaces of hands and fingers, until hands are dry. Follow manufacturer's recommendations regarding the volume of product to use.
- Soap and water—Wet hands first with water, apply an amount of product recommended by the manufacturer, and rub hands together vigorously for at least 15 seconds, covering all surfaces of hands and fingers. Rinse hands with water and dry thoroughly with a disposable towel. Use towel to turn off the faucet.
- Multiple-use cloth towels of the hanging or roll type are not recommended for health care facilities.

CHOOSING A HAND-HYGIENE PRODUCT

- Consider efficacy of the antiseptic agents against pathogens.
- Consider how acceptable the products are to personnel who use them (accessibility, ease of use, minimal irritation, etc.). Refer to Chapter 8 for more information about specific products.
- In cases where there is a use of a soap dispenser, soap should not be added to a partially empty container, because the practice of "topping off" can lead to bacterial contamination.

SKIN CARE

- Hand lotions should be provided to minimize the occurrence of dermatitis associated with frequent hand decontamination.

OTHER ASPECTS OF HAND HYGIENE

- Keep natural nail tips less than 1/4 inch long.
- Do not wear artificial fingernails or extenders when having direct contact with patients at high risk.
- Change gloves between patients; do not wash the same gloves between patients.

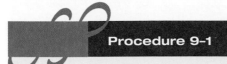

Procedure 9–1   Gloving Technique

1. Decontaminate hands using soap and water or an alcohol-based hand rub.
2. When hands are dry, slip fingers of one hand into clean glove.
3. Pull taught with the other hand so that there is no slack or bagginess of the gloves at the fingertips. (Fig. 9-1a ■)

4. Do the same with the other hand.
5. After the procedure, turn gloves inside out as you remove them. (Fig. 9-1b ■)
6. Discard them with biohazardous materials.

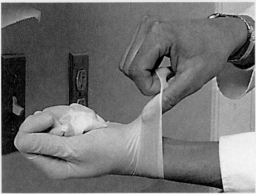

Figure 9–1a

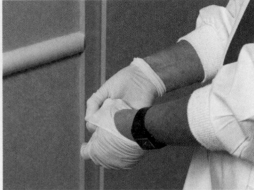

Figure 9–1b

■■■■■ ASSESSING, IDENTIFYING, AND APPROACHING THE PATIENT

TEST REQUISITIONS

Laboratory test requests are usually transmitted electronically or in the form of a paper-based requisition. Electronic (computer-generated) requests contain the same required information as paper requisitions. In either case, the requisition should contain the following information:[5]

1. Patient's identification (name, identification/registration number, date of birth)
2. Types of tests to be performed
3. Date of test
4. Room number and bed, if applicable
5. Name of the physician or legally authorized person who ordered the tests
6. Test status (timed, STAT, fasting, etc.)
7. Billing information (optional)
8. Special precautions (potential bleeder, faints easily, latex sensitivity, etc.)
9. Clinical information, when appropriate
10. Source of specimen, when appropriate

When requisitions are received in a centralized laboratory department, computer-generated labels may also serve as the requisition, as indicated in Figure 9–2 ■. The numerous types, colors, and styles of labels (e.g., bar-coded labels) and requisitions are discussed in Chapter 7.

Figure 9–2. Requisition Forms

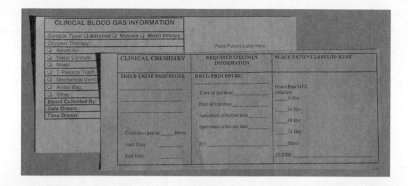

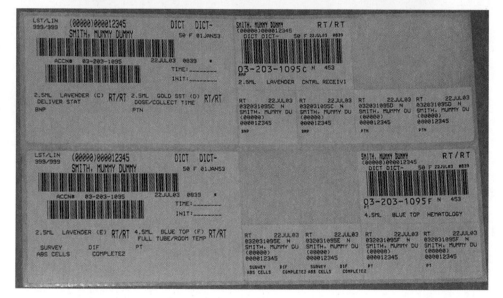

Paper or electronic requisitions should include all of the following components:[5]

Patient identification information (name, registration number and location, or a unique confidential specimen code)

Name and address (if different than that of the receiving lab) of the physician or legally authorized person ordering the test

Tests requested

Time and date of specimen collection when appropriate

Source of specimen, when appropriate (important for microbiology, surgical pathology, etc.)

Clinical information, when appropriate

Requisitions are courtesy of The University of Texas M.D. Anderson Cancer Center, Houston, Texas, and obtained with permission.

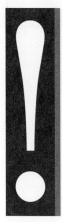

Clinical Alert

Use of gloves does not eliminate the need for hand hygiene, nor does good hand hygiene eliminate the need for gloves. *Both* hand hygiene and gloves should be used before and after each patient.

Regardless of whether the requisitions are computer generated or multipart paper forms, the health care worker should be familiar with the forms and with the procedures for generating, printing, and using the requisition forms properly. Collection requests should be checked prior to the venipuncture procedure to ensure that there are no discrepancies or duplicates in the test orders.

PATIENT IDENTIFICATION PROCESS

Positive patient identification is the most crucial responsibility for which a phlebotomist is held accountable. The 2003 National Patient Safety Goals and Recommendations set by the Joint Commission on Accreditation of Healthcare Organizations include improving "accuracy of patient identification." Their recommendations suggest using "at least two patient identifiers (neither to be the patient's room number) whenever taking blood samples or administering medications or blood products."[6] Correct patient identification is critical to accurate laboratory results upon which clinical decisions are made by physicians, nurses, and other members of the health care team. Patient identification errors can occur either at the time of phlebotomy or as the specimen is being prepared for testing, for example, after centrifugation when the specimen is divided into aliquots. The process of identifying patients varies slightly based on the patient's location (inpatient or

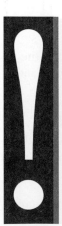

Clinical Alert

If phlebotomists care for patients who are at high risk of acquiring infections, artificial nails should be avoided and natural nails should be less than one quarter of an inch long.[3]

Box 9–2	Preventing Needlestick Injuries

Data compiled from various studies by the Centers for Disease Control and Prevention (CDC) indicate that needlestick injuries occur due to the following reasons:[4]

- The type and design of the needle device used
- Recapping a needle
- Transferring body fluids between containers
- Failing to properly dispose of used needles in puncture-resistant sharps containers

WHAT EMPLOYERS CAN DO:

- Analyze needlestick and sharps-related injuries in the workplace to identify hazards and injury trends.
- Set priorities/strategies for prevention by researching national information about risk factors and intervention efforts.
- Ensure that staff are trained properly in the safe use and disposal of needles, as well as in universal precautions.
- Modify work practices that pose needlestick injury hazards.
- Promote safety awareness in the work environment.
- Provide high-risk employees with free hepatitis B vaccinations
- Establish procedures and encourage timely reporting of all needlestick or sharps-related injuries.
- Evaluate the success of the needlestick prevention program and modify the exposure control plan accordingly.

WHAT EMPLOYEES CAN DO:

- Avoid use of needles where safe alternatives are available.
- Help the employer select, evaluate, and use safety devices.
- Avoid recapping needles.
- Before beginning a procedure, plan for safe handling and needle disposal.
- Assist in coordinating specimen collections to reduce the number of times needles are used on a patient.
- Promptly dispose of used needles in the proper sharps disposal containers.
- Report all needlestick and other sharps-related injuries promptly to ensure follow-up care and to allow for tracking the hazards in the workplace.
- Tell employer about hazards from needles that are observed in the work environment.
- Participate in bloodborne pathogen training and follow infection prevention practices such as hepatitis B vaccination.

outpatient or emergency room), the type of patient (pediatric or adult), whether the patient is conscious or unconscious, and the available information at the time (armband or picture identification).

Inpatient Identification

Hospitalized patients (except those just entering an emergency room) must wear an identification bracelet indicating the first and last names and a designated hospital number (often called a unit number). Hospital identification numbers help hospital personnel to distinguish between patients with the same first and/or last names.

Information on the identification bracelet may also include the patient's room number, bed assignment, and physician's name. A three-way match should be made with the identi-

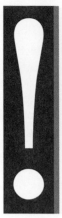

Clinical Alert

If the health care worker does not understand the test ordered, a supervisor, a laboratory technologist, or a nurse should be consulted prior to the phlebotomy procedure. Knowing which tests are requested helps the health care worker to prepare the patient appropriately and to collect the specimen in the appropriate tubes and in the correct order. Failure to do so results in preanalytical errors, misleading test results, and repeated venipunctures for the patient.

fication bracelet, the test requisition, and the patient's statement of his or her name, birthday, or address.

Identification of Patients Who Are Sleeping

A patient who is sleeping should be awakened before collecting the blood, and the patient identity verified as previously stated. Verbal information should be compared with the information on the requisition and the identification bracelet.[2]

Identification of Patients Who Are Unconscious, Mentally Incompetent, or Do Not Speak the Language

A nurse, relative, or friend may identify patients who are unconscious, mentally incompetent, comatose, or cannot speak the phlebotomist's language by providing the patient's name, address, and identification number and/or birth date. Again, this information should

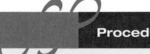

| Procedure 9–2 | The Basics of Patient Identification |

Patient identification involves *at least 3 steps*:

1. After greeting a conscious patient (Fig. 9–3 ■), ask the patient to *state his or her full name and birth date.* (You may also request the patient's address and ID number.)

2. Compare the information stated with the information on the laboratory *test requisitons.*

3. Confirm the information (from steps 1 and 2) with another source of reliable, *verifiable identification* (e.g., printed identification number, hospital identification bracelet, driver's license, nurse, parent).

Refer to Figure 9–2 and Chapter 7 for more information about requisitions.

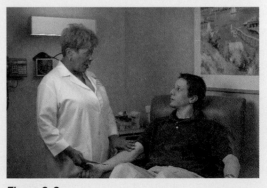

Figure 9–3

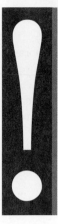

Clinical Alert

There are special cases that involve patients with severe burns or in isolation, in which the identification is attached to the patient's bed, rather than the arm. These are the only circumstances in which a phlebotomist may use a bed-labeled identification tag to confirm identity. This step should be followed up by a nurse's confirmation and appropriate documentation. Normally, a name card on the bed or door should never be used for confirming identity, because the tags are sometimes not changed in a timely manner when patients are discharged and new patients are admitted.

be compared with the information on the requisition to confirm identity. Any discrepancy should be reported to a supervisor.[1,2]

Identification of Infants and Young Children

It is preferable to use the same identification procedures for both children and adults; however, it is not always practical or feasible. A nurse or relative may identify an infant or child by providing the name, address, and identification number, and/or birth date. This topic will be covered in greater detail in Chapter 12, "Pediatric Procedures."

Emergency Room Patient Identification

Because all patients must be positively identified, patients who come to the emergency room (ER) unconscious and/or unidentified pose a situation where the phlebotomist must be particularly careful. The National Committee on Clinical Laboratory Standards (NCCLS) suggests that a temporary master identification (e.g., hospital number attached to the patient's body by wristband or other suitable device) may be provided until a positive

Clinical Alert

The health care worker should *not* ask, "Are you Ms. Doe?" because an ill patient on medication may mistakenly utter something, nod, or answer yes. Consequently, the best tactic is to ask, "What is your name?" and let the patient reply. The patient must be correctly identified by his or her identification bracelet. If the patient does not have an identification bracelet, the nurse responsible for the patient must be asked to make the identification. In such cases, the situation and the nurse's name should be documented on the requisition and/or electronically. Specimens should not be collected until a positive identification can be made and documented. Drawing blood from the wrong patient can lead to serious consequences such as incorrect treatment or therapy, and it is a violation for which the health care worker may be counseled or dismissed.

Clinical Alert

Phlebotomists should never collect a specimen from a patient whose identity is not confirmed or assured. If there is a discrepancy in the identification process, the specimen should not be obtained until identity can be verified. Discrepancies should be reported. Patient identification errors can be life-threatening and pose significant liability to both the phlebotomist who makes the error, and to the health care facility who employs him or her. The phlebotomist should never base identity, on records or charts placed on the patient's bed or equipment. Identity errors occur because of inaccurate requisitions, mixed-up paperwork, or failure to follow identification procedures. All discrepancies should be reported to a supervisor.

Box 9–3   Patient Identification Self-Assessment

Patients frequently have the same or similar last name. Common ones are Smith, Jones, and Johnson. As a self-assessment exercise, pretend you are tired and at the end of a busy work shift. Reflect on the names listed below and think about how you would react if any of these patients appeared together for venipuncture at the same time:

Betsy Johnson and Betty Johnston

P. Garcia and J. C. Garza

Jan Cheung and Jen Chang

John Riley and Jon Reilly

Consider how important each step of the identification process is in these (and all) situations. Next, come up with your own list of names that you are familiar with. "Tune-in" your eyes and ears to notice different spellings and verbal pronunciations of these names. Remember that language differences and/or accents may cause one name to sound like another, therefore resulting in misunderstandings. However, if the identification process is followed carefully and thoroughly, mistakes can be prevented. All discrepancies in the identification process should be reported to a supervisor.

Box 9–4   Advances in Identification Systems

New technology continues to provide enhancements to identification methods. One- and two-dimensional bar-code technologies enable more information to be encoded. Bar codes are quick, accurate, cost-effective and widely used for patient and specimen identification and tracking. Wireless technology such as radio frequency identification (RFID), which uses radio waves to transmit data, has the potential of holding more information than a single linear bar code. Essentially, each patient has a penny-sized "tag" that accompanies the specimen throughout the laboratory and uploads information as the tag is scanned at various points in the testing process.[7] Also, a microchip wristband is available that stores up to 80 pages of information about a patient. At each step, information is entered or retrieved from the chip for record keeping. It can also be erased and reused.[8] Each new identification system must be evaluated by the health care facility for accuracy, usefulness for the end user, cost-effectiveness, training involved, compatibility with existing computer technology, ease of updating records, access and security issues, failure rates, and ability to ensure privacy.

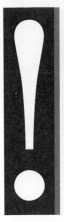

Clinical Alert

Patients who are semiconscious, comatose, or sleeping may jerk unexpectedly during the blood collection process, particularly as the needle is inserted.[2]

identification can be made. Refer to Box 9–5 for the NCCLS recommendations in dealing with these situations.

Outpatient/Ambulatory Patient Identification

Ambulatory patients are normally called to a blood collection area from a waiting room. (When calling a patient's name in the waiting room, phlebotomists must be careful to state only the name and not to reveal any confidential clinical information. Alternative methods for dealing with patients in a waiting room may involve the use of a numbering system.) Thus, ambulatory patient identification may be slightly more time-consuming because the patients have to walk into the specimen collection area first, and they usually lack an armband, which would provide an easy visual check. (While not the majority, some ambulatory clinics issue identification bracelets to patients.) Many clinics, however, distribute identification cards to patients before any specimens are collected. If this is the case, and the patient has the card available, positive identification can occur in the same manner as with hospitalized patients. These cards can also be used to make an imprinted label for the specimen if an Addressograph machine is used. If the patient does not have a patient identification armband or card, it is strongly recommended that another form of identification (e.g., driver's license or ID card with photograph) be checked and documented prior to specimen collection. Again, the identification process would involve verbally asking for name,

Box 9–5	NCCLS Recommendations for Identification of ER Patients Who Are Unconscious and/or Unidentified

- Assign a master identification number (temporary) to the patient in accord with institutional policy).
- Select the appropriate test request forms and record with master identification number.
- Complete the necessary labels either by hand or by computer and apply the labels to the test request forms and specimens.
- When a permanent identification number is assigned to the patient, make sure the temporary identification number is cross-referenced to the permanent number to ensure correct identification and correlation of patient and test result information.[1]

address, and/or birth date. The verbal information is compared with the requisition and any other form of identity available.

PHYSICAL DISPOSITION OF THE PATIENT

Factors related to the physical or emotional disposition of the patient often have an impact on the blood collection process or the integrity of the specimen. As mentioned in previous chapters, this relates to the preanalytical phase of laboratory testing. If the phlebotomist is aware of a variable that might affect the laboratory test or the patient encounter, she or he may be able to prepare more adequately for the venipuncture. Sometimes the phlebotomist can get clues about the patient's disposition upon entering a hospital room. For example, if there is an empty food tray by the patient's bedside, it is likely that the patient has eaten recently, and a notation about the nonfasting condition should be made after confirming the observation with the patient. At other times, a clue about something unusual may come after talking to the patient or after the identification process has taken place. Phlebotomists should use keen listening skills, direct observation of the situation, and make professional judgments about what modifications or documentation is needed to complete the specimen collection procedure. Refer to Box 9–6.

Many patient variables can influence test results, including those listed in Box 9–7. Effects of these and other preanalytic factors on blood collection are discussed in more detail in Chapter 11.

APPROACHING THE PATIENT

In addition to being prepared with the proper equipment and supplies and safety precautions, the health care worker must be emotionally prepared. Such preparation involves adopting a professional appearance and behavior, as well as exercising good communication skills, both as a listener and as a speaker. (Refer to Chapter 1 for more information about professional behavior, dress codes, and communication skills.)

Box 9–6   Factors Affecting the Patient's Disposition

- **Diet, alcohol, exercise, and/or smoking**—Many body substances are affected by the ingestion of foods and beverages (particularly alcohol), and by smoking. Therefore, it is important to note whether the patient has been fasting or not, if the patient seems intoxicated, or if the patient has smoked a cigarette. Diet and alcohol intake have an effect on coagulation activation in people with diabetes and other populations. Smoking elevates plasma fibrinogen, von Willebrand factor, coagulation factors, thrombin generation, and platelet activation. Moderate ethanol intake inhibits platelet reactivity. Vigorous physical activity leads to coagulation activation so patients should rest in a comfortable position for 15 to 30 minutes prior to the specimen collection procedure.[9]

- **Stress**—Excessively anxious or emotional patients may need extra time to calm down prior to, during, or after the procedure. The phlebotomist should deal professionally with these emotional needs based on the patient's age, gender, and cultural sensitivities. (Refer to Chapter 1 for more details on communication, and Chapters 11 and 12 for age-related issues.) Stress has also been linked to changes in the coagulation and fibrinolytic systems.[5]

- **Age**—Elderly patients have fragile, more "difficult" veins from which to choose the venipuncture site. (Refer to Chapter 14 for more details about the treatment of elderly patients.)

- **Weight**—Obese patients may require special equipment such as a large blood pressure cuff for the tourniquet or a longer needle to penetrate through fatty tissues to the vein.

> ### Box 9–7   Patient Variables That Affect Laboratory Test Results
>
> Phlebotomists are not expected to evaluate the patient for *all* aspects of these variables prior to each specimen collection procedure. However, they are expected to intervene and act responsibly with patient issues in their scope of practice as it relates to the specimen collection process. Actions may include documenting a situation, adjusting the patient to be in a more comfortable position, selecting alternative supplies for the procedure, transporting a specimen a in a certain manner, and/or seeking guidance from a supervisor about how to proceed. Whatever the case, the listed variables can introduce preanalytical variability.[5,9]
>
> Age and gender
>
> Blood type
>
> Circadian and seasonal rhythms
>
> Diet and exercise
>
> Smoking and alcohol intake
>
> Medications
>
> Intravenous lines or vascular access devices
>
> Menstrual cycle, pregnancy, menopausal status
>
> Emotional stress and psychiatric disorders

Several professional and courteous behaviors and phrases can help make the patient–health care worker encounter a smooth interaction. The first of these is a polite knock on the patient's door prior to entering the patient's room. The health care worker should introduce him- or herself and state that he or she is from the laboratory and has come to collect a blood sample. Sometimes, the health care worker may need to explain to the patient that the physician ordered the laboratory test or tests. The health care worker may also need to explain the procedure as supplies are being set up or as gloves are put on. During setup, the specimen collection tray should not be placed on the patient's bed or eating table. As supplies are being readied and the vein is being palpated, the health care worker may try to alleviate some of the patient's fears. It may be reassuring if the phlebotomist purposefully shows the patient that the supplies are "new" and "unused." Chapter 1

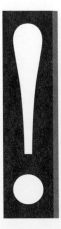

Clinical Alert

If a physician or nurse is consulting with the patient when the phlebotomist enters the room, the specimen collection procedure should be delayed until the consultation is completed. The **physician-patient relationship** has priority over a phlebotomy procedure unless the request is for a timed or stat specimen. In this case, the phlebotomist may ask permission to proceed.

Box 9–8   Typical Health Care Worker/Patient Interaction

The following scenario depicts a phlebotomist and patient interaction just prior to the blood collection. It begins when the phlebotomist knocks on the patient's door and slowly enters the room.

Health care worker: Good morning. I am Ms. Smith from the laboratory. I have come to collect a blood sample.

Pause to give the patient an opportunity to speak. If the lights are off or dimmed, explain that you need to turn the lights on. Doing so gives the patient a moment to adjust to the idea of bright lights if he or she has been asleep.

Health care worker: What is your name, please? (In general, it is not wise to ask a patient "How are you?" because most patients in the hospital do not feel well.)
Patient: I am John Jones.
Health care worker: May I please see your identification (ID) armband?

Check armband against laboratory requisitions and patient's verbal identification. If all three match, proceed.

Health care worker: This will take only a few minutes.
Patient: Will it hurt?
Health care worker: It will hurt a little, but it will be over soon. Please allow me to look at your arm veins.

Proceed with the remainder of the procedure, maintaining a highly professional atmosphere and a respectful attitude.
For certain tests, you may need to ascertain whether the patient has been fasting.

Health care worker: Mr. Jones, when was the last time you ate or drank anything? (Do not use the term fast because some patients may not understand it completely.)

As supplies are being "readied," the health care worker could demonstrate that she is opening a new needle. She should also inquire about latex-sensitivity if using latex products (gloves or tourniquet).

Health care worker: Mr. Jones, please notice that I will be using a new needle to collect your blood sample.

At the end of the procedure, say the following:

Health care worker: Thank you, Mr. Jones.

---

covers verbal and nonverbal cues for detecting apprehension in patients. Box 9–8 presents a typical scenario of a health care worker–patient interaction.

Refer to Figures 9–4 ■ and 9–5 ■ and Chapter 8 for more information about blood collection chairs. A slight rotation of the patient's arm or hand may help expose a vein and prevent it from rolling as the needle is inserted. The visibility of veins varies with each individual's skin color, weight, physiologic conditions, gender, and physical features (Refer to Figure 9–6 ■). Therefore, the health care worker must rely on the sense of touch (palpation) to locate the vein. A pillow, or an arm-resting device may be used for arm support of a weak, bedridden patient or for ambulatory patients to adjust to a more comfortable position. If there are no other suitable arm supports, the patient's free wrist can be used to cushion the arm being punctured. Collection equipment and supplies should be placed in

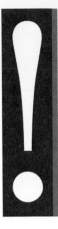

Clinical Alert

Proper positioning is important to both the health care worker and the patient for a successful venipuncture or skin puncture, and efforts to make sure that the patient is comfortable are worthwhile. Patients should not stand or sit on high stools during the procedure because of the possibility of fainting. A reclining (supine) position is preferred; however, sitting in a sturdy, comfortable chair with arm supports is also acceptable. The health care worker can position him- or herself in front of the chair to protect the patient from falling forward in the event of fainting. The patient should not have anything (e.g., food, chewing gum, or a thermometer) in their mouth during the venipuncture procedure.

an accessible spot where they are unlikely to be disturbed by the patient. The phlebotomist can then palpate and trace the path of veins with an index finger.

EQUIPMENT SELECTION AND PREPARATION
SUPPLIES FOR VENIPUNCTURE

Supplies for venipuncture differ according to the method used (i.e., evacuated tube system or winged infusion/butterfly system, or syringe method) and the tests that have been ordered. Supplies common to most methods of blood collection are the following:

- Gloves
- Tourniquet
- Alcohol pads or other skin disinfectants
- Non alcohol cleansers if blood alcohol levels are requested
- 1–10% povidone iodine pads or chlorhexidine disinfectants if blood cultures are requested.
- Bandages or gauze pads
- Glass microscope slides
- Needles with single-use, evacuated tube holders and winged infusion sets
- Plastic capillary tubes with tube sealer
- Syringes and syringe transfer devices
- Blood collection tubes
- Laboratory requisitions or labels
- Marking pens
- Puncture-proof sharps container

Supplies should be readily available and selected just prior to the procedure. Supplies are discussed in more detail in Chapter 8.

POSITIONING OF THE PATIENT AND VENIPUNCTURE SITE SELECTION

It is important to choose the least hazardous site for blood collection by skin puncture or venipuncture. Several techniques can facilitate the selection of a suitable site. For details about the positions and locations of veins, refer to Figures 9–7 ■, 9–8 ■, and 9–9 ■.

Figure 9–4. Blood Collection Chairs

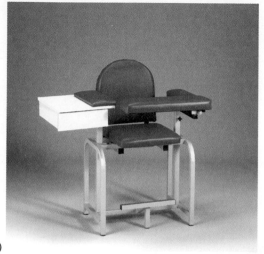

(a)

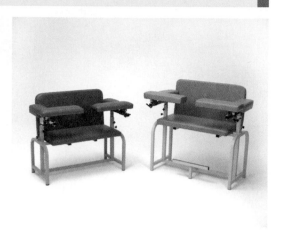

(b)

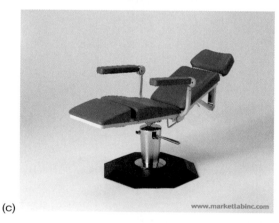

www.marketlabinc.com

(c)

a. Extra-tall chairs are advantageous for the phlebotomist because they eliminate "stooping over" a chair during the procedure. It should be used for patients who have greatest mobility and are not likely to loose balance or have trouble getting in or out of the chair.

b. Extra-wide chairs for large and/or obese patients.

c. Recliner-style chair.

Courtesy of Clinton Industries, Inc., and MarketLab, Inc., Kentwood, Michigan, 800-237-3604, www.marketlab.com, with permission.

Figure 9-5. Devices to Assist in Positioning the Patient and Supplies

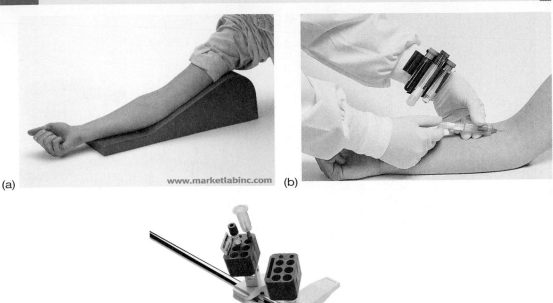

(a)

www.marketlabinc.com

(b)

(c)

a. A phlebotomy wedge is used to stabilize and cushion the arm in a comfortable position.

b. This tube holder fits on the phlebotomist's wrist to keep blood collection tubes immediately available during and after the procedure.

c. This tube holder provides a temporary and easy-to-access device that holds the tubes in an upright position.

Courtesy of Clinton Industries, Inc., and MarketLab, Inc., Kentwood, Michigan, 800-237-3604, www.marketlab.com, with permission.

The most common sites for venipuncture are in the antecubital area of the arm just below the bend of the elbow. This is where the median cubital, cephalic, and basilic veins lie close to the surface of the skin and are most prominent. The median cubital, often referred to as the median vein, is the most commonly used vein for venipuncture because it is the easiest to obtain blood from and has been reported to be less painful;[10] the second choice of vein should be the cephalic vein, which lies on the outer edge of the arm; and the third choice should be the basilic vein, which lies on the inside edge of the anticubital fossa area. The basilic vein is in close proximity to the median nerve and the brachial artery so the other choices are usually preferable.

Palpating the anticubital area usually helps the health care worker get an idea of the size, angle, and depth of the vein. The patient can assist in the process by opening and closing

Figure 9–6. Individual Vein Variations in the Hand and Arm

Visible vein patterns are dramatically different among individuals. Phlebotomists learn to visualize but, more importantly, feel the veins prior to venipuncture.

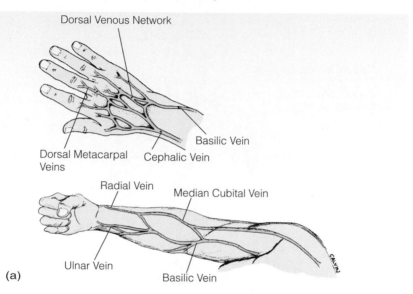

(a)

a. A typical human arm labeled with prominent veins.

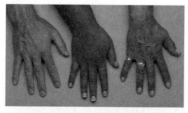

(b)

b. Dorsal hand veins show up in different locations and in varying degrees of visibility in the three hands. The first is a young adult white male; the other two are African American females, one young adult and one middle-aged. Note the variability in skin tones as well.

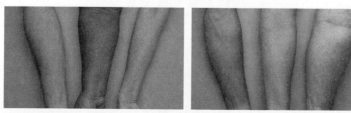

(c)

c. These six arms are all of different aged adults with varying skin tones, muscle mass, fatty tissue, and bone structure. Note that in the arms with more muscle mass and fatty tissue, the veins are hardly visible at all. In these cases, the phlebotomist must rely on feeling the vein rather than seeing it.

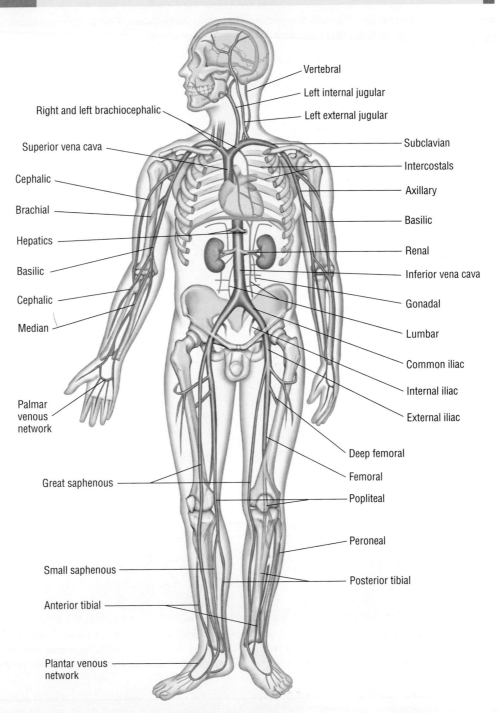

Figure 9–7. An Overview of the Venous System

Figure 9–8. Venous Drainage of the Abdomen and Chest

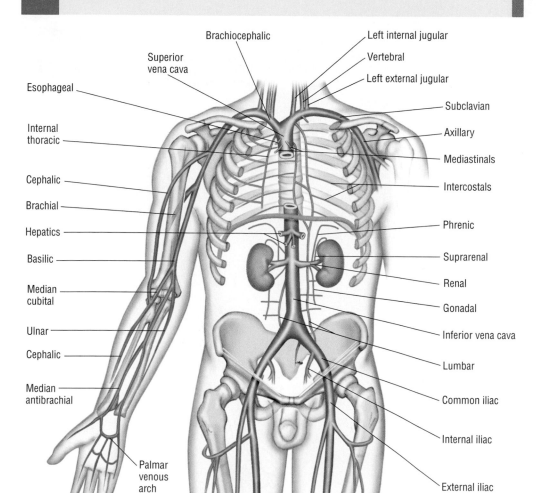

Brachiocephalic

Superior vena cava

Esophageal

Internal thoracic

Cephalic

Brachial

Hepatics

Basilic

Median cubital

Ulnar

Cephalic

Median antibrachial

Palmar venous arch

Left internal jugular

Vertebral

Left external jugular

Subclavian

Axillary

Mediastinals

Intercostals

Phrenic

Suprarenal

Renal

Gonadal

Inferior vena cava

Lumbar

Common iliac

Internal iliac

External iliac

the fist tightly.[1] It is important to remember that veins may also be used for transfusion, infusion, and therapeutic agents. Thus, sometimes physicians request that veins have restricted use ("reserved") for those purposes only.

Veins on the dorsal side of the hands or wrists (i.e. the back side), are acceptable venipuncture sites if the median cubital, cephalic, or basilic veins are inaccessible. Veins in the wrist or ankle tend to move, or roll aside, as the needle is inserted; therefore, it may be helpful to have the patient extend the foot or hand into a position that helps hold the vein taut (see Fig. 9–10 ■).

Ankle and foot veins (on the dorsal, or upper, side) should be used *only* if arm veins have been determined to be unsuitable. Arm veins are sites preferred over foot or ankle veins

Figure 9-9. Veins Arteries, and Nerves of the Arm

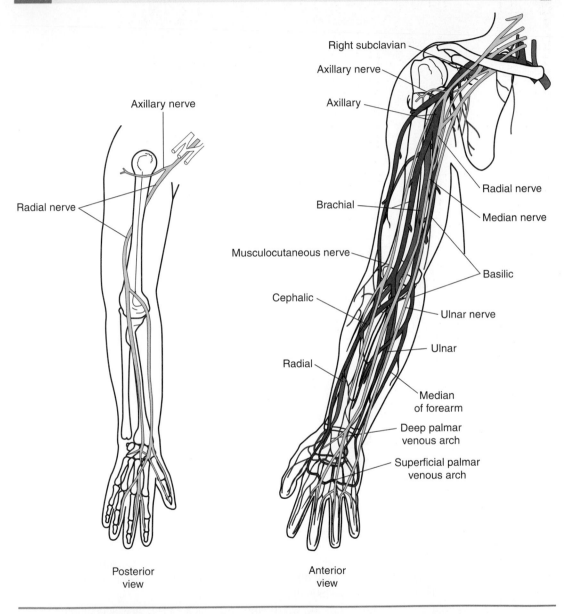

Posterior
view

Anterior
view

because coagulation and vascular complications tend to be more troublesome in the lower extremities, especially for diabetic patients. Some hospitals do not allow health care workers to use the lower extremities (foot and ankle) for blood-sampling sites. Other hospitals allow sampling from these sites only after permission is granted from the patient's physician. Venipuncture in small veins is facilitated by the use of a 21- to 25-gauge safety butterfly needle.

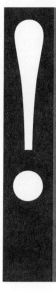

Clinical Alert

Nerve damage during a venipuncture is rare but has been known to occur due to excessive needle probing, sudden movements of the patient, etc. Serious damage can occur if a nerve is accidently punctured or nicked during the venipuncture procedure. If the patient complains of severe pain during the procedure, the needle must be removed *immediately* and the procedure discontinued, and assistance should be sought from a nurse or supervisor. Only a physician can evaluate whether or not nerve damage has occurred. Nevertheless, the incident should be documented. Figure 9–9 depicts the proximity of nerves in relation to the veins.

It is also important to know that arteries do not feel like veins. Arteries pulsate, are more elastic, and have a thick wall. Accidental arterial puncture may result in excessive bleeding and hematoma formation. If the phlebotomist believes she has punctured an artery, the needle should be removed immediately, direct pressure should be applied to the site for at least 5 minutes or until bleeding has stopped.[1] A supervisor or nurse should be notified.

WARMING THE PUNCTURE SITE

Warming the puncture site helps facilitate phlebotomy by increasing arterial blood flow to the area and, in some cases, by making the veins more prominent. Several warming devices are available commercially that are quick and easy to activate and provide localized heat to the potential venipuncture area (Refer to Figure 9–11 ■).

Another method is to use a clean towel or a washcloth heated to about 42°C. When the warm towel is wrapped around the site for 3 to 5 minutes, the skin temperature can increase several degrees. The wrap can be encased in a plastic bag to help retain heat and keep the patient's bed dry. The health care worker may leave the warm wrap on the patient while he or she collects specimens from other patients, and then return to the original patient after several minutes.

Clinical Alert

Reasons for not using the patient's arm veins include the following:

- Intravenous (IV) lines in both arms
- Burned or scarred areas
- Areas with a hematoma
- Cast(s) on arm(s)
- Thrombosed veins (Thrombosed veins lack resilience, feel much like a rope cord, and roll easily.)
- Edematous arms (swollen area due to excessive amounts of tissue fluids)
- Partial or radical mastectomy on one or both sides

Figure 9–10. Dorsal Hand Veins

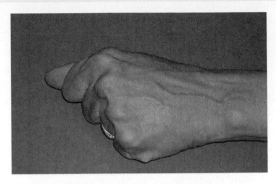

Hand veins are more prominent if the hand is held taut.

Clinical Alert

For hand vein punctures, the posterior, or dorsal, surface of the wrist (the back of the hand) should be used. Do *not* use the anterior side or the palmar venous network in the wrist, because nerves lie very close to the palmar venous network and can easily be injured by needle probing.

Clinical Alert

Patients who have had mastectomies often have lymph nodes removed from the same surgical area. Without lymph vessels to remove fluid, swelling occurs on the affected side of the body. Thus, blood should not be withdrawn from the mastectomy side unless approved by the physician.[11]

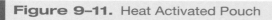

Figure 9–11. Heat Activated Pouch

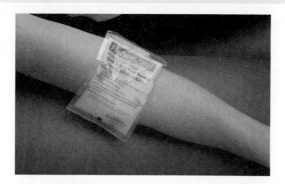

TOURNIQUET APPLICATION

A tourniquet or blood pressure cuff makes veins more prominent and easier to puncture by causing venous filling: the tourniquet slows down blood flow toward the heart so it gathers in the veins.[1] A soft rubber tourniquet about 1 inch (2.5 cm) wide and about 15 to 18 inches (45 cm) long is most comfortable for patients, affordable, and easy to use for phlebotomists. Tourniquets come in a variety of colors, as shown in Procedure 9–3.

DECONTAMINATION OF THE PUNCTURE SITE

Once the site is selected, it should be decontaminated with a gauze pad soaked in 70 percent isopropanol (isopropyl alcohol), or with a commercially packaged alcohol pad. This prevents microbiological contamination of the patient and the specimen. The health care worker should rub the site, working in concentric circles from the inside out. If the skin is particularly dirty, the process should be repeated with a new alcohol pad. The health care worker should also decontaminate his or her own gloved finger if he or she intends to palpate the site again. The site should be air-dried.

Povidone–iodine (Betadine) or iodine preparations are primarily used for drawing blood for blood gas analysis and blood cultures (see Chapter 14, "Arterial, Intravenous (IV), and

! Clinical Alert

The tourniquet should not be left on for more than 1 minute, because it becomes uncomfortable and causes hemoconcentration—that is, increased blood concentration of large molecules, such as proteins, cells, and coagulation factors. The patient may be asked to clench and unclench the fist only a few times because excessive clenching also results in hemoconcentration. If no vein becomes apparent, or "pops up," the patient may be asked to dangle the arm for 1 to 2 minutes to allow blood to fill the veins to capacity, then the tourniquet may be reapplied and the area palpated again. The health care worker should never stick a vein unless it can be felt. It is better to defer the patient to someone else who can search for the vein than to take a blind chance.

Procedure 9–3   Use of a Tourniquet

1. A clean latex-free tourniquet should be used (Fig. 9–12a ■).

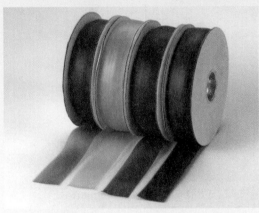

Figure 9–12a Courtesy of MarketLab, Inc., Kentwood, MI, 800-237-3604, www.marketlab.com

2. Stretch the ends of the tourniquet around the patient's arm about 3 inches (7.6 cm) above the venipuncture area (antecubital area). Both ends of the tourniquet can be held in one hand while the other hand tucks in a section next to the skin and makes a partial loop with the tourniquet (Fig. 9–12b ■).

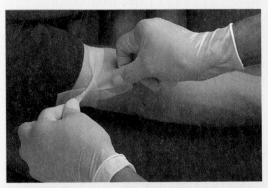

Figure 9–12b

3. The tourniquet should be tight but not painful to the patient. It should not be left on more than 1 minute. It should *not* be placed over sores or burned skin; however, depending on the policies of each health care facility, it may be placed over a hospital gown sleeve or a piece of gauze.

4. When it is time to release the tourniquet, the partial loop should allow for easy release by the health care worker. For patient comfort and to obtain a good specimen it should be released while the phlebotomist is getting supplies ready to perform the initial puncture, especially if the process takes longer than 1 minute. The tourniquet should then be reapplied and released after the puncture when blood has begun to flow into the collection tubes. During the venipuncture, the health care worker should be able to release the tourniquet with one hand because the other hand will be holding the needle and tubes.

5. Once released it can remain loosely on the arm or surface of the work area (e.g., bed or blood collection chair) until the procedure is completed (Fig. 9–12c ■).

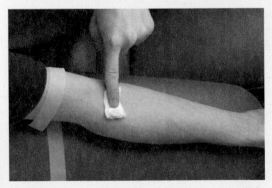

Figure 9–12c

Clinical Alert

The decontaminated area should never be touched with any nonsterile object. The alcohol should be allowed to dry (approximately 30 to 60 seconds) or should be wiped off with sterile gauze or cotton after the site is prepared; otherwise, the puncture site will sting, and the alcohol may interfere with test results, such as blood alcohol levels. Blowing on the site to hasten the drying process is not advised because doing so may recontaminate the site.

Special Collection Procedures"). For some patients, iodine causes skin irritation. Efforts should be made to remove iodine from the skin with sterile gauze or alcohol after decontamination, because excess iodine can interfere with some laboratory tests. For patients who are allergic to both iodine and/or alcohol, chlorohexidine has been reported as an alternative skin decontaminant with removal of excess solution using sterile saline.[12]

▄▄▄▄ VENIPUNCTURE METHODS

EVACUATED TUBE SYSTEM AND
WINGED INFUSION SYSTEM, OR BUTTERFLY METHOD

NCCLS recommends that venipuncture specimens be collected with a system that enables blood to flow directly into the tubes.[1] Evacuated tube systems and winged infusion systems are widely available, equipped with safety devices and comply with this recommendation. Procedure 9–4 on pp. 272–274 demonstrates a basic venipuncture technique.

Phlebotomists should note that while the procedural steps for the puncture are the same for the evacuated tube system and the winged-infusion system, there may be different steps to follow as the tubes are acutally filled. Since the tubing from the winged infusion system contains air, it will underfill the first evacuated tube by 0.5 mL, thus affecting the additive-to-blood ratio. Therefore, a red-topped nonadditive tube should be filled prior to any tube with additives. After the first tube, the order of the tube draw should be the same as other methods. When tubes for coagulation are the only ones to be collected, it is suggested that a "dummy" tube be collected and discarded. This fills the tubing with blood so that the correct additive-to-blood ratio is obtained for the following coagulation tube. When using the winged infusion system, each tube should be held horizontally or slightly down to avoid transfer of additives from one tube to the next. It is also suggested that small evacuated collection tubes (i.e., 13 × 75 mm or 4 ml) be used with winged infusion sets to avoid collapsing fragile veins. If using a syringe attached to the Luer adapter, a small syringe, such as 5 or 10 ml, should be used for the same reason. Usually a 21- or 23-gauge needle is better than a 25-gauge needle because the small diameter may lead to hemolysis as the specimen is withdrawn. For an infant, however, the 25-gauge needle is the best choice (for small veins).

Procedure 9-4   Performing a Venipuncture

Supplies:

Gloves

Evacuated specimen tubes

Needles (for evacuated tube holders and winged-infusion/butterfly sets)

Tube holders

Tourniquet

70% isopropyl alcohol pads

Gauze pads

Blood culture decontamination kits (if blood cultures are requested)

Bandages

Venipuncture can be accomplished by using either an evacuated tube system or a winged-infusion/butterfly needle system. The steps listed below are typical for either venipuncture system.

1. After greeting and identifying the patient, decontaminate hands, don gloves, and prepare equipment, preferably in the presence of the patient. Offer to answer any questions for the patient. (Fig. 9–13a ■)

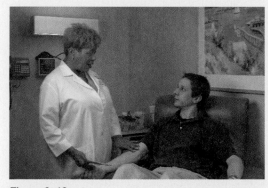

Figure 9–13a

2. Prepare equipment according to the manufacturer's instructions, including attaching a needle onto the appropriate holder. For an evacuated tube system, the most commonly used, the needle is threaded directly onto the tube holder. For a winged-infusion or butterfly apparatus, the smaller needle (1/2 to 3/4 inch in length and

21–25 guage in diameter) comes attached to a thin tubing with a luer adapter which, in turn, must be attached to a tube holder.

3. Position the patient's arm slightly bent, in a downward but comfortable manner. Apply the tourniquet and check for potential sites by palpating the vein. Feel for the median cubital vein first (it is usually bigger and anchored better); the cephalic vein (depending on its size) is the second choice (it does not roll and bruise as easily as the basilic); and the basilic vein is third choice. If a suitable vein is not felt, remove the tourniquet and try the other arm or other sites mentioned in the text. Remember, do not leave the tourniquet on for more than 1 minute. Choose a vein that feels the fullest. Other strageties to improve vein selection include warming the site and lowering the arm further in a downward position. (Fig. 9–13b ■)

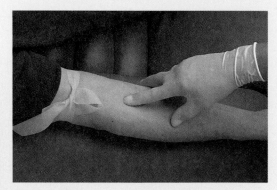

Figure 9–13b

4. Select the site and decontaminate the patient's skin with an alcohol pad in a circular motion from in to outside. Allow it to air dry and do not blow on it. Ask the patient to "please close your fist" to make veins more prominent and easier to puncture. Vigorous hand exercise or "pumping" should be avoided because it affects some laboratory values. Never say "this will not hurt"; simply mention to the patient that he or she will "feel a stick" or say, "please remain still while I begin the procedure, you will feel a slight prick." Be mindful that from

Procedure 9-4 *(continued)*

this step forward a patient may feel faint and/or lose consciousness. (Fig. 9–13c ■)

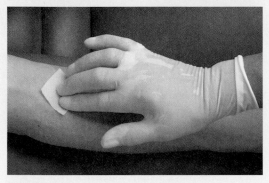

Figure 9–13c

5. Hold the patient's arm below the site, pulling the skin tightly but comfortably with the thumb. Remove the needle cap carefully so as not to touch anything that would contaminate it. If it does touch any surface that is not sterile, replace it with a new needle assembly and discard the old one. Hold the needle assembly in one hand while the thumb of the other hand anchors the vein 1-2 inches below the puncture site. Position the needle so that it is parallel or running in the same direction as the vein. Insert the needle quickly, with the bevel side up, and at a 15-30 degree angle with the skin. A slight "pop" should be felt as the needle enters the vein. (Fig. 9–13d ■)

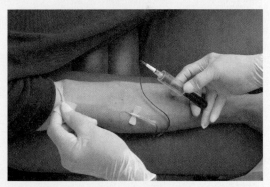

Figure 9–13d

6. If blood does not flow, palpate gently above the puncture to feel for the vein and possibly reorient the needle slightly. Do not probe!

7. As the blood begins to flow, instruct the patient to open his/her fist, and release the tourniquet. (The tourniquet can be left on until after the tubes have filled if it appears that blood flow is slow, however always remove it before withdrawing the needle.) Carefully push an evacuated tube into the holder so that the tube closure is punctured by the inside needle and blood can enter. Orient the tube in a downward position so as to avoid any possibility of backflow. (Fig. 9–13e ■)

Figure 9–13e

8. Allow the blood to flow into the tube until it stops so that the proper dilution of blood to additive can occur. Watch carefully to see when the blood flow ceases. If multiple sample tubes are to be collected, remove each tube from the holder with a gentle twist-and-pull motion and replace it with the next tube. (During tube transfer be mindful of these key issues: hold the needle apparatus firmly and motionlessly so that the needle remains comfortable and in the vein during tube changes, follow the correct order of draw, and remember that blood stops flowing between tube changes because of the inner needle design which

continued

Procedure 9–4   *(continued)*

allows a sleeve to block flow if it is not in use.) Experienced phlebotomists can gently mix/invert a full tube in one hand while holding the needle apparatus and waiting for another tube to fill. Some phlebotomists switch hands to use a dominant hand during tube exchange. Whatever the case, find the approach that is most reliable and comfortable for both patient and phlebotomist.

9. When all tubes have been filled and removed from the holder, withdraw the needle, and hold a gauze pad over the site. (Fig. 9–13f ■)

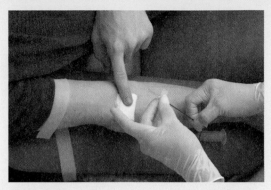

Figure 9–13g

11. Apply pressure until the bleeding has stopped. Label specimens appropriately (patient's first and last name, identification number, date, time of collection, and phlebotomists initials). Dispose of contaminated supplies and equipment. Double-check to make sure that the bleeding has stopped and apply a bandage, if appropriate. Thank the patient for cooperating and depart with all specimens and remaining supplies. (Fig. 9–13h ■)

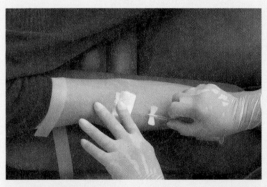

Figure 9–13f

10. Activate the safety device according to the manufacturer's instructions. This may involve resheathing/covering the needle once it has been withdrawn or rotating a device that renders the needle blunt prior to withdrawal from the vein. Instruct the patient to apply pressure to the site using the gauze. (If necessary, continue gentle inversion of the specimen tubes for complete mixing of additives with the blood. Remember do not shake the tubes.) (Fig. 9–13g ■)

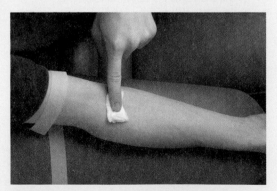

Figure 9–13h

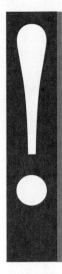

Clinical Alert

A winged infusion system, butterfly needle assembly, or scalp needle set can be used for certain patient populations or for particularly difficult venipunctures. This type of method may be useful in the following circumstances:

- Patients with small veins (hand or wrist)
- Pediatric patients
- Geriatric patients
- Patients having numerous needlesticks (e.g., cancer patients)
- Patients in restrictive positions (e.g., traction, severe arthritis)
- Patients who are severely burned
- Patients with fragile skin and veins
- Patients who specifically request it because they feel it is less painful
- Short-term infusion therapy.

Health care workers should be extra cautious as the butterfly needle apparatus is removed from the patient because it tends to hang loose on the end of the tubing, and may sometimes recoil back unexpectedly. Therefore, the safety device that is built into the system should be activated immediately. Use of winged infusion or butterfly systems requires training and practice, but they are widely used because patients report that they are less painful than other methods. Use of this system may be more hazardous for health care workers than the use of conventional needles. Failure to activate the safety devices correctly as described by the manufacturers may result in a higher incidence of needlestick injuries.

SYRINGE METHOD

Syringes are *not* routinely used for venipuncture. Reasons for this include many safety concerns and issues of accidental cross-contamination of anticoagulants if the blood specimen is injected into multiple evacuated tubes using the same needle and syringe. If the syringe method is to be used, recommendations are as follows:[1]

- Use a syringe with a safety device.
- Before the needle is inserted, the plunger should be moved back and forth to allow for free movement and to expel all air.
- The same approach to needle insertion should take place as is used for the evacuated tube method.
- Once the needle is in the vein, the syringe plunger can be drawn back slowly until the required amount of blood is drawn. (It may be helpful to turn the syringe slightly so that the graduated markings are visible.)
- Care must be taken not to accidentally withdraw the needle while pulling back on the plunger and not to pull hard enough to cause hemolysis (i.e., rupture of the cells) or collapse of the vein.
- After tourniquet release and collection of the appropriate amount of blood, the entire needle assembly should be withdrawn quickly and the safety device should be activated immediately, depending on the manufacturer's specifications.

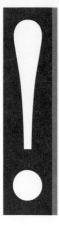

Clinical Alert

When all tubes have been filled, the needle should be carefully but quickly withdrawn. Depending on the needle manufacturer's instructions the safety device should be activated. To minimize hazards, a syringe transfer device must be use to move the sample from the syringe into the tubes.

- The needle or winged collection set should be removed and discarded appropriately.
- Evacuated tubes for testing should be immediately filled using a syringe transfer device.
- The tubes should fill until flow stops; there is no need to push the plunger to expel blood.
- Tubes should be filled in the same order as for the evacuated tube method.

BANDAGE FOR THE PUNCTURE SITE

A dry, sterile gauze should be applied with pressure to the puncture site for several minutes or until bleeding has ceased. If the patient has a free hand, he or she may be asked to apply the pressure. The patient's arm may be kept straight, slightly bent at the elbow, or elevated slightly above the heart. A bandage should be applied, and the patient should be instructed to leave it on for at least 15 minutes. If the patient continues to bleed, the phlebotomist should apply pressure her- or himself until the bleeding stops. A gauze bandage can then be applied, and the patient should be instructed to leave it on for at least 15 minutes. If the patient continues to bleed, a nurse and/or supervisor should be notified.

PROPER DISPOSAL

All disposable or contaminated equipment should be discarded into appropriate containers. Paper and plastic wrappers can be thrown into a wastebasket. Needles and lancets should not be thrown into a wastebasket, however, but into a sturdy, punctureproof, disposable

Clinical Alert

The phlebotomist should not panic if blood does not flow immediately after the puncture is made. The following suggestions may help:[1]

- Change the needle position *slightly, but do not probe;* that is, pull *gently* outward, push *gently* forward, or rotate so that the bevel is positioned in the vein. These should be minute movements so as to minimize the risk of complications.
- Replace the tube with another evacuated tube in case the first one is defective.
- Attempt the collection from another site but do not make more than 2 attempts.

Refer to Chapter 11 for more information about complications during the blood collection procedure.

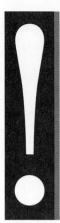

Clinical Alert: Use Once and Discard Immediately

Needles, lancets, syringes, and other bloodletting devices—"sharps"—that are capable of transmitting infection from one person to another should be used only *once,* then immediately discarded. Sharps must be discarded in puncture-resistant containers that are easily accessible, located in areas where they are commonly used, and have proper warning labels. "Shearing" or "breaking" of contaminated sharps is illegal and strictly prohibited. Bending, recapping, or removing contaminated needles is not acceptable practice.

OSHA also suggests that blood tube holders should be used only once due to the potential needlestick hazards associated with the double-ended needle at and after disposal.[13]

container to be autoclaved or incinerated. Any items that have been contaminated with blood should be disposed of in biohazardous disposal containers as explained in the universal precautions (Refer to Chapter 5, "Infection Control" and Chapter 8, "Blood Collection Equipment.")

ORDER OF TUBE COLLECTION

Multiple blood assays are often ordered on patients. There are guidelines for delivery of blood into the proper collection tubes based on the method of venipuncture used, the types of tubes or additives needed for testing, and specific manufacturer's instructions. A specified "order of draw" is important in reducing the effects of additive carry-over cross-contamination from one tube to the next. Carry-over of additives can cause erroneous laboratory results. Each laboratory should document their practices and provide continuing education about the order of draw.

Box 9-9	Order of Draw for Blood Collection Tubes

Revised "order of draw" recommendations from the National Committee for Clinical Laboratory Standards (NCCLS) were published in 2003. They recommend the following specific order when collecting blood in multiple tubes (either glass or plastic) via the evacuated method or the syringe transfer method:[1,14]

1. Blood culture tubes (yellow closure) or blood culture vials. Blood cultures are always drawn first after special skin decontamination procedures to decrease the possibility of bacterial contamination. (The procedure for collection of blood cultures is discussed in Chapter 13 in greater detail.)

2. Coagulation tube (sodium citrate) (light blue closure)

3. Serum tube, with or without clot activator, with or without gel (red, speckled closure). (Glass, nonadditive serum tubes can be filled before the coagulation tube. However, plastic serum tubes containing a clot actiator may interfere with coagulation tests.)

4. Heparin tube (green closure) with or without gel plasma separator

5. EDTA tube (purple/lavender closure)

6. Glycolytic inhibition tube (potassium oxalate/sodium fluoride or lithium iodoacetate/heparin) (gray closure)

> **Box 9–10   A Note about Manufacturers of Blood Collection Tubes**
>
> As mentioned in previous chapters, there are numerous manufacturers of blood collection tubes and related supplies including, but not limited to, Becton Dickinson Vacutainer Systems, *Preanalytical Solutions,* and Greiner. These companies maintain websites (www.bd.com and www.vacuette.com, respectively) that provide updates and recommendations on new devices and how to use them. (Refer to Chapter 8 for other sources.) For example, Becton Dickinson provides color charts for their recommended order of draw. Generally speaking, they follow the NCCLS guideline but include additional information on specific additive tubes that are available from their company. It is important for laboratories to stay updated on specific procedural modifications that relate to the products that they buy.

SPECIMEN IDENTIFICATION AND LABELING

No foolproof method exists for labeling specimens. However, firmly attached, completed labels should be attached *prior* to leaving the patient. Labels must accompany all blood specimens.

ASSESSING THE PATIENT BEFORE LEAVING

Before leaving the patient's side, the phlebotomist must

- Check the puncture site to make sure that the bleeding stopped;
- Apply an adhesive bandage if the patient is agreeable;

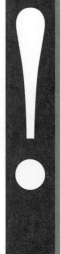

Clinical Alert: Special Considerations for Coagulation Testing

- The coagulation specimen should be the second or third tube drawn when multiple tubes are collected.
- Whenever coagulation tests (prothrombin time, PT, partial thromboplastin time, PTT) are the sole tests ordered, accurate results can be obtained using one tube.[9] (Until recently most phlebotomy practices required that at least one other tube of blood be drawn and discarded before the coagulation test specimen so as to diminish contamination with tissue fluids that could initiate the clotting sequence.) Each health care worker should use the procedure adopted by his or her own facility. However, if coagulation studies are the *only* tests ordered, and a *winged infusion (butterfly) system* is to be used for collection, a "discard" tube should be collected before drawing the citrate tube. This is the only way to rid the specimen of the air in the winged infusion tubing. If this air in the "dead space" enters the citrate tube, it causes an inaccurate blood to citrate ratio.
- Since coagulation tests require a specific plasma concentration of sodium citrate, "overfilling" the tube causes artificial results indicating short clotting times.
- If a tube is "underfilled" the opposite occurs and artificial results indicate prolonged clotting times.
- Immediately after collection coagulation tubes should be mixed gently to prevent clotting in the tube. However, an excessive number of inversions or vigorous mixing can lead to platelet activation and shortening of clotting times when tested.[1,9,15,16,17]

Box 9–11   Other Issues Related to Filling the Blood Collection Tubes

- *During the venipuncture procedure, care should be taken so that the additive or anticoagulant present in one tube does not come into contact with the multisample needle as the tubes are changed.* To minimize transfer of anticoagulants from tube to tube, holding the tube horizontally or slightly downward during blood collection is recommended. If an anticoagulant is inadvertently carried into the next tube it may cause erroneous test results. For example, it is recommended that blood for serum iron be drawn before other specimens with chelating anticoagulants (e.g., EDTA). This will avoid interference in testing the serum iron level. Also, electrolyte determinations include measurement of potassium (K) and sodium (Na). Since the chelating anticoagulant EDTA is usually bound to potassium as EDTA (K_3) or to sodium (Na) as EDTA (Na_2), it is important to collect specimens that require EDTA after a specimen is collected in heparin for electrolytes. The K_3 and Na_2 from the EDTA may falsely elevate the patient's K or Na values.

- *Be attentive to the "fill" rate and volume in each tube.* This is discussed more fully in Chapter 8. Evacuated tubes with anticoagulants must be filled to the designated level for the proper mix of blood with the anticoagulant ie., the blood-additive ratio. "Partial-fill" tubes are available when it is suspected that the blood specimen will not be adequate.

- Although the use of a syringe should be restricted to special cases, occasionally a large volume (more than 20 mL) of blood needs to be drawn using a syringe. Closures on the tubes should not be removed, and a safety-syringe-shielded transfer device should be used to transfer the blood into the tubes. *In order to prevent accidental needlesticks, the tubes should not be held by hand during the transfer.*

- Occasionally, especially when large amounts of blood are collected in a syringe, there is a possibility that some of the blood may be clotted. If clotting occurs in the needle, it can be carefully removed from the hub of the syringe, the top can be removed from the tube, and then the blood can be carefully expelled into the tube. Again, it is suggested that the tube be filled by letting the blood run gently, not forcefully, down the inside of the tube to avoid hemolysis. If two syringes of blood have been withdrawn, NCCLS recommends taking blood from the second syringe for coagulation studies.[1]

Box 9–12   Labels for Blood Specimens

Specimens should be labeled (using adhesive and/or barcoded labels) immediately at the patient's bedside or ambulatory setting prior to leaving the patient. Laboratory procedure manuals should contain explicit instructions on labeling requirements, and supervisors should spend ample time not only training new employees in correct identification and labeling practices, but also observing as they perform the steps.

The phlebotomist may write directly on the container. Commercial collection tubes may have affixed blank labels for this purpose. Similarly, hospitals often use computer-generated labels for collection tubes; however, capillary tubes, microcollection tubes and vials, or other containers without labels must be identified, either by labeling them directly with a permanent felt-tipped pen, wrapping an adhesive label around them, or placing them into a larger labeled test tube for transport. In some cases, small computerized adhesive labels with printed information are available with and detachable from the requisition form.

Specimen labels should consistently include the following information:[1,2]

1. Patient's full name

2. Patient's identification number

3. Date of collection

4. Time of collection

5. Health care worker's initials

6. Patient's room number, bed assignment, or outpatient status (optional)

Clinical Alert

Tubes should not be prelabeled, because if they are then not used, they may be erroneously picked up and used for another patient. Also, a different health care worker may complete the venipuncture if the initial health care worker is unsuccessful. In that case, the prelabeled tubes may display the initials of the first health care worker and, therefore, be inaccurate. In addition, if the prelabeled tubes are not used, tearing off the old or unused label may be difficult because of the adhesive; thus, either a new label (from a different patient) would have to be placed on the tube with a partially torn label, or the unused tube would have to be discarded. Either option is unsatisfactory, messy, and wasteful.

- Ensure that all tubes are appropriately labeled;
- Decontaminate hands again;
- Remove or appropriately discard supplies and equipment that were brought in; and
- Thank the patient.

The specimen can then be transported in an appropriate container. Considerations for specimen transportation and handling are covered in Chapter 7.

 ## PRIORITIZING PATIENTS

In the course of a day's work at a busy hospital or clinic, a health care worker may have to make decisions about the order in which blood work is obtained. Priorities must be set and adhered to, whether they concern the order in which certain blood tests are drawn on a particular patient or which patients are to be drawn first from among a group. If these distinctions are not made properly, test results can be affected and interpretation of the results may be difficult.

Clinical Alert

- The health care worker should always decontaminate hands, thank the patient, and ensure that all the information on the label is complete and correct before leaving the patient's hospital room or before drawing blood from another clinic outpatient.
- The date and time are necessary information because physicians need to know exactly when the specimen was drawn so that they may correlate results with any medications given or with changes in the patient's condition. Requisition forms only indicate the date and time when a laboratory test was ordered, rather than the date and time when it was collected.
- The health care worker's initials are necessary to help clarify questions about the specimen if any arise during laboratory processing or testing.

Box 9-13   Other Ideas for Improving Venipuncture Practices

All members of the health care team members should strive to reduce the total number of daily phlebotomies and the amount of blood collected daily. One study done in a surgical intensive care unit (SICU) reported daily blood losses of up to 29.5 mL prior to implementing improvement measures. After reorganizing test practices, blood loss volumes decreased by 12.5 mL.[18] A few suggestions include:

- Coordination of laboratory requests among *all* staff physicians working with the patient to reduce duplicate and triplicate laboratory orders.
- Nurses and ward secretaries could organize laboratory orders as much as possible to avoid sending frequent requests minutes apart.
- When orders are transcribed or entered into the computer, all should be requested at the same time.
- Possible modifications to laboratory testing panels and better education of physicians to be aware of all the tests on each laboratory panel.
- The laboratory could be notified when multiple timed tests are ordered. For example, if a patient needs a hemoglobin test at 2:00 P.M. and a glucose test at 3:00 P.M., coordinating the times and drawing both specimens during one venipuncture may be possible.
- Reassessment of STAT test orders to make sure they are clinically necessary.
- Therapeutic drug monitoring should be coordinated among laboratory, nursing, and pharmacy personnel.
- The laboratory should be aware of patient transfers.
- Slogans can be developed for their health care personnel regarding phlebotomy:
  - A stick in time saves nine.
  - For their sake, let's stick together.

Box 9-14   Other Specimen Collection Issues for Possible Inclusion in Policies/Procedures

- Number of times that a patient can be punctured. (Generally, a health care worker should not puncture a patient more than twice before calling for a second opinion.)
- Number of times that a patient can be punctured in one day. Coordinated efforts should minimize the number of patient venipunctures.
- The total volume of blood that can be drawn daily from a patient, especially for infants and children. (Refer to Appendix 6 for more information.)
- Clinical information provided to the patient by the phlebotomist is usually restricted to very basic information about the tests that have been ordered. It should be emphasized that the patient's physician ordered the tests.
- Procedures for documenting a patient's refusal to have blood collected. All patients have a right to refuse treatment. The phlebotomist can explain to the patient that laboratory results are used to help the physician make an accurate diagnosis, establish proper treatment, and monitor the patient's health status, and that the patient's cooperation would be greatly appreciated. If the patient continues to refuse, the phlebotomist must remain professional and acknowledge his or her right to refuse. Documentation of the refusal should be made and the patient's physician notified.
- Guidelines for specimen rejection. Refer to Box 9-15.

Box 9-15   Factors for Specimen Rejection

- Discrepancies between requisition forms and labeled tubes (names, dates, times)
- Unlabeled tubes
- Inadequate volume of blood
- Hemolyzed specimens (except for tests in which hemolysis does not interfere)
- Specimens in the wrong collection tubes
- Specimens that were improperly transported (chilled or unchilled)
- Anticoagulated specimens that contain blood clots
- Use of outdated equipment, supplies, or reagents
- Contaminated specimens
- A timed sample drawn at the wrong time or with the time recorded incorrectly[19,20]

When a problem arises, the appropriate investigational channels should be followed. The health care worker who drew the specimen and his or her supervisor should try to solve the problem initially. Errors should be acknowledged and documented with corrective actions. Other personnel may be involved as needed. Communication, honesty, and ethical professional behavior are the keys to an efficient and reliable health care environment. Chapter 11 addresses complications in blood collection.

TIMED SPECIMENS

If a test is ordered to be drawn at a particular time, the health care worker is responsible for drawing the blood as near to the requested time as possible. The most common requests for timed specimens are for glucose level determination, for which blood should be drawn 2 hours after a meal. The glucose value in the blood is constantly changing, so the blood must not be drawn too early, which yields a falsely elevated result, or too late, which yields a falsely normal result.

Timed specimens are also crucial for therapeutic drug monitoring (TDM). The laboratory results taken from blood samples for TDM are used in establishing a patient's drug dose. More specifically, TDM is used for the following reasons:[21,22]

- Monitor or confirm overdose.
- Determine the dosage of a medication.

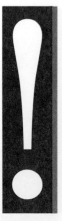

Clinical Alert

Bandages are not recommended for infants or very young children because of possible irritation and the potential of swallowing or aspirating the bandage if it comes off.

- Establish a baseline measurement after a patient has begun or changed to a new drug therapy.
- Check to see that a drug is not interacting with a drug the patient is already taking.
- Check to see if a drug is influenced by the patient's habits; e.g., smokers clear theophylline faster than in nonsmokers, so their serum drug levels will be lower.
- After a change in the patient's kidney, liver, or GI functions.
- Within 6 hours after a seizure recurrence (when using antiepileptic drugs).
- When drug toxicity is suspected: some drugs have a narrow therapeutic window such that the amount needed to benefit the patient is often close to the toxic amount.
- When the patient is noncompliant with the prescribed medications, a physician may need the serum level to confirm that the patient has not taken the drug or has not taken it as prescribed.
- If a patient's condition is not improving after drug therapy, the serum drug level may be subtherapeutic, so a change in dose may be needed.

When a patient is taking a drug orally, blood samples for TDM are drawn right before he or she takes the next dose. This is called the "trough" sample because it is usually when the drug is at a low concentration in the patient's serum. "Peak" samples are collected for some intravenous (IV) drugs, for example, antibiotics such as amikacin, gentamicin, and tobramycin, and after IV loading doses of drugs such as phenytoin. "Peak" drug levels represent the highest drug concentration in the patient's blood. Other drugs such as digoxin and lithium take a long time to reach a steady state in the patient's body. Therefore, blood collection should be delayed until the drug reaches the steady state and should be coordinated with the nursing and pharmacy staff to ensure proper timing.[21] Until recently, TDM required that the specimen be collected in tubes that did not contain gel separators because some gels absorbed certain drugs, thus causing falsely lowered results. Other studies indicated that if the samples are processed promptly, some of the effects of gel interference could be minimized, and that acrylic based gels did not exhibit absorption problems that are linked to silicone or polyester gels. More recently, manufacturers have improved these types of additives, nevertheless, it is important to check with the tube manufacturers for specific information on each of their products.[21,23]

SPECIMENS FOR HORMONES AND RENIN

Certain natural hormone levels, such as cortisol, also increase and decrease with the time of day. For instance, a sample of blood taken at 8:00 A.M. shows the highest value for cortisol during the day, whereas a sample taken at 8:00 P.M. usually shows approximately two thirds the value of the morning sample. Therefore, if a health care worker has difficulty obtaining a blood specimen on a patient at 8:00 A.M., someone else should try as soon as possible thereafter, or the test may be canceled until the following day at the discretion of the attending physician. Obtaining a specimen at noon for cortisol level determination may give the physician little information on which to base treatment.

Aldosterone, another hormone, requires the patient to be in a recumbent position for at least 30 minutes prior to blood collection. Serum or plasma can be used in the analyte determination, but heparin or EDTA should be the anticoagulant if plasma is preferred. Because glass interferes in the aldosterone determination, the collecting container should be made of plastic.

Blood collection for a renin-activity test requires an anticoagulated blood specimen from the patient after a 3-day special diet, and also documentation about whether the patient was in an upright or supine (prone) position when blood was drawn. For this analyte, the blood should be collected from a peripheral vein (e.g., antecubital vein).

FASTING SPECIMENS

Fasting specimens require that blood be taken from a patient who has abstained from eating and drinking anything (except water) for a particular period of time. Care should be taken that the patient is not unduly inconvenienced by an order for fasting blood tests. Fasting levels of glucose, cholesterol, and triglycerides are used for diagnosis and monitoring. If the phlebotomist finds that a patient has not been fasting, the physician should be consulted to determine whether a nonfasting level will be of benefit. The requisition should then indicate that the patient is non-fasting.

STAT SPECIMENS

STAT, or emergency, specimens mean that they should be acted on immediately because the patient has a medical condition that must be treated or responded to as a medical emergency. When blood work is ordered "STAT," the specimen must be drawn, delivered to the laboratory, and analyzed without delay.

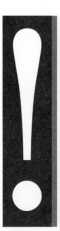

Clinical Alert

Laboratory analyses of drug levels are often used to reevaluate drug dosages. If blood samples are drawn at inappropriate times, that is, before the drug has reached equilibrium, or if the "peak" level is erroneously reported as the "trough" level, the wrong dosage will be used to calculate a new dose. It is possible that the patient may then receive an incorrectly calculated dosage. This could be life threatening. TDM requires careful coordination among all members of the health care team, including the physician and the laboratory, nursing, and pharmacy staff members. The time of day, for example, morning versus evening, that blood is collected can have an effect on carbamazepine, cyclosporine, lithium, and theophylline.[21] Again, coordinating the timing with interdisciplinary staff members so as to be consistent from day to day will ensure accurate results.

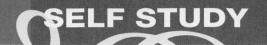

SELF STUDY

KEY TERMS

butterfly system

decontaminated

evacuated tube system

fasting blood tests

hand hygiene

hemoconcentration

hemolysis

National Committee for Clinical
  Laboratory Standards (NCCLS)

"peak"

physician–patient relationship

STAT

supine

syringe method

therapeutic drug monitoring (TDM)

tourniquet

"trough"

winged infusion system

STUDY QUESTIONS

The following questions may have more than one answer.

1. A patient may be identified by which of the following means?
   a. patient's chart
   b. nurse
   c. patient's armband
   d. ward clerk

2. Identification procedures for outpatients may include asking for which of the following?
   a. photo identification
   b. birth date
   c. address
   d. identification by a family member

3. The most common sites for venipuncture are in which of the following areas?
   a. the dorsal side of the wrist
   b. the antecubital area of the arm
   c. the middle finger
   d. the middle forearm

4. Palpating the venipuncture site serves what purpose(s)?
   a. provides an indication of the size of the vein
   b. distracts the patient from the discomfort of the procedure
   c. provides an indication of the depth of the vein
   d. helps the phlebotomist determine at what angle to insert the needle

5. Using a butterfly needle is beneficial for:
   a. heel puncture
   b. veins in the wrist or hand
   c. geriatric patients
   d. patients who are burned

6. What effect does warming the site have on venipuncture?
   a. prevents veins from rolling
   b. makes veins stand out
   c. causes hemoconcentration
   d. increases localized blood flow

7. How long should the tourniquet be placed around the patient's arm?
   a. approximately 4 minutes
   b. until the needle is removed
   c. until the entire venipuncture is completed
   d. no more than 1 minute

8. What is the best angle for needle insertion during venipuncture?
   a. 5 degrees
   b. 30 degrees
   c. 45 degrees
   d. 80 degrees

9. What is the suggested order of draw using the evacuated tube system for the following specimens?
   a. blood culture
   b. lavender-topped tube
   c. light-blue-topped tube
   d. red-topped tube

10. Containers for the disposal of needles and syringes should have which of the following features?
    a. be puncture resistant
    b. be labeled with a "biohazard" sign
    c. have yellow and black markings
    d. contain antiseptic solution

References

1. National Committee for Clinical Laboratory Standards (NCCLS): Procedures for the Collection of Diagnostic Blood Specimens by Venipuncture, Approved Standard, 5th Edition, H3-A5. Wayne, PA: NCCLS, December, 2003.

2. National Committee for Clinical Laboratory Standards (NCCLS): Procedures and Devices for the Collection of Diagnostic Capillary Blood Specimens, Approved Standard, H4-A5. Wayne, PA: NCCLS, 2004.

3. Centers for Disease Control and Prevention: Morbidity and Mortality Weekly Report: Guideline for hand hygiene in health-care settings, October 25, 2002; 51(16), www.cdc.gov/handhygiene/.

4. Department of Health and Human Services, National Institute for Occupational Safety and Health (NIOSH): Preventing needlestick injuries in health care settings. Publication No. 2000-108, November 1999, www.cdc.gov/niosh/2000-108.html, accessed 10/5/03, (4676 Columbia Parkway, Cincinnati, OH 45226-1998, 1-800-35-NIOSH)

5. College of American Pathologists, LAP Inspection Checklists, Laboratory General, Collection Manual, March 2003, www.cap.org, accessed 6/22/03.

6. Joint Commission on Accreditation of Healthcare Organizations: Joint Commission Announces National Patient Safety Goals, News Release Archives, www.jcaho.org/news+room/news+release+archives/npsg.htm, March 5, 2003.

7. The Observatory: Radio frequency technology in the lab. *Med Lab Observ,* February 2000: 8–9.

8. Erwin, J: Keeping track, Patient wristbands hold medical records. *Healthweek,* August 1998; 17: 8.

9. Lawrence, JB: Preanalytical variables in the coagulation laboratory. *Laboratory Medicine,* January 2003; 1: 34, 49–57.

10. Jackson, S: Caution: Entering the danger zone, Proper vein selection is key in successful venipunctures. *Advance for Medical Laboratory Professionals,* March 24, 2003: 10.

11. Faber, V, Gingrich, DP: Tips for drawing blood from a mastectomy arm. *Adv Med Lab Professionals,* June 2000; 5: 4.

12. Ernst, D: Iodine disinfectant for infants. *Medical Laboratory Observer,* July 2003: 54, www.mlo-online.com.

13. Occupational Safety and Health Administration: *Re-Use of Blood Tube Holders, Standard Interpretations,* June 12, 2002, www.osha.gov.

14. Becton Dickinson Vacutainer Systems: *Preanalytical Solutions,* www.bd.com, accessed Feb 20, 2004.

15. Gottfried, EL, Adachi, MM: Prothrombin time and activated partial thromboplastin time can be performed on the first tube. *Am J Clin Pathol,* 1997; 107(6): 681–683.

16. Yawn, BP, Loge, C, Dale, J: Prothrombin time: One tube or two. *Am J. Clin Pathol,* 1996; 105(6): 794–797.

17. Adcock, DM, Kressin, DC, Marlar, RA: Are discard tubes necessary in coagulation studies? Lab Med, 1997; 28(8): 530–533.

18. Saxena, S, Belzberg, H, Chogyoji, M, et al: Reducing phlebotomy losses by streamlining laboratoy test ordering in a surgical intensive care unit. *Laboratory Medicine,* October 2003; 34(10): 728–732.

19. Richael, JL, Naples, MF: Creating a workable specimen rejection policy. *Med Lab Observ,* March 1995: 37–42.

20. National Committee for Clinical Laboratory Standards (NCCLS): Procedures for the Handling and Processing of Blood Specimens, Approved Guideline, H18-A2. Villanova, PA: NCCLS, 1994.

21. Warner, AM: Pitfalls in monitoring therapeutic drugs. *Laboratory Medicine,* 1997; 28(10): 653–663.

22. Sayers, J, Friedman, M: How clinicians use therapeutic drug monitoring. *Lab Med,* 1997; 28(8): 524–538.

23. Pruett, S: Tips from the clinical experts: Gel separator tubes for TDM. *Med Lab Observ,* January 1999.

Procedures for Collecting Capillary Blood Specimens

CHAPTER OBJECTIVES

Upon completion of Chapter 10, the learner is responsible for the following:

1. Describe reasons for acquiring capillary blood specimens.
2. Identify the proper sites for performing a skin puncture procedure.
3. Explain why controlling the depth of the incision is necessary.
4. Describe the procedure for making a blood smear.
5. Explain why capillary blood from a skin puncture is different from blood taken by venipuncture.

 MediaLINK

Access the accompanying CD-ROM to explore a wide variety of review questions and interactive activities for this chapter, including multiple choice, true/false, and video exercises.

◼◼◼◼ INDICATIONS FOR SKIN PUNCTURE

Skin punctures are particularly useful for both adult and pediatric patients when small amounts of blood can be obtained and adequately tested.

It is crucial to withdraw only the smallest amounts of blood needed for laboratory testing from neonates, infants, and children so that the effects of blood-volume reduction are minimal. A 10 mL blood sample, which could be tolerated by most adults, would represent 5 to 10 percent of the total blood volume in a neonate's body.[1] Sample sizes and procedures for obtaining specimen collections from children are in Appendix 6, and pediatric topics are covered in Chapter 12.

Skin punctures are used also when the following conditions occur in adult patients:[1]

- Severe burns
- Obesity
- Thrombotic tendencies
- Fragile veins (e.g., in geriatric patients)
- When veins are being "saved" for therapy (e.g., for oncology patients)
- Home testing (e.g., blood glucose screening)
- Point-of-care testing

Sometimes a skin puncture cannot be used because testing may require larger amounts of blood; swollen sites may be causing interstitial fluids to dilute the blood; the patient may be dehydrated; and/or a patient may have poor peripheral circulation. Specific tests for which skin punctures are not recommended include coagulation studies (because of the interstitial fluid), blood cultures, and erythrocyte sedimentation rate (ESR) determinations.

◼◼◼◼ COMPOSITION OF CAPILLARY BLOOD

The composition of capillary blood acquired by skin puncture is significantly different from that of venous blood acquired by venipuncture. It is composed of blood from:

- arterioles
- venules
- capillaries
- intracellular and interstitial (tissue) fluids

Clinical Alert

Venipuncture in children, especially infants, can be hazardous and difficult because of the risk of complications, such as anemia, cardiac arrest, hemorrhage, venous thrombosis, reflex arteriospasm, gangrene of an extremity, damage to surrounding tissues or organs, infections, and injuries from restraining the child during the procedure.[1]

The exact proportions in a capillary blood specimen from these sources is not known; however, the amount of arterial blood will be greatest, because the arterial pressure in the capillaries is stronger than the venous pressure. Therefore, skin puncture blood is actually more like arterial blood than venous blood.

BASIC TECHNIQUE FOR COLLECTING DIAGNOSTIC CAPILLARY BLOOD SPECIMENS

Many of the steps used for the venipuncture procedure also apply to skin puncture. Basic steps include the following:

1. Greeting and identifying the patient
2. Upholding hand-hygiene and gloving techniques
3. Preparing supplies and the microcollection device
4. Positioning the patient
5. Verifying diet restrictions and that the patient does not have latex allergies
6. Selecting the site and warming it, if necessary
7. Cleaning the site
8. Opening the sterile puncture device within view of the patient
9. Performing the puncture
10. Obtaining the specimen
11. Applying gentle pressure to the wound using a clean gauze pad
12. Discarding the lancet in a puncture-resistant biohazard container
13. Labeling the specimen and preparing it for transportation
14. Assuring that bleeding has stopped, and thanking the patient before leaving.

PREPARATION FOR SKIN PUNCTURE

Skin puncture procedures involve the same preparation steps as discussed for venipuncture procedures. These issues were discussed previously in greater detail in Chapter 9. It is *imperative* that phlebotomists review the details of these steps because they are essential responsibilities. Such steps include:

- Being emotionally prepared
- Exercising standard precautions
- Practicing the correct hand-hygiene techniques
- Utilizing gloves
- Greeting the patient to put him or her at ease
- Ensuring proper patient identification in a variety of situations
- Positioning the patient in a safe, comfortable bed or reclining chair
- Asking about his or her dietary condition (i.e., fasting state)
- Asking about latex sensitivity
- Asking about hand preference or dominance

SUPPLIES FOR SKIN PUNCTURE

As mentioned in Chapter 8, "Blood Collection Equipment," supplies for skin puncture include the following:

- Disposable gloves
- Automatic puncture devices

- Disinfectant pads
- Sterile bandages or prepackaged gauze pads
- Glass microscope slides
- Diluting fluids
- Plastic microcollection tubes or plastic-coated capillary tubes
- Capillary tube sealers or closures
- Laboratory request slips or labels
- A marking pen
- A puncture-proof biohazard discard container

SKIN PUNCTURE SITES

Skin puncture in adults and older children most often involves one of the fingers. The fleshy, central palmar surface of the distal phalanx (fingertip section) of the third (middle) finger or fourth (ring) finger of the nondominant hand is the preferred site for puncture. The puncture should be made at the thickest part of the finger (not the sides or extreme tip where the tissue is not as thick).[1] Refer to Figure 10–1 ■.

For infants less than 1 year old, or neonates, the recommended site for skin puncture is the lateral or medial plantar surface of the heel.[1] Refer to Chapter 12 for further information regarding pediatric phlebotomies.

WARMING THE SKIN PUNCTURE SITE

Warming the skin puncture site helps facilitate phlebotomy by significantly increasing arterial blood flow to the area. Capillary specimens from warmed sites can be described as "arterialized." Several "easy to use" methods of warming are commercially available (refer to Chapter 9), but a heated surgical towel or a washcloth heated with warm water to 42°C will not burn the skin and is acceptable. When the towel is wrapped around the site for 3 to 5 minutes, the skin temperature can increase several degrees and arterial blood flow can increase up to sevenfold.[1]

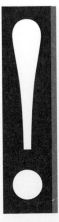

Clinical Alert

Phlebotomists are at risk of injury if glass capillary tubes shatter. Therefore, regulatory agencies have recommended the use of capillary blood collection devices that are less likely to break. These include nonglass capillary tubes, glass capillary tubes wrapped in puncture-resistant film, and products that avoid the step of pushing tubes into sealant putty.

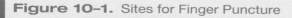

Figure 10–1. Sites for Finger Puncture

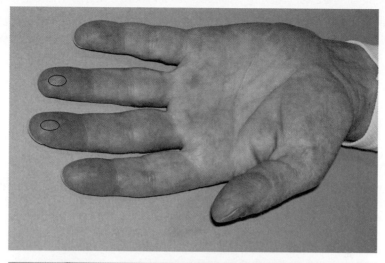

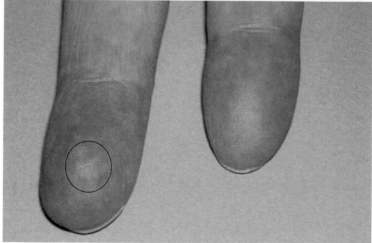

1. The fleshy surface of the distal segment of the third (middle) finger or fourth (ring) finger are the preferred sites. Note the circled areas.

2. The puncture should be made across the fingerprints at the thickest part of the finger (not the sides or extreme tip).

CLEANSING THE SKIN PUNCTURE SITE

The skin puncture site should be cleaned with 70 percent aqueous solution of isopropanol and allowed to thoroughly dry before being punctured, because residual alcohol causes rapid hemolysis and may contaminate glucose determinations. Also, alcohol may sting the patient and prevent formation of rounded drops of blood, which are best for making blood smears on microscopic slides. Povidone–iodine (Betadine) preparations are not

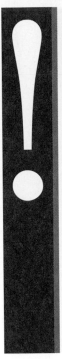

Clinical Alert

The following sites are *not generally recommended* for routine skin punctures:[1]

- Earlobe (Even though the earlobe is still used by some, it is not a preferred site due to possible interference with pierced earrings; also, because of the site's close proximity to the eyes, a puncture device may cause undue anxiety to a patient)
- Central arch area of an infant's heel and posterior curve of the heel (due to risk of injuring nerves, tendons, cartilage, and bone)
- Fingers of a newborn or infant less than one year old (due to the risk of hitting the bone and causing infections).[2]
- The fifth (pinky) finger (because the tissue of this finger is considerably thinner than that of the others and there is a risk of hitting the bone)
- The thumb (because it has a pulse)
- The index (pointer) finger (because it may be more sensitive or it may be callused)
- Swollen or previously punctured sites (because accumulated fluid may contaminate the specimen and the site may be bruised, thus causing more pain if it is punctured again)
- Fingers on the side of a mastectomy (because removal of lymph nodes during surgery may result in excessive lymph fluid on the side of the surgery; consult with the ordering physician in the case of a bilateral mastectomy)

recommended for disinfecting skin puncture sites because they can falsely elevate potassium, phosphorus, or uric acid determinations.[1]

■■■■■ SKIN PUNCTURE PROCEDURE

Microcollection by skin puncture involves many of the same steps used during venipuncture. If the phlebotomist is performing a heel stick, the infant's heel should be held firmly, with the forefinger at the arch of the foot and the thumb below and away from the puncture site (see Chapter 12). If a finger stick is being performed, the patient's finger should be held firmly, with the phlebotomist's thumb away from the puncture site (see Procedure 10–1 and Figures 10–1 ■ and 10–2 ■).

Retractable puncture devices are currently available on the market and are recommended in place of the manual sterile lancet, a nonretractable device (see Chapter 8 for more information about devices and microcollection tubes).[1] Phlebotomists should understand and follow the manufacturer's directions for use of each device. Puncture devices are made to control for variable depth and length depending on the patient's age and weight. The average depth of skin puncture should be 2 to 3 mm for adults, and no more than 2.0 mm for small children and infants, to avoid injuring the bone. Laser devices are also available as skin puncture alternatives. They provide a smaller hole (about 250 mm wide and 1 to 2 mm deep).

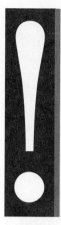

Clinical Alert

If the bone is repeatedly punctured, it can lead to osteomyelitis, which is an inflammation of the bone due to bacterial infection.

ORDER OF COLLECTION

The order of filling microcollection tubes with capillary blood is different than for venipuncture. If multiple laboratory tests have been ordered, the "order of collection" should be as follows:[1]

- EDTA specimen for hematology tests
- Other tubes with additives
- Nonadditive tubes

BLOOD FILMS FOR MICROSCOPIC SLIDES

Procedure 10–2 demonstrates the procedure for making blood smears on microscopic glass slides for performing white blood cell differentials. Also, blood spot testing for newborn screening is covered in Chapter 12.

MICROHEMATOCRIT

The packed cell volume, PCV or microhematocrit, can be collected directly into a capillary tube containing heparin. The tube should be filled at least two thirds full, and be sealed at one end as soon as it is filled.

Clinical Alert

Manual, nonretractable lancets are not recommended for acquiring capillary specimens; however, in some facilities their use is still in practice (e.g., those that are not subject to OSHA regulations). If a sterile lancet is used, it should be carefully removed from its packaging. (If the lancet accidently touches clothing or brushes against the countertop, it is no longer sterile, and a new device should be opened and used.) Manufacturer's directions should be followed. The finger or heel should be held so as to prevent sudden jerky movements during the puncture. If applicable, remove the protective shield or cap from the lancet. The puncture should be in one continuous movement, perpendicular to the skin. As soon as the lancet has penetrated it's full depth, it should be quickly removed and immediately discarded into a puncture-proof biohazard sharps container.

Procedure 10-1　Skin Puncture Procedure Using a Retractable Device

1. Remember the following supplies: gloves, prepackaged gauze (2 × 2 or 3 × 3 inches), alcohol swabs, commercial puncture device, sterile lancets, pipettes, plastic capillary tubes, microcollection tubes, diluting fluids, marking pen or pencil, and bandages. Exercise standard precautions, including the use of hand hygiene and gloves. Greet and identify the patient.

2. Choose a finger that is not cold, cyanotic, or swollen. If possible, the stick should be at the tip of the third or fourth finger of the nondominant hand.

3. Gently massage a few times from base to tip to aid blood flow. If the patient's hands are cold, wrap one of them in a warm towel for 3 to 5 minutes, use a commercially available warming device, or ask the patient to wash their hands in warm water before the puncture is performed.

4. With an alcohol swab (70 percent isopropanol), cleanse the ball of the finger. Allow to air-dry. (Fig. 10–2a ■)

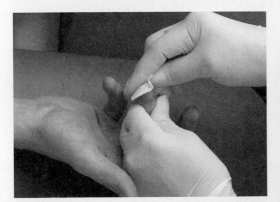

Figure 10–2a

5. Remove the puncture device and/or lancet from its packaging and follow the manufacturer's instructions. Hold the patient's finger firmly (or heel, in the case of an infant) with one hand. With the other hand position the puncture device on the site.

6. Activate the release mechanism on the retractable safety puncture device. The cut should be oriented across the fingerprints to generate a large, round drop of blood. If the puncture is made along the lines of (i.e., parallel to) the fingerprint, the blood tends to run down the finger. (Fig. 10–2b ■)

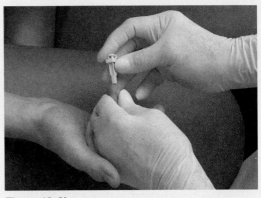

Figure 10–2b

7. Wipe the first drop of blood away with clean gauze. (Fig. 10–2c ■)

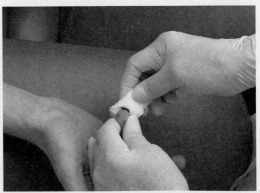

Figure 10–2c

8. A second drop will form and should be collected when touched by the tip of the microcollection device. The blood will flow into the

Procedure 10–1 *(continued)*

tube by capillary action whereby blood flows freely into the tube on contact, without suction. If the blood becomes jammed in the collection top, a gentle tap on a hard surface will usually dislodge it so the blood can flow freely again to the bottom of the tube. (Fig. 10–2d ■)

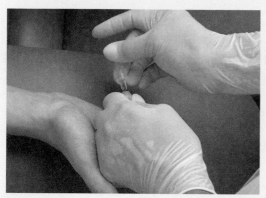

Figure 10–2d

9. Gently apply pressure to the finger and hold the puncture site in a downward position to encourage a free flow of blood, thereby getting the proper amount of blood. Do not use excessive milking/massaging of the finger, or forceful scooping-up of blood because it may result in excess tissue fluid and/or hemolysis of the specimen.

10. Each type of microcollection has different tube and blood volume requirements. Follow the appropriate manufacturer's instructions. Containers with additives should be inverted gently to mix the blood with the additives. Microcollection tubes should be carefully and safely sealed with a sealant or with other commercially available devices. When filling the capillary tubes, the phlebotomist must not allow air bubbles to enter the tubes, because air bubbles can cause erroneous results in many laboratory tests. Blood flow is better and air bubbles

are less likely if the puncture site is held downward and gentle pressure is applied.

11. Blood smears can also be made from subsequent drops of blood.

12. Using a clean gauze pad, apply pressure to the site until bleeding has stopped. (If collecting blood from an infant's heel the gauze pad should be applied and the heel should be elevated until bleeding stops.) (Fig. 10–2e ■)

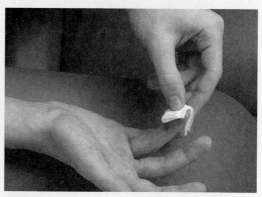

Figure 10–2e

13. Label the specimens and/or outside containers.

14. Remove gloves, dispose of gloves in a puncture-resistant biohazard container, and perform hand hygiene.

15. Assure that bleeding has stopped and thank the patient before leaving with specimens and remaining supplies.

Notes:

• A free flow of blood is essential to obtain accurate test results. Do not use excessive squeezing or massaging to obtain blood.

• If the sample is not adequate and blood has stopped flowing from the puncture site, a new sterile lancet may be used to repuncture at a *different* site.

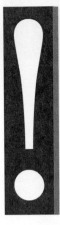

Clinical Alert

Microcollection tubes must be adequately filled and gently mixed to prevent clotting. Excessive amounts (overfilling) can cause clot formation; inadequate amounts (underfilling) can cause cells to change morphologically because of too much anticoagulant.[1]

BLOOD PH AND BLOOD GAS DETERMINATIONS

The site must be warmed prior to collecting capillary blood for pH and blood gas determinations. This increases arterial blood flow to the area. The heparinized capillary tubes must not contain air bubbles and must be quickly sealed after inserting a mixing flea, because the exposure of blood to air (even for short periods of 10 to 30 seconds) can cause significant changes in laboratory values.[3] This is covered in greater detail in Chapter 14.

LANCET DISPOSAL, LABELING THE SPECIMEN, AND COMPLETING THE INTERACTION

Used disposable lancets should be placed into a rigid, puncture-resistant biohazard container with a lid. All tubes must be appropriately labeled immediately after collection and mixing, and the information on the labels confirmed. Several tubes may be placed together in a larger labeled container. All supplies and equipment that were brought in should be removed or discarded appropriately. Hand hygiene, as mentioned in previous chapters, must be performed after contact with each patient. Before leaving the patient's side, the phlebotomist must check the puncture site to make sure that the bleeding has stopped, and then thank the patient. An adhesive bandage may be applied. Such bandages are not recommended for infants or young children, however, because of possible irritation and the potential of swallowing or aspirating a bandage.

Procedure 10-2   Blood Films for Microscopic Slides

1. Blood smears should be made from fresh drops of blood. Perform the finger puncture in the usual way, wiping the first drop of blood away. The slide can be touched to the second drop at approximately 1/2 to 1 in. (1.3 to 2.5 cm) from the end of the slide. (Fig. 10–3a ■)

3. When the blood spreads almost to the edges, the spreader slide should be quickly and evenly pushed forward at an angle of approximately 30 degrees. Do not press downward. The only downward pressure should be the weight of the spreader slide. (Fig. 10–3c ■)

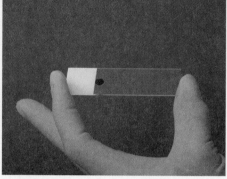

Figure 10–3a

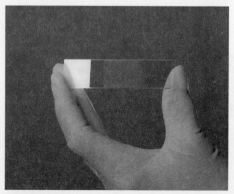

Figure 10–3c

2. Place the second (spreader) slide in front of the drop of blood and the pull it slowly into the drop, allowing blood to spread along the width of the slide. (Fig. 10–3b ■)

4. Allow the slide to air dry, i.e., do not blow on it. (Fig. 10–3d ■)

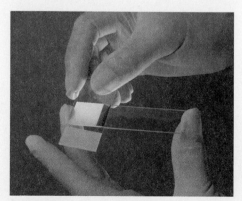

Figure 10–3b

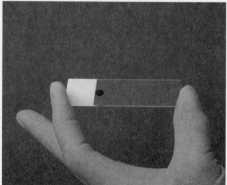

Figure 10–3d

continued →

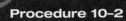

Procedure 10-2   *(continued)*

5. Blood flims should have a feathered edge, as shown in the first slides. It has a visible curved edge that thins out smoothly and resembles the tip of a bird's feather, and it covers approximately half the surface of the glass slide. (Fig. 10–3e ■)

6. The last four blood flims are unacceptable for analysis. No ridges, lines, or holes should be visible in the smear. Errors are often the result of too large a drop, too long a delay in making the smear, blowing on the slide, or using a chipped slide.

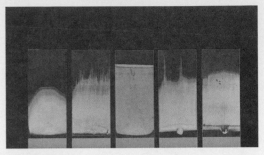

Figure 10–3e

Clinical Alert

Hemolysis of the capillary blood specimen can cause erroneous laboratory results and is usually preventable if good technique is maintained. A phlebotomist can cause hemolysis by:[1]

- Not removing residual alcohol at the puncture site
- Excessive milking of the finger
- Excessive mixing of the specimen

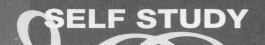

KEY TERMS

arterialized capillary blood
capillary action
cyanotic
differentials
feathered edge

interstitial (tissue) fluid
osteochondritis
osteomyelitis
peripheral circulation

■■■■ STUDY QUESTIONS

The following may have more than one answer.

1. Which of the following are not sites for skin puncture?
   a. wrist
   b. vein
   c. ankle
   d. heel

2. Controlling the depth of lancet insertion during skin puncture prevents which of the following?
   a. puncturing a vein
   b. bacterial contamination
   c. excessive bleeding
   d. osteomyelitis

3. A finger puncture should involve which of the following steps?
   a. puncturing parallel to fingerprint
   b. collecting the first drop
   c. puncturing across the fingerprint
   d. wiping away the first drop

4. Skin puncture is useful for patients who have which of the following conditions?
   a. obesity
   b. burns
   c. fragile veins
   d. thrombotic tendencies

5. Which fingers are used most often for skin puncture?
   a. thumb
   b. second, or index, finger
   c. third or fourth finger
   d. fifth, or pinky, finger

6. Test(s) for which skin puncture cannot be used are:
   a. routine hematology tests
   b. blood cultures
   c. coagulation studies
   d. erythrocyte sedimentation rate (ESR) determinations

7. Capillary blood is more like arterial blood than venous blood for which of the following reasons?
   a. the skin has more arterioles
   b. arterial pressure is stronger in capillaries
   c. more arterial blood flows in capillaries
   d. venous pressure is greater in capillaries

8. Plastic microcollection tubes should be filled with blood in which of the following ways?
   a. using a syringe to fill the tube
   b. allowing tube to fill by itself using capillary action
   c. using suction to pull blood into the tube
   d. using the tube to scoop droplets off the skin carefully

9. Alcohol should be allowed to dry completely prior to skin puncture:
   a. to prevent stinging
   b. to prevent dilution of sample
   c. to prevent lysis of red blood cells
   d. to allow formation of a round drop of blood

10. The best angle for using two glass slides to make a blood smear is approximately:
    a. 10 degrees
    b. 15 degrees
    c. 30 degrees
    d. 90 degrees

References

1. National Committee for Clinical Laboratory Standards (NCCLS): Procedures and Devices for the Collection of Diagnostic Capillary Blood Specimens, Approved Standard, 5th ed. H4-A4. (940 West Valley Road, Suite 1400, Wayne, PA 19087-1898): NCCLS, 2003.
2. Phelan, SE: Fingersticks on children. *Lab Med,* 1999; 30(9): 569–570.
3. National Committee for Clinical Laboratory Standards (NCCLS): Procedures for the Collection of Arterial Blood Specimens, Approved Standard, 3th ed. H11-A3. (940 West Valley Road, Suite 1400, Wayne, PA 19087-1898): NCCLS, 1999.

Preanalytical Complications in Blood Collection

11

CHAPTER OBJECTIVES

Upon completion of Chapter 11, the learner is responsible for the following:

1. Describe preanalytical complications related to phlebotomy procedures.

2. Explain how to prevent and/or handle complications in blood collection.

3. List at least five factors about a patient's physical disposition that can affect blood collection.

4. List examples of substances that can interfere in clinical analysis of blood constituents and describe methods used to prevent these interferences.

MediaLINK

Access the accompanying CD-ROM to explore a wide variety of review questions and interactive activities for this chapter, including multiple choice, true/false, and video exercises.

▮▮▮ OVERVIEW

Preanalytical variables that are important to phlebotomists are categorized in Box 11–1. As mentioned in other chapters, preanalytical variables are particularly crucial to phlebotomists because most of them can be controlled by the phlebotomist. Often when a blood collection error occurs it could have been prevented with precautionary measures or proper documentation. Occasionally, however, patient complications during or after the blood collection procedure are unavoidable. If so, the health care worker must be knowledgeable of methods that will decrease the negative impact of the complication to the patient, to the quality of the blood sample, to the phlebotomist, or to all three. This chapter covers patient complications and preanalytical variables that are often reported, but the list is not exhaustive. Phlebotomists must be able to assess unusual situations and/or patient conditions and determine when to contact a supervisor for additional expertise or assistance.

▮▮▮ COMPLICATIONS ASSOCIATED WITH PATIENT ASSESSMENT AND PHYSICAL DISPOSITION

Blood specimens used to determine the concentrations of body constituents such as glucose, cholesterol, triglycerides, electrolytes, proteins, etc., should be collected when the patient is in a basal state—that is, in the early morning, approximately 12 hours after the last ingestion of food. The results of laboratory tests on basal state specimens are most reliable. However, several factors, including diet, exercise, emotional stress, obesity, menstrual cycle, pregnancy, diurnal variations, posture, tourniquet application, and chemical constituents (alcohol or drugs), can cause changes in the basal state. Phlebotomists need to have a general understanding of these effects and their relationship to laboratory testing.

DIET

To ensure that the patient is in the basal state, the physician must require the patient to fast overnight. The term "fasting" refers to abstinence from nutritional support such as food and beverages (except water). The required time period necessary for abstaining varies with the test procedures to be performed. Before collecting a specimen, the health care worker should ask the patient if he or she has eaten. Blood composition is significantly altered after meals and consequently is unsuitable for many clinical chemistry tests. If the patient has eaten recently but the physician still needs the test, the word "nonfasting" must be documented on the requisition and/or directly on the specimen.

When giving dietary instructions, gaining the patient's cooperation is important and is determined by the professional behavior and the competence of the health care worker. Inadequate patient instructions can cause mistakes in specimen collection. Casual instruc-

Box 11–1	Variables Important in Specimen Collection

- Patient assessment and physical disposition
- Test requests
- Specimen collection
- Specimen transport
- Specimen receipt in the laboratory[1]

tions are apt to be taken lightly by the patient or even forgotten. If the phlebotomist has to explain fasting restrictions to a patient, the instructions should be thorough and clear, with emphasis on the important points of the procedure. Some patients assume that the term "fasting" refers to abstaining from food and water. Abstaining from water can result in dehydration, which can alter test results. Thus, the health care worker must ensure that the patient understands all the requirements. Written instructions are also helpful, if available.

If a procedure involves some discomfort or inconvenience, the patient should be informed. For example, if blood is to be drawn for a timed blood glucose level determination, the patient needs to fast for 8 to 12 hours. The health care worker can inform the patient that several specimens will be collected at timed intervals and that he or she may drink water, but that coffee, chewing gum, and tea should be avoided because they cause a transitory fluctuation in the blood sugar level.

OBESITY

More than half of adult patients in the United States are overweight. A healthy body weight is based on body mass index (BMI), and for adults the BMI range is 20 to 25 kg/m^2.[3] Obese patients (i.e., patients with an unhealthy accumulation of body fat, or a body mass index of greater than 30 kg/m^2) generally have veins that are difficult to visualize and/or palpate. (Refer to Chapter 9 to view examples of different arm veins.) If the vein is not accessed when first punctured, the health care worker must be careful not to probe excessively with the needle, because doing so ruptures red blood cells (RBCs), increases the concentration of intracellular contents, and releases some tissue-clotting factors. Usually the patient him- or herself knows where the "best site" is for venipuncture, so it is helpful to check with the patient prior to selecting the site.

DAMAGED, SCLEROSED, OR OCCLUDED VEINS

Obstructed, or occluded, veins do not allow blood to flow through them; sclerosed, or hardened, veins are a result of inflammation and disease of the interstitial substances. Patients' veins that have been repeatedly punctured often become scarred and feel hard when palpated. Because blood is not easily collected from these sites, they should be avoided.

Clinical Alert

Prolonged fasting and/or unsupervised fasting to loose weight can cause health hazards including electrolyte disturbances, cardiac dysrhythmias, and—occasionally—death.[2]

Box 11-2   **Practice Giving Instructions**

Write out the instructions you would give a patient that needs to fast prior to a blood collection procedure. Try to think of the all the most unusual questions that the patient might ask about eating or drinking.

Practice giving the instructions to a friend or coworker. Practice your communication techniques by double checking that they completely understand; ask them specific questions about their comprehension of the fasting process; and ask them to give a friendly and constructive critique of your instructions.

ALLERGIES

Some patients are allergic to iodine, alcohol, or other solutions used to disinfect a puncture site. If a patient indicates that he or she is allergic to a solution, all efforts should be made to use an alternative method. (Chlorohexidine has been reportedly used as an alternative to decontaminate skin. After application, it can be wiped off with sterile water.[4] In addition, some patients are allergic to latex. Latex-free tourniquets, gloves, and bandages must be used for patients who have this allergy.

EXERCISE

Effects of exercise on laboratory tests can be categorized as either short-term effects (reported in marathon runners and endurance athletes) or long-term effects (due to exercise training programs). Studies suggest that it is hard to separate the two effects because most endurance athletes go through extensive training programs. In either case, the effects of exercise on laboratory tests depends on intensity, duration, and frequency of the exercise and the individual's genetic factors, ethnicity, age, gender, hormonal status, and body weight.[5]

Many studies about the effects of exercise are inconclusive and/or contradictory, but better data is surfacing as exercise is incorporated more often into daily lives. In general, moderate or excessive exercise has an effect on laboratory test results, but it is up to the physician to interpret the effects. Exercise also has some effects on hemostasis (i.e., some reports indicate that physical exercise activates coagulation, fibrinolysis, and platelet formation; however, other reports cite conflicting results or no changes in measured hemostatic parameters).[5]

Box 11-3   **Marathon Runners**

In a study of 37 marathon runners, laboratory results showed increases in glucose, total protein, albumin, uric acid, calcium, phosphorous, BUN, creatinine, total and direct bilirubin, ALT, AST, and alkaline phosphatase 4 hours after the marathon. No change was measured in sodium, potassium, and osmolality after 4 hours, while magnesium, chloride, carbon dioxide, and globulin results decreased. Laboratory results for BUN, creatinine, uric acid, ALT, AST, and direct bilirubin remained elevated 24 hours after the race, but glucose, total protein, albumin, globulin, calcium, phosphorous, total bilirubin, and alkaline phosphatase returned to baseline. There was also an increase in white blood cell count, neutrophilia, monocytosis, and decreased lymphocytes. Platelets, hemoglobin, MCH, MCHC, and RDW were elevated at 4 and 24 hours, while the hematocrit, RBC, and MCV decreased. The hematocrit returned to baseline after 24 hours.[6]

STRESS

Patients are often frightened, nervous, and overly anxious, especially prior to blood collection. These emotional stresses can cause a transient elevation in the white blood cell (WBC) count, a transient decrease in serum iron levels, and abnormal hormone (e.g., cortisol, aldosterone, renin, thyroid-stimulating hormone [TSH], prolactin) values. Also, mental anxiety can increase blood concentrations of albumin, fibrinogen, glucose, cholesterol, and insulin.[7] In one report, newborns who had been crying violently had WBC counts that are 140 percent above resting baseline counts. Even mild crying was shown to increase WBC counts 113 percent. These elevated counts return to baseline values within 1 hour. Therefore, whenever possible, blood samples for WBC counts should be taken approximately 1 hour after a crying episode.[8] Anxiety that results in hyperventilation also causes acid–base imbalances, increased lactate levels, and increased fatty acid levels.[9]

DIURNAL RHYTHMS AND POSTURE

Diurnal rhythms, which are body fluid fluctuations during the day, cause some hormone levels to decrease in the afternoon (e.g., cortisol, adrenocorticotropic hormone [ACTH] TSH, T4 plasma renin activity, aldosterone, insulin, iron), whereas eosinophil counts increase. Thus, collecting specimens during the designated time periods is important for proper clinical evaluation.

Posture changes are also known to vary laboratory test results of some chemical constituents (e.g., aldosterone and plasma renin activity). This consideration is important when inpatient and outpatient results are being compared. Thus, blood collection should be performed under standardized posture conditions. Changing from a supine (or lying) position to a sitting or standing position causes body water to shift from intravascular to interstitial compartments (in tissues). Certain larger molecules cannot filter into the tissue; therefore, they concentrate in the blood. Enzyme, protein, lipid, iron, and calcium levels are significantly increased with changes in position.[10,11] For example, when the patient's sample is collected while he or she is standing, total cholesterol results will be approximately 10 percent higher, triglycerides 12 percent higher, and HDL cholesterol 7 percent higher than in samples collected when the patient is lying down. The standard position for these blood collections is with the patient sitting.[12] These effects can be more pronounced in patients with congestive heart failure and hepatic disorders.

AGE

Laboratory test results vary considerably during the stages of life: infancy, childhood (pediatric population), adulthood, and older adulthood (geriatric population). For example, blood cholesterol and triglyceride values increase as a person ages. Various hormone levels, such as estrogen and growth hormone (GH) levels, decrease in geriatric women. GH levels are also decreased in geriatric men.

MASTECTOMY

Patients who have undergone a mastectomy (i.e., surgical removal of the breast) often have resulting lymphedema on the side of the surgery. The stagnant flow of tissue fluid in the area may make the patient more prone to infections; therefore, the lymphedematous limbs should be protected from cuts, scratches, burns, and blood drawing.

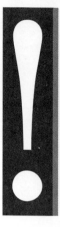

Clinical Alert

Venipuncture should never be performed on the same side as that of a mastectomy (unless approved by the physician), since the patient is more susceptible to infection and some chemical constituents in the blood may be altered. Also, the pressure from the tourniquet could lead to injuries in a patient who has had this type of surgery. If the patient has had a double mastectomy, the back of the hands or finger sticks are alternative methods. However, *the physician should always be involved in determining suitable sites.*

EDEMA

Some patients develop edema (i.e., an abnormal accumulation of fluid in the intercellular spaces) because of reasons other than a mastectomy (e.g., heart failure, renal failure, inflammation, malnutrition, bacterial toxins, etc.). This swelling can be localized or diffused over a larger area of the body. The health care worker should avoid collecting blood from these sites, because veins in these areas are difficult to palpate or locate, and the specimen may become contaminated with fluid. Again, consultation with the physician is needed to determine if and where a blood specimen should be taken.

MENSTRUAL CYCLE

Women normally begin menstruation during puberty (9 to 17 years of age). The menstrual flow lasts between 3 and 7 days and contains normal, hemolyzed, or sometimes agglutinated red blood cells, disintegrated endometrial cells, and glandular secretions. The average blood loss ranges from 44 to 80 ml but may be lessened (if the patient is using oral contraceptives) or increased (if the patient has an intrauterine device, IUD). Menstrual blood loss is the single most common cause of iron-deficiency anemia in women.[2] This fact reinforces the issue that phlebotomists need to be careful not to withdraw more blood than is absolutely necessary so as not to increase the negative effects of additional blood loss during venipuncture.

MEDICATIONS

Blood being collected to determine levels of medications should, in most cases, be collected just prior to the next dose. There are hundreds of medications available, each of which has particular pharmacokinetics (i.e., characteristics related to a drug's metabolism and action, e.g., time needed for absorption, duration of action, distribution in the body, and method of excretion). Some drugs taken orally reach maximum effective serum concentrations slower than if administered by IV. Or a drug may be absorbed faster if taken on an empty stomach. Therefore a phlebotomist must be knowledgeable of the institutional procedures and/or what the health care team (nursing, laboratory, pharmacy, and physician) requires in terms of when the specimen is to be collected and any additional information needed to help interpret the test results. This may involve notations of the drug name and the time and dates that the drug was administered, in addition to other required information. Refer to Chapter 9 for more information on therapeutic drug monitoring.

INTERFERENCE OF DRUGS AND OTHER SUBSTANCES IN BLOOD

Many prescribed drugs can interfere with clinical laboratory determinations or can physiologically alter the levels of blood constituents measured in the clinical laboratory. The interference of drugs and other substances is so complicated and dependent on the chemical procedures used that only general recommendations are described in this section. Consequently, physicians must work closely with pharmacy and laboratory staff to rule out laboratory test results that are altered because the patient is taking medication.

Drugs administered to alleviate an illness can induce physiologic abnormalities in one or more of the following systems: hepatic, hematologic, hemostatic, muscular, pancreatic, and renal. The erroneous results may sometimes obscure the clinical diagnosis. Drugs or drug metabolites in blood can also directly cause falsely decreased or falsely elevated values in laboratory analyses. If the patient must be maintained on medication that may cause interferences in laboratory assays, it is helpful if the medication name can be documented on the laboratory request. Ideally, when interference of medications cannot be avoided by using different laboratory assays, the physician should have medications discontinued if possible. Assays should be repeated when false laboratory values are suspected.[13]

Another way that some drugs, including over the counter (OTC) drugs such as aspirin, affect specimen collection is in causing the patient to bleed excessively. The most common

---

Box 11-4	Drug Interference

Interference from medications usually causes falsely elevated values when the true values are in the normal range or the subnormal range. Some drugs, such as acetaminophen (Tylenol) and erythromycin, can increase serum AST and bilirubin levels and, thus, falsely create a clinical interpretation of hepatic dysfunction without the true presence of an abnormality.[14]

Oral medication and intravenous medications or dyes can interfere with laboratory test results. For example, the results of laboratory tests (blood creatinine, cortisol, and digoxin) are affected by the intravenous fluorescein dye administered during angiography.[15] Consequently, the phlebotomist who collects blood in a cardiology section needs to be alert to this potential for laboratory test interference. If collecting blood from a patient who just had a dye injection, this information must be communicated promptly to the specimen collection supervisor.

Chemotherapeutic drugs used in cancer treatment can lead to a decrease in blood cellular elements and, thus, their metabolic and immunologic processes.

Various medications are toxic to the liver, causing acute hepatic necrosis and a subsequent increase in the concentration of blood liver enzymes, such as alanine aminotransferase (ALT), alkaline phosphatase (ALP), and LD.[13] The production of globulins and clotting factors is decreased in patients with drug-induced hepatotoxicity. Patients should also be monitored for a possible electrolyte imbalance and elevation of blood urea nitrogen (BUN) levels. Antihypertensive agents given for a long period to lower high blood pressure can lead to kidney damage if the patient is not monitored closely.

Pancreatitis can be caused by corticosteroids, estrogens, and diuretics, which cause elevations of serum amylase and lipase values. Aspirin causes hypobilirubinemia (a decrease in bilirubin) by expelling bilirubin from the plasma to the surrounding tissue cells.[16]

side effect in patients being treated with anticoagulant drugs such as warfarin or heparin (for management of acute coronary syndromes) is abnormal bleeding.[2] Thus, phlebotomists should take extra care in assuring that the bleeding has stopped after the collection procedure.

In addition to medications, other substances such as smoking may affect several laboratory tests' results. Through the action of nicotine from the tobacco, the blood concentrations of glucose, growth hormone, cholesterol, and triglyceride increase. Alcohol consumption also can skew laboratory tests' results, especially hematology results.

The health care worker collecting the blood specimen is the link between the clinical laboratory and the patient. Laboratory tests are often ordered without knowledge of the drugs taken or inhaled (e.g., nicotine) or consumed (e.g., alcohol) by a person. Yet, as discussed previously, these drugs will lead to falsely elevated or decreased values. Sometimes during blood collection a patient will mention that he or she has taken over-the-counter drugs, such as Tylenol, or that he or she has just smoked a cigarette. It is important for the health care worker to communicate the patient's name and the possible drug interference to the clinical laboratory supervisor in charge of specimen collection. The supervisor can then communicate with the attending physician and determine whether the medication or drug will interfere in the laboratory assays. The follow-up communication can lead to better patient management and care.

THROMBOSIS

Thrombi are solid masses derived from blood constituents that reside in the blood vessels. A thrombus may partially or fully occlude a vein (or artery), and such occlusion will make venipuncture more difficult.

Clinical Alert: Burned or Scarred Areas

Areas that have been burned or scarred should be avoided during phlebotomy. Burned areas are very sensitive and susceptible to infection, and veins under scarred areas are difficult to palpate. Collecting specimens from these sites can be very painful.

INFECTIONS

It should always be remembered that many patients have transmittable diseases (e.g., hepatitis) that could be passed from one patient to another. (For precautionary techniques, refer to Chapter 5, "Infection Control," and Chapter 6, "Safety and First Aid.")

VOMITING

Sometimes the thought or sight of blood before or during blood collection leads to vomiting. If this reaction occurs, have the patient take deep breaths and use a cold compress on his or her head. Also, inform the patient's physician of this complication.

OTHER FACTORS AFFECTING THE PATIENT

Many other factors can affect laboratory test results. Gender and pregnancy have an influence on laboratory testing; thus, reference ranges are often noted according to gender.

Geographic factors, such as altitude, temperature, and humidity, also affect baseline values. Collecting blood during home health care visits may entail traveling to regions other than the location of the laboratory. Thus, geographic information may need to be provided on the laboratory requisition or on the specimen in order to be considered in the patient's tests results.

▬▬▬ COMPLICATIONS ASSOCIATED WITH TEST REQUESTS AND IDENTIFICATION

IDENTIFICATION DISCREPANCIES

Improper identification is the most dangerous and costly error a phlebotomist can make, because it can be life threatening. As mentioned in previous chapters, identification should include a match between the patient's identification, his or her verbal confirmation, and the test requisition. Bed labels, water pitchers, or door charts should not be used as a patient identifier. Even armbands are not completely reliable.[17] Refer to Chapter 9 for more details on identification procedures in various circumstances. Sometimes a phlebotomist is the first to detect a discrepancy between a name on the requisition and the name that the patient verbalizes or the name on the armband. In these cases, the discrepancy should be reported to a supervisor and/or nurse and may result in the prevention of other errors related to that patient.

TIME OF COLLECTION

Timing factors can affect test results. In some cases, such as testing drug levels, the timing of the collection must coincide with when the dosage was given. Refer to Chapter 9 for further discussion of therapeutic drug monitoring. Early morning specimens are most commonly requested in hospital settings because a fasting specimen is preferred (since reference ranges are based on fasting specimens). If a phlebotomist is running late, the specimen might be collected *after* an inpatient has eaten breakfast, and would require a special notation about his or her "nonfasting" condition.

REQUISITIONS

Checking the requisition to match the laboratory tests requested with the appropriate type of collection tube is essential to minimize the amount of blood withdrawn from each patient. Too much blood loss because of excessive specimen removal can result in anemia.

COMPLICATIONS ASSOCIATED WITH THE SPECIMEN COLLECTION PROCEDURE

TOURNIQUET PRESSURE AND FIST PUMPING

Laboratory test results can be falsely elevated or decreased if the tourniquet pressure is too tight or is maintained too long. The pressure from the tourniquet causes biological analytes to leak from the tissue cells into the blood, or vice versa. For example, plasma cholesterol, iron, lipid, protein, and potassium levels will be falsely elevated if the tourniquet pressure is too tight or prolonged. Significant elevations may be seen with as short as a 3-minute application of the tourniquet (the recommended time for tourniquet application is no longer than 1 minute at a time).[10] In addition, some enzyme levels can be falsely elevated or decreased because of tourniquet pressure that is too tight or prolonged. Also, pumping of the fist before venipuncture should be avoided because it leads to an increase in the plasma potassium, lactate, and phosphate concentrations.

FAILURE TO DRAW BLOOD

Several factors may cause the health care worker to "miss the vein." These factors include not inserting the needle deep enough, inserting the needle all the way through the vein, holding the needle bevel against the vein wall, or losing the vacuum in the tube (as demonstrated in Figure 11–1 ■). During needle insertion, the phlebotomist's gloved index finger can be used to help locate the vein. The needle may need to be moved or withdrawn somewhat and redirected. In the geriatric patient, the vein may be "tough" during needle entry and may roll; such rolling can cause the needle to slip to the side of the vein instead of properly puncturing it. Thus the health care worker must securely anchor the vein prior to blood collection.

On occasion, a test tube will have no vacuum because of a manufacturer's error, the age of the tube, or tube leakage after a puncture. Consequently, an extra set of tubes should be readily available in case this should happen during venipuncture. Also, needles for evacuated tube systems have been known to unscrew from the barrel during venipuncture. If this happens, the tourniquet should be released immediately and the needle removed.

FAINTING (SYNCOPE)

Syncope is the transient (and frequently sudden) loss of consciousness due to a lack of oxygen to the brain and results in an inability to stay in an upright position. Patients usually recover their orientation quickly, but injuries (e.g., abrasions, lacerations) often result from falling to the ground. Syncope may be caused by a variety of things including hypoglycemia, hyperventilation, cardiac, neurologic, or psychiatric conditions, or medications.[2] Many patients become dizzy and faint ("get weak in the knees") at the thought or sight of blood. Also, patients who have donated blood recently and/or fasting patients frequently become faint. Consequently, the health care worker should be aware of the patient's condition throughout the collection procedure. This can be done by asking ambulatory patients if they tend to faint or if they have ever previously fainted during blood collections. If so, they should be moved from a seated position to a lying position. Even for an ambulatory patient without a history of fainting, it is still extremely important to use a blood collection chair with a "locked" armrest to avoid the possibility of a fall if he or she faints. If a seated patient feels faint, the needle should be removed, the patient's head should be lowered be-

Figure 11–1. Needle Positioning and Failure to Draw Blood

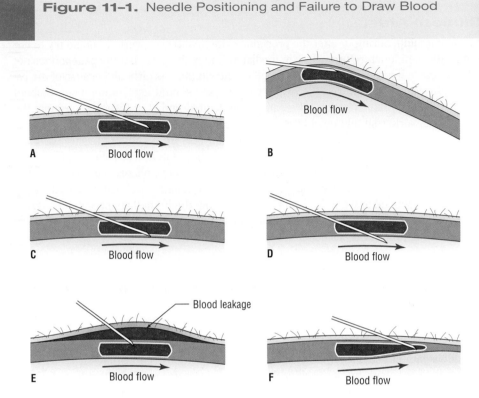

A. Correct insertion technique; blood flows freely into needle. B. Bevel on vein upper wall does not allow blood to flow. C. Bevel on vein lower wall does not allow blood to flow. D. Needle inserted too far. E. Needle partially inserted, which causes blood leakage into tissue. F. Collapsed vein.

tween the legs, and the patient should breathe deeply. If possible, the health care worker should ask for help and move the patient to a lying position. Talking to patients can often reassure them and divert their attention from the collection procedure. Bed-bound patients also experience fainting, or syncope, during blood collection, though rarely. In any case, the health care worker should stay with the patient at least 15 minutes until he or she recovers or until a nurse or physician takes over. A wet towel gently applied to the forehead or a glass of juice or water may help the patient feel better.

HEMATOMAS

When the area around the puncture site starts to swell, usually blood is leaking into the tissues and causing a hematoma.

PETECHIAE

Petechiae, small red hemorrhagic spots appearing on a patient's skin, indicate that minute amounts of blood have escaped into skin epithelium. This complication may be a result of a coagulation abnormality such as thrombocytopenia, that is, low platelet count, and should

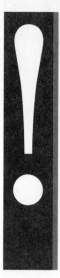

Clinical Alert

If a patient faints during or after the procedure, the health care worker should try to terminate the venipuncture procedure immediately and make sure that the patient does not fall or become injured. Sometimes, controlling the situation is difficult because of the patient's physical size; however, the health care worker should use common sense about the safest position for a patient. If a patient has fainted and is in a secure position, the health care worker should quickly request assistance from the nursing staff or a physician. A patient who has fainted should recover fully before being allowed to leave and should be instructed not to drive a vehicle for at least 30 minutes. Patients often think they recover very quickly, and after they try to stand up, they collapse again—with a possible injury. An incident report must be filed with the health care facility regarding the fainting incident and any injuries as a result of the fall, the immediate precautions taken, and what instructions were provided to the patient to prevent the possibility of long-term complications (e.g., a car accident after the fainting incident).

be a warning that the patient's puncture site may bleed excessively. Petechiae also occur during febrile illnesses.

EXCESSIVE BLEEDING

Normally a patient usually stops bleeding at the venipuncture site within a few minutes. Patients on anticoagulant therapy and/or those taking high dosages of arthritis medication or other medication, however, may bleed for a longer period. As mentioned above, coagulation abnormalities can also cause excessive bleeding. Thus, anytime a venipuncture is performed, pressure must be applied to the venipuncture site until the bleeding stops.

NEUROLOGICAL COMPLICATIONS

If the health care worker accidentally inserts the needle all the way through the vein, he or she may hit the nerve below the vein. If this happens, the patient will most likely have a sharp, electric tingling (and painful) sensation that radiates down the nerve. The tourni-

Clinical Alert

A hematoma can occur when the needle has gone completely through the vein, the bevel opening is partially in the vein, or not enough pressure is applied to the site after puncture. This swelling results in a large bruise after several days (Figure 11–2 ■). If a hematoma begins to form, the tourniquet and the needle should be removed immediately, and pressure should be applied to the area for approximately 2 minutes. If the bleeding continues, a nurse should be notified.

Figure 11–2. Patient's Hematoma After Venipunctures

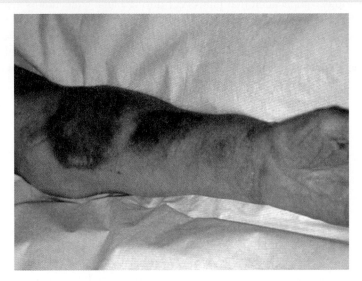

Source: Johnson & Johnson Medical Division, Ethicon, Inc., 1997. Used with permission of the copyright owner.

quet should be released immediately, the needle removed, and pressure held over the blood collection site. An incident report on the occurrence should be completed and given to the supervisor.

INTRAVENOUS THERAPY

Every time a catheter is used, vein damage occurs. Circulatory blood is rerouted to collateral veins and can result in hemoconcentration. Consequently, patients on intravenous (IV) therapy for extended periods often have veins that are palpable and visible but damaged or

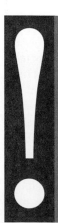

Clinical Alert

The health care worker must not leave the patient until the bleeding stops or a nurse takes over to assess the patient's situation. In rare instances, the phlebotomist may accidentally puncture an artery instead of a vein. These cases require that pressure be applied as quickly as possible to stop the bleeding and that a nurse and/or supervisor be notified as soon as possible.

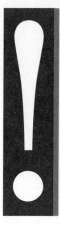

Clinical Alert

A rare but serious complication that may occur during blood collection is a seizure. If a patient begins to have a seizure, the health care worker should immediately release the tourniquet, remove the needle, move the patient to a lying position if they have not fallen already, attempt to hold pressure over the blood collection site, and call for help from the nursing station. No attempt should be made to place anything in the patient's mouth unless the health care worker is experienced and authorized to do so.

occluded (blocked). Whenever a patient has an IV line, the arm with the IV line should not be used for venipuncture because the specimen will be diluted with IV fluid. Instead, the other arm or another site should be considered. Alternatively, sometimes the nurse or the physician can disconnect the IV line and draw blood from the line that is already inserted. In this situation, the first few milliliters of the specimen should be discarded to remove the IV fluid, and a note should be made on the laboratory requisition that this step was performed. (Refer to Chapter 13 for more detailed information about blood collection from intravenous lines.)

HEMOCONCENTRATION

Hemoconcentration, the increased concentration of larger molecules and formed elements in the blood is caused by several factors, including prolonged (i.e., longer than 1 minute) tourniquet application; massaging, squeezing, or probing a site; long-term IV therapy; and sclerosed or occluded veins. All of these practices and/or sites for venipuncture should be carefully avoided.

HEMOLYSIS

Hemolysis results when RBCs are lysed, hemoglobin is released, and serum, which is normally straw colored, becomes tinged with pink or red. If a specimen is grossly hemolyzed, the serum appears very dark red. Hemolysis can be caused by improper phlebotomy techniques, such as using a needle that is too small, expelling the blood vigorously into a tube, shaking or mixing tubes vigorously, performing blood collection before the alcohol has dried at the collection site, or pulling a syringe plunger back too fast (although syringes are not recommended for routine use). Hemolysis may also be the result of physiological abnormalities (e.g., sickle cell diseases, exposure to drugs or toxins, artificial heart valves, some infections, etc.).[2] Hemolysis causes falsely increased results for many analytes, including potassium, magnesium, iron, lactate dehydrogenase, phosphorus, ammonia, and total protein.[1] Hemolysis also shows decreased RBC count, hemoglobin, and hematocrit. These problems can easily be prevented with appropriate handling. The health care worker should document the fact if he or she notices that a specimen is hemolyzed.

COLLAPSED VEINS

Veins collapse when blood is withdrawn too quickly or forcefully during venipuncture, especially when blood is being collected from smaller veins (see Figure 11–1F) and/or the veins of geriatric patients. Thus the phlebotomist should use an evacuated tube with a smaller volume and/or a smaller needle size during the collection process on patients with smaller veins and/or geriatric patients. A collapsed vein should not be probed with the needle.

TURBID OR LIPEMIC SERUM

After the cells have settled or have been separated from the serum it is normally clear, light yellow, or straw colored. Turbid serum appears cloudy or "milky" and can be a result of bacterial contamination or high lipid levels in the blood. Turbidity is primarily caused by ingestion of fatty substances, such as meat, butter, cream, and cheese, or can occur when a lipid supplement is included in parenteral nutrition preparations. If a patient has recently eaten fatty substances, he or she may have a temporarily elevated lipid level, and the serum will appear lipemic, or cloudy. Because lipemic serum does not represent a basal state and may indicate some chemical abnormalities, documentation about the appearance of the serum may be useful to the physician.

IMPROPER COLLECTION TUBE

Phlebotomists should learn which common laboratory tests require which collection tubes. However, there are so many possible laboratory tests and tubes available that they should also be familiar with how and where to seek information (electronically via laboratory reference manual, etc.) about test and tube requirements that they are unfamiliar with. An example of an blood specimen collected in the wrong tube would be as follows: green-topped tubes containing lithium heparin are not suitable for a patient's lithium studies because laboratory values will be falsely high suggesting that the patient has a toxic level of lithium when he or she really does not.

◼◼◼◼ COMPLICATIONS ASSOCIATED WITH SPECIMEN TRANSPORT

Methods for transporting specimens, including how to transport specimens that require chilling, are covered in Chapter 7. Equipment such as pneumatic tube systems should be carefully evaluated and selected prior to use. Couriers who transport specimens should be knowledgeable of all precautions and special transporting techniques as noted below.

CHILLED TRANSPORT

Specimens that should be kept cool should not be placed directly on ice, but instead in an icy water slurry (mixture of ice and water). Ammonia and renin are examples of analytes that deteriorate rapidly if not chilled.

EXPOSURE TO LIGHT

Bilirubin deteriorates rapidly if exposed to light and needs to be shielded from light by covering the tube with aluminum foil.

◼◼◼◼ COMPLICATIONS ASSOCIATED WITH SPECIMEN RECEIPT IN THE LABORATORY

PROCESSING DELAYS

Specimens should be transported to the laboratory for processing as soon as possible because delays can significantly affect laboratory results. Table 11–1 describes time limits for common laboratory tests. In addition, if serum or plasma stays in contact with cells for prolonged periods, significant changes in laboratory values occur.

Clinical Alert

Patients on oral anticoagulant therapy (e.g., warfarin, heparin) require constant monitoring by physicians, using coagulation test results. In recent years adverse events and deaths were linked to coagulation testing errors related to the PT (prothrombin time) and the INR (international normalized ratio, a value calculated from the PT and a reagent-specific number, the international sensitivity index (ISI).

One factor that affects the INR is the concentration of sodium citrate in the collection tube. Sodium citrate concentrations of 3.2 percent are now recommended for most coagulation studies. Another factor that affects the PT (and thus the INR) is the length of time and how a specimen should be stored. Studies have shown varying effects of storage; however, NCCLS guidelines state that uncentrifuged specimens for PT/INR or centrifuged plasma left on the cells in the tube that are stored at various temperatures from 2 to 24 degrees should be run within 24 hours from the time the sample was collected. However, if the patient is on anticoagulant therapy, the PT results may vary between the time of collection and after storage.

One author recommends that "all specimens should be treated as if they were the last specimens that could be obtained from the test subject without having to recollect the sample. If another assay is required, such as an APTT or factor assay, the prolonged storage times of >4 hours would possibly render the specimen compromised and require the patient to have a second venipuncture. This increases time and expense for all concerned".[18,19] A third factor that causes variability in coagulation testing are the "partial-draw tubes" that withdraw 1.8 or 2.7 mL of blood versus the conventional 4.5 mL draw. Since the partial-draw tubes fill more slowly, reports suggest that platelets have more time to become activated, thus releasing factors that would compromise coagulation test results.[18,19,20] Therefore, each laboratory must carefully establish its own protocols for coagulation specimen collection, processing, and testing, and phlebotomists should follow the protocols precisely.

TABLE 11–1. Time Delays for Common Laboratory Testing[17,18,19,20]

Common laboratory tests are listed below if their results exhibit significant changes due to time delays. Even though some analytes may be stable for longer periods, NCCLS suggests that cells be removed/separated from serum or plasma within 2 hours of collection. The results of some of the tests included below change significantly if the cells remain in contact with the plasma or sera.

LABORATORY TEST	ACCEPTABLE TIME DELAY AND/OR METHOD OF STORAGE*	EFFECTS OF PROLONGED DELAY
Acid Phosphatase		Decreased level if left in contact with cells
ALT and AST	After cell separation can be stored 24 hours at 22°C	
Ammonia	Deteriorates quickly; requires chilling	Increased level if left in contact with cells
Bilirubin	Protect from light	Begins to deteriorate after 1 hour of exposure to light
Calcium		Decreased level if left in contact with cells
Coagulation Studies	Can be kept at room temperature up to 4 hours	After 4 hrs, PTT is unreliable.
	May be frozen up to 21 days at −70°C	PT is stable unopened up to 48 hours at room temperature, but refrigeration may increase results.
		(Data from numerous studies are variable on times and temperatures for specimen storage. Each laboratory must carefully establish their own protocols.)
CO_2		Decreased level if left in contact with cells.
Creatinine	After cell separation can be stored 24 hours at 22°C	Increased level if left in contact with cells
Glucose	After cell separation can be stored 2 hours at 22°C	Decreased level if left in contact with cells
Hematology Studies	Refrigerate up to 24 hours at 4°C for cell counts and cell morphology. For sedimentation rates use unrefrigerated within 4 hours or within 12 hours if refrigerated at 4°C. Reticulocytes are stable up to 6 hours at room temperature, or 72 hours if refrigerated.	
Ionized Calcium	After cell separation can be stored 2 hours at 22°C	Decreased level if left in contact with cells
Iron		Increased level if left in contact with cells
LDH	After cell separation can be stored 24 hours at 22°C	Increased level if left in contact with cells
Magnesium	After cell separation can be stored 4 hours at 4°C	Increased level if left in contact with cells
Phosphate		Increased level if left in contact with cells
Phosphorous	After cell separation can be stored 24 hours at 22°C	Increased level if left in contact with cells
Potassium	After cell separation can be stored 2 hours at 22°C	Increased level if left in contact with cells

*Room temperature is considered about 22°C, and refrigeration is about 4°C.

SPECIMEN REJECTION

Each department or section in the clinical laboratory should establish its own guidelines for specimen rejection. In general, the factors shown in Box 11–5 should be considered. In all of the cases listed below, the resulting effects are negative: the patient has to undergo another venipuncture; there is loss of critical data for the physician to make clinical decisions upon; there are costly and inefficient uses of work time; and legal risks are more pronounced. All these circumstances should be avoided through diligent practices and adherence to standards.

When a problem arises, the appropriate investigational channels should be followed including supervisory and/or management staff. Communication and honesty are the keys to an efficient and reliable health care environment.

Box 11–5   Criteria and Complications Leading to Blood Specimen Rejection

Anticoagulated blood-containing clots

Contaminated specimen

Discrepancies between requisition form and labeled tube (e.g., names, dates, times)

Excessive delays in processing the specimen

Hemolyzed specimen (except for tests in which hemolysis does not interfere)

Improper specimen transportation or storage (e.g., blood gas specimen not transported in slurry of ice water)

Improper blood collection tube (the correct additive is a requirement for specific tests)

Inadequate specimen identification (e.g., tubes are not labeled or erroneously labeled)

Insufficient quantity (volume) of blood in collection tube (e.g., too little blood results in excessive additives within the tube; too much blood dilutes the additive so as to make it ineffective)

Lipemic specimen

Nonfasting specimen

Outdated/expired equipment, supplies, or reagents (e.g., because vacuum decreases in old blood collection tube; silicon coating tends to break down with age; etc.)

Variation in patient's posture (because the level of aldosterone, for example, changes depending on whether the patient is sitting or lying for blood collection)

Unlabelled tube(s)

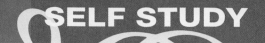

SELF STUDY

KEY TERMS

basal state

diurnal rhythms

fasting

hematoma

hemoconcentration

hemolysis

hypobilirubinemia

lipemic

lymphostasis

mastectomy

menstrual cycle

obesity

occluded veins

petechiae

sclerosed veins

supine

syncope

thrombi

turbid

STUDY QUESTIONS

The following questions may have more than one answer.

1. Which of the following factors result in failure to draw blood during venipuncture?
   a. losing the vacuum in the tube
   b. tying the tourniquet too tightly
   c. inserting the needle through the vein
   d. puncturing a sclerosed vein

2. Hematomas during venipuncture result from which of the following?
   a. needle bevel is against vein wall
   b. needle bevel is partially inserted in the vein
   c. needle is occluded
   d. patient has coagulation problems

3. Which of the following causes hemoconcentration?
   a. long-term IV therapy
   b. lengthy tourniquet application
   c. excessive needle probing
   d. sclerosed or occluded veins

4. Which of the following is a solid mass derived from blood constituents and can occlude a vein (or an artery)?
   a. hemolyzed RBC
   b. hemolyzed WBC
   c. thrombus
   d. triglyceride

5. If blood is to be drawn for a timed blood-glucose-level determination, the patient must fast for how long?
   a. 4 to 6 hours
   b. 6 to 8 hours
   c. 8 to 12 hours
   d. 14 to 16 hours

6. Which of the following laboratory test results are affected most if the patient is not fasting?
   a. AST and CPK
   b. triglycerides and glucose
   c. cortisol and testosterone
   d. complete blood cell (CBC) count and prothrombin time

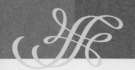

7. An abnormal accumulation of fluid in the intercellular spaces of the body that is localized or diffused is referred to as:

   a. hemoconcentration   c. atherosclerosis

   b. edema   d. hemolysis

8. If a patient is taking high doses of Tylenol, which of the following analyte results is most likely to be affected?

   a. serum bilirubin   c. blood glucose

   b. CPK   d. blood cholesterol

9. If the tourniquet is applied for longer than 3 minutes, which of the following analytes will most likely become falsely elevated?

   a. potassium   c. GGT

   b. bilirubin   d. parathyroid hormone

10. Emotional stress, such as anxiety or fear, can lead to alterations of which of the following analytes?

   a. serum iron   c. cortisol

   b. WBCs   d. RBCs

References

1. National Committee for Clinical Laboratory Standards (NCCLS): Procedures and Devices for the Collection of Diagnostic Capillary Blood Specimens, Approved Standard, 5th ed. H4-A4. (940 West Valley Road, Suite 1400, Wayne, PA 19087-1898): NCCLS, 2003.

2. Venes, D: *Taber's Cyclopedic Medical Dictionary,* 19th ed. Philadelphia: FA Davis Company, 2001.

3. Weight Watchers: Welcome brochure. (175 Crossways Park West, Woodbury, NY 11797-2055, 1800-651-6000) www.weightwatchers.com, 2000.

4. Ernst, D: Iodine Disinfectant for Infants, Tips from the Clinical Experts. *Medical Laboratory Observer,* July 2003: p.54, www.mlo-online.com.

5. Foran, SE, Lewandrowski, KB, Kratz, A: Effects of Exercise on Laboratory Test Results, *Laboratory Medicine,* October 2003; 34(10): 736–742.

6. Kratz, A, Lewandrowski, KB, Siegel, AJ, et al: Effect of marathon running on hematologic and biochemical laboratory parameters, including cardiac markers. *Am Journal of Clinical Pathology,* 2002; 118: 856–863.

7. Guder, WG, Narayanan, S, Wisser, H, et al.: *Samples: From the Patient to the Laboratory.* Germany: Git Verlag Pub, 1996.

8. Becton-Dickinson and Company: *Blood Specimen Collection by Skin Puncture in Infants.* East Rutherford, NJ: Becton-Dickinson and Company, 1982.

9. Statland, BE, Winkel, P: Preparing patients and specimens for laboratory testing. In Henry, JB (ed), *Clinical Diagnosis and Management by Laboratory Methods.* Philadelphia: WB Saunders, 1991.

10. Statland, BE, Winkle, P, Bokelund, H: Factors contributing to intra-individual variation of serum constituents: Effects of posture and tourniquet application on variation of serum constituents in healthy subjects. *Clin Chem,* 1974; 20: 1513.

11. Dale, J: Preanalytical Variables in Laboratory Testing. *Laboratory Medicine,* 1998; 29: 540–545.

12. McNamara, JR: Cardiovascular disease: Laboratory testing adds important information to risk profile. *Clin Lab News,* 2000; 26(10): 12–16.

13. Young, DS: *Effects of Drugs on Clinical Laboratory Tests,* 5th ed. Washington, DC: AACC Press, 2000.

14. Sherlock, S: Progress report: Hepatic reaction to drugs. *Gut,* 1979; 20: 634.

15. Elin, RJ, Bloom, JN, Herman, DC, et al.: Interference by intravenous fluorescein with laboratory tests. *Clin Chem,* 1989; 35(6): 1159.

16. Routh, J, Paul, W: Assessment of interference by aspirin with some assays commonly done in the clinical laboratory. Clin Chem, 1976; 22: 837.

17. Ernst, DJ: *Eliminating Preanalytical Errors in Specimen Collection.* Presented at 2002 Texas Phlebotomy Conference, Lubbock, TX, September 21, 2002.

18. McGlasson, DL: Laboratory Variables That May Affect Test Results in Prothrombin Times (PT)/International Normalized Ratios (INR). *Laboratory Medicine,* February 2003; 34(2): 124–129.

19. National Committee for Clinical Laboratory Standards (NCCLS): Collection, Transport, and Processing of Blood Specimens for Coagulation Testing and General Performance of Coagulation Assays, Approved Standard, H21-A3. (940 West Valley Road, Suite 1400, Wayne, PA 19087-1898): NCCLS, 1998.

20. National Committee for Clinical Laboratory Standards (NCCLS): Procedures for Handling and Processing of Blood Specimens, Approved Standard, H18-A2. (940 West Valley Road, Suite 1400, Wayne, PA 19087-1898): NCCLS, 1999.

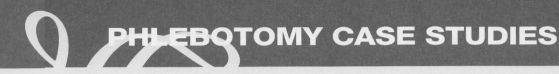

Ambulatory Health Care Collections

Ms. Jeanne Peterson is a health care provider who contracts with two community hospitals to make home health care visits. This morning as she arrived at Lake Mountain Hospital late due to an early winter snowstorm, she noticed she had seven home visits. She quickly threw blood collection equipment in her lockable container and hurried to her first patient, Ms. Verle Ragsdale, an 82-year-old African American woman, who has type II diabetes with myocardial complications. Her physician had requested a complete chemistry profile and protime, in addition to a physical examination. After Ms. Peterson checked Ms. Ragsdale's vital signs, she decided to collect Ms. Ragsdale's blood with a winged infusion blood collection set due to the fragility of her veins. She prepared the site for blood collection and after opening a 25-gauge safety winged infusion needle set, she inserted the needle into the patient's vein in her hand and first collected blood in a light blue–topped tube for the protime, followed by blood collection into a red speckled–topped vacuum tube. After completing the physical exam and blood collection, she labeled the tubes, discarded the biohazardous blood collection items in her biohazardous disposal container, and left Ms. Ragsdale's home with the collected blood and health care equipment, including the blood collection items.

Next, she traveled over the slippery, snow-covered roads to the home of Mr. Ben Sadler, a 32-year-old white hemophiliac who had acquired hepatitis C from a blood transfusion years earlier. His physician had requested a liver profile. Ms. Peterson introduced herself to Mr. Sadler and prepared her blood collection supplies and equipment for blood collection for Mr. Sadler. As she checked Mr. Sadler's veins, she decided to use a butterfly needle in Mr. Sadler's lower arm due to the sclerosed veins in the antecubital fossa area on both arms. She looked for a blood collection set in her supplies but only found a 23-gauge needle, separate tubing, and a separate Luer Lok. She put the pieces together and found a needle holder assembly and red-speckled collection tube. After attaching the various pieces, hoping they would work together, she prepared Mr. Sadler's arm for blood collection. She inserted the needle into his vein and as she pushed the tube onto the needle holder assembly, the Luer-Lok became disengaged and splattered blood over Ms. Peterson's laboratory coat and into her face. She immediately pulled the tourniquet off of Mr. Sadler's arm, pulled the needle out of his vein, cleaned the area around him, and ran to his bathroom to wash the blood from her face and eyes.

Questions

1. Did the health care provider use the proper order of draw for Ms. Ragsdale's laboratory tests? Explain.
2. Was the proper blood collection procedure used for obtaining blood from Ms. Ragsdale? Explain.

3. Was the proper blood collection procedure used for obtaining blood from Mr. Sadler? Explain.

4. What preventive measures could the phlebotomist have taken to avoid the negative outcome with Mr. Sadler? Why might the following phrase be appropriate in this case, "an ounce of prevention is worth a pound of cure"?

Venipuncture Site Selection

The medical laboratory technician, Sara Wong, went to collect blood from a 65-year-old hospitalized patient, Mary McDonald. Mrs. McDonald was a diabetic. She had recently undergone a partial mastectomy on her right side. The area around the mastectomy appeared swollen. She had an IV going just below the antecubital area of her left arm. The ordered tests were CBC, differential, and electrolytes. Sara carefully selected a site and was successful on the first attempt to collect the blood samples.

Questions

1. What would be the preferred site and method of choice for the phlebotomy procedure for this patient?

2. Explain why other sites were eliminated.

3. What special documentation (if any) might be helpful for this phlebotomy procedure?

4. List several techniques that can facilitate the selection of a suitable site.

Finding the Right Site

A 68-year-old woman, Mrs. Triplet, comes for her annual check up to the oncology clinic. After her visit with her doctor, she is sent to the laboratory to have some "routine" blood specimens collected. The phlebotomist correctly identifies her, prepares the site, supplies, and equipment and inquires about which arm Mrs. Triplet prefers to have the puncture performed on. Mrs. Triplet says, "Well, it doesn't really matter to me but I had my mastectomy done 5 years ago on this side and they usually stick me over here," as she points to her left arm.

Questions

1. How should the phlebotomist proceed?

2. Why would a mastectomy make any difference in site selection?

3. Does the length of time after a mastectomy make any difference?

Tricky Complications with an IV

A 76-year-old male veteran was hospitalized for surgery to remove a brain tumor. He had an IV with chemotherapy drugs in one arm and the other arm had been amputated above the elbow due to war injuries. The phlebotomist, Betty Booboo, was sent to collect blood for chemistry tests. After testing, the physician called the laboratory supervisor requesting that the electrolytes be repeated because of hyponatremia (i.e., low sodium level). He explained the patient's condition. The laboratory supervisor immediately called Betty to ask about the site she used for blood collection. As a result the patient's specimen was re-collected and the new samples were re-tested.

Questions

1. Why was the sodium value falsely low?
2. What blood collection sites should be considered in this scenario?
3. What other steps could Betty have taken to avoid another venipuncture to the patient?

Answers for all case study questions can be found in Appendix 12.

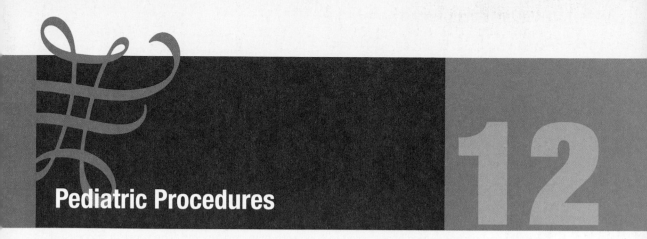

Pediatric Procedures

CHAPTER OBJECTIVES

Upon completion of Chapter 12, the learner is responsible for the following:

1. Describe fears or concerns that children in different developmental stages might have toward the blood collection process.

2. List suggestions that might be appropriate for parental and health care worker behavior during a venipuncture or skin puncture.

3. Identify puncture sites for a heelstick on an infant and describe the procedure.

4. Describe the venipuncture sites for infants and young children.

5. Discuss the types of equipment and supplies that must be used during microcollection and venipuncture of infants and children.

6. Describe the procedure for specimen collection for neonatal phenylketonuria (PKU) and metabolic screening.

 MediaLINK

Access the accompanying CD-ROM to explore a wide variety of review questions and interactive activities for this chapter, including multiple choice, true/false, and video exercises.

Collecting blood from a pediatric patient requires much expertise and knowledge. Not all pediatric phlebotomies are finger sticks, so the novice health care worker must have additional knowledge specific to pediatric anatomy and physiology. Children are not just little adults and should not be treated as such. There are differences that relate to anatomy and physiology in children. The health care worker needs to be familiar with special types of equipment that are available, observe the various techniques as they are performed by a health care worker experienced in pediatric phlebotomy, and practice the techniques to develop the necessary skills. The health care worker will also need to develop competence in relating psychologically with children of various ages and developmental stages.

Performing venipunctures on young patients is technically and emotionally challenging for the health care worker because of their small size and because children are less emotionally and psychologically prepared to cope with pain and anxiety. Therefore, a successful outcome requires the use of good interpersonal skills in preparing the child and the concerned, apprehensive parents.[1,2]

With proper training in technique and an understanding of pediatric developmental characteristics, the delicate task of collecting blood from a frightened child need not cause fear or dread in the health care worker. Phlebotomy skills should be perfected on older children first, then when confidence is attained, venipunctures can be attempted on younger children. When learning the techniques, the health care worker should remember to ask for help if needed and allow adequate time to develop the necessary skills. Many pediatric hospitals employ Child Life specialists who are trained in helping children cope with hospitalization and painful procedures. If a Child Life specialist is available he or she can play an important role in assisting the child and parent through the procedure.[3]

■■■■■■ AGE-SPECIFIC CARE CONSIDERATIONS

Age-specific care considerations are shown in Table 12–1. It describes not only the fears and concerns of the pediatric patient at various ages, but also suggests parental involvement, comfort measures, and provides competencies and tips for the phlebotomist.

■■■■■■ PREPARING CHILD AND PARENT

The timing of the preparation depends on the child's age; generally, the younger the child, the closer the explanation should be to the time of the procedure.[3]

Preparing the child and the parent for the blood collection procedure involves the following steps:

1. A calm, confident approach is the first step in limiting the anxiety of the patient and parent and obtaining their cooperation. Introduce yourself. Be warm and friendly, establish eye contact, and show that you are concerned about the child's health and comfort. When you interact with a pediatric patient and his or her parent, you should instill a sense of trust and confidence.
2. Correctly identify the patient. JCAHO Patient Safety Goal 1 states, "Improve the accuracy of patient identification; use at least two patient identifiers."[4] The patient should have an identification bracelet with name and hospital number or birth date. Verify the correct name and hospital number or name and birth date. A hospitalized infant usually has the identification bracelet on his or her ankle. Newborns that are not yet

TABLE 12–1. Age-specific Care Considerations and Competencies for Phlebotomists

AGE	FEARS AND CONCERNS	COMMUNICATION	COMFORT	SAFETY	PARENT BEHAVIOR
0–6 months	• Totally dependent on and trusts parents and other adults	• Introduce yourself to caregiver • Explain procedures	• Keep patient warm • Warm site of puncture if needed • Parent may hold child • Use very gentle approach • Use of a distraction, such as light pen, key ring, or bell, may minimize fear	• Keep side rails up during procedure • Do not leave any supplies or discarded items on bed • Encourage parent to hold or cuddle infant after procedure • Use appropriate microcollection supplies and equipment	• Parent may hold child as an aid to the phlebotomist and to provide comfort
6–12 months	• Fear of strangers • Fear of separation from parent • Limited language use	• Introduce yourself to caregiver • Talk slowly to infant • Try to make eye contact with infant	• Keep patient warm • Warm site of puncture if needed • Allow familiar health care worker to perform procedure • Allow parent to be in close proximity • Allow child to use pacifier, hold teddy, blanket, or other comforting items	• Do not separate from caregiver unless absolutely necessary • Keep side rails up • Do not leave any supplies or discarded items on bed • Encourage parent to hold or cuddle infant after procedure • Use appropriate microcollection supplies and equipment	• Parent may assist by holding, explaining to, and comforting the child • Parent may help identify comforting toy

(continued)

TABLE 12–1. Continued

AGE	FEARS AND CONCERNS	COMMUNICATION	COMFORT	SAFETY	PARENT BEHAVIOR
1–3 years	• Self-centered • Fear of injury • Fear of long separation from parent	• Introduce yourself to both child and caregiver • Child will understand simple commands and may choose to cooperate • Take it slowly, do not rush patient, he or she needs time to think about your requests • Allow child to touch supplies but dispose if they become contaminated • Ask parent to also explain procedure in familiar terms	• Keep patient warm • Warm site of puncture if needed • Allow familiar health care worker to perform procedure • Allow parent to be in close proximity	• Try not to separate from parent unless absolutely necessary. If needed, reinforce that it is only for a short period of time • Keep side rails up • Do not leave supplies or discarded items on bed • Use appropriate microcollection supplies and equipment	• Parent may assist by holding, explaining to, and comforting the child • Parent may help identify comforting toy • Encourage parent to praise child after procedure • Allow child to use pacifier, hold teddy, blanket, or other comforting items
3–5 years	• Self-centered • Fear of injury • Enjoys pretending and role playing	• Introduce yourself • Talk to child in simple terms • Allow child to touch equipment • Try using familiar cartoon characters (Disney, Sesame Street) in the explanation • Perhaps use toys to demonstrate procedure	• Allow child to have familiar things or people near by • Give child time to verbalize his or her fears	• May tolerate separation from parent • Able to recognize danger and obey simple commands • Needs close supervision • Keep side rails up • Do not leave supplies or discarded items on bed	• Parent may be present to provide emotional support and to assist in obtaining the child's cooperation • Encourage praise for bravery

Age	Behaviors / Characteristics	Strategies	Equipment / Procedure	Parent Presence
6–12 years	• Less dependent on parents • Fear losing self-control • More willing to participate • Tries to be Independent • Curious	• Introduce yourself • Child may be interested in health concepts, "why" and "how" • Explain "why" the blood is needed • Involve child in the procedure • Child may pretend he or she is the doctor and will "help" with the procedure • Provide tokens for bravery • Try not to embarrass the child but offer them a comforting toy or familiar object • Take it slowly, allow time for repeat questions • Allow child some input on decisions (e.g., color of bandage, etc.)	• Use appropriate microcollection supplies and equipment	• Child may ask parent to leave room
13–17 years	• Actively involved in anything concerning the body • More independent • Embarrassed to show fear • Needs privacy • May act hostile to mask fear	• Introduce yourself • Use adult vocabulary, do not "talk down" • Explain procedure thoroughly • Ask if he or she would like to help with the procedure • Ask what might make them more comfortable • Allow time for questions or to handle supplies • Maintain privacy • Take extra time for explanations and or preparation • Offer them the opportunity to have parent close by • Give them time to recover after the procedure if they have cried • Use same strategies as adult	• Use appropriate collection supplies and equipment depending on the size of the individual and the physical and emotional tolerance to procedure • Side rails should be left up after procedure • Do not leave supplies or discarded items on bed • Use appropriate microcollection supplies and equipment	• Child may not want parent to be present
Children with special problems or mental disabilities	• Fears are similar to the behaviors of the developmental level • Need relaxed, gentle approach	• Use strategies that are appropriate for the developmental stage	• Use strategies that are appropriate for the developmental stage	• Use strategies that are appropriate for the developmental stage

named are usually identified by their last names (e.g., Baby Boy Smith, Baby Girl Jones) and identification number. If the mother is still in the hospital after delivery, the baby may wear an identification band that is cross-referenced to the mother. Keeping identifications straight is always crucial, but especially so when specimens from twin babies must be collected and labeled.

3. Find out about the child's past experience with blood collections. Ask whether the child has ever had blood collected. The child and the parent can then tell about their experiences with past procedures and provide you with valuable information about the approaches that worked effectively for them and those that were not as successful.

4. Develop a plan. Ask the parent how cooperative his or her child will be. Parents are excellent predictors of their child's behavior and possibility for distress. Usually, the younger child with poor venous access will experience more distress. A successful plan involves not only the parent's suggestions about what will be most helpful but also the health care worker's knowledge of pediatric phlebotomy techniques. If possible, allow the child to have some control by offering a choice of which arm or finger he or she prefers blood to be taken. After assessing the experiences, anxieties, and fears of the parent and the child, use the procedure for that will provide the best possible success.

5. Place yourself at the child's eye level to explain and demonstrate the procedure (Figure 12–1 ■). When explaining what you will be doing, use words appropriate for the child's age. Children interpret words literally, so be careful of your choice of words. Use of a doll, puppet, or stuffed animal in the demonstration can help you relate to the child in a nonthreatening manner. If the child has a favorite doll, blanket, or toy, he or she should be encouraged to hug it for comfort and support.

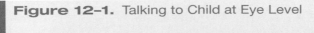

Figure 12–1. Talking to Child at Eye Level

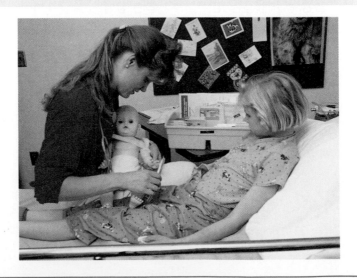

6. Establish guidelines. Tell the child and the parent that the procedure will most likely be successful on the first attempt. If not, it will be attempted only once more by another health care worker who will complete the procedure.

7. Be honest when a child asks if the puncture will hurt. Tell the child that if the procedure hurts too much, it can be momentarily stopped, but that the quicker the procedure is performed the less painful it will be. Instruct the child to say when he or she feels the pain or "hurt." The child should be told that saying "ouch" or making faces is acceptable, but that he or she must make an effort to keep the arm absolutely still. Reassure the child that the blood will be collected as quickly as possible so that the pain will be brief.[3]

8. Encourage parent involvement. Research demonstrates that parental presence and behavior can have the most beneficial effect on the child's anxiety and behavior during the procedure.[3] Explain how the parent can assist by holding, distracting, and soothing their child during the procedure. Some parents, however, may be reluctant to participate because they do not want to be a part of a procedure that will cause their children pain. If the parent does not wish to assist but is willing to be in the room, ask him or her to maintain eye contact with the child to reduce stress. Each parent's ability to assist must be assessed. If after discussing his or her role the parent is still reluctant to be in the room, his or her wishes should be respected. If the parent does not wish to participate, you may ask a Child Life specialist or nurse to assist.

The following parental behaviors and examples will have a positive effect on relieving the child's distress.[2,5]

Behaviors	Examples
Distraction	"Look at Mommy"; "Tell the nurse about your doll"
Emotional support	Hugging, stroking hair, patting, and talking in a soothing voice
Explanation	"We need to take a tiny bit of blood from your finger"; "You will feel a little prick"; "Mommy will help you hold your arm still so that we can finish quickly"
Positive reinforcement	"You did a great job in holding your arm still!"

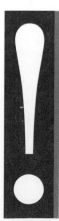

Clinical Alert

It is not unusual for a sick or injured child to act younger than he or she really is. If a child who is 6 behaves like a 3 year old, the health care worker should use strategies appropriate for a 3 year old.[5]

PSYCHOLOGICAL RESPONSE TO NEEDLES AND PAIN

Children especially fear needles, and an emotionally distraught child has difficulty separating fear from actual pain. Children 1 to 2 years of age may react as intensely to painless procedures, such as taking a temperature, as to those that actually do cause pain. Children 3 to 5 perceive pain as a punishment for bad behavior. They may react aggressively, especially if restrained. Children 6 to 10 are more likely to relate pain to past experiences. Many children perceive that a "shot," or needle, hurts more than anything else that has ever happened to them. Nevertheless, with proper preparation, the child and the parent can develop coping skills to help alleviate the fear and thereby diminish the "hurt."

DISTRACTION TECHNIQUES

Children over three respond well to distraction techniques to help them cope and lessen distress. Distraction helps the child refocus on a more pleasant experience. A parent, another health care worker, or Child Life specialist can provide the distraction. Some examples of distraction are blowing bubbles, pinwheels, counting, reading a book or looking at a video, listening to music, singing, or talking in a gentle voice about something enjoyable. School-age children may respond to strategies such as picturing themselves in a pleasant setting or participating in the procedure.[2,5]

ROOM LOCATION

For psychological reasons, the best room location for a painful procedure is a treatment room away from the child's bed or playroom. For a hospitalized child, the bed should be a safe, secure place to rest and sleep, not a place associated with pain. If the child shares a room with another child, performing the procedure at the bedside can be upsetting to the roommate as well. If the child cannot be moved to a treatment room, privacy should be maintained by drawing a curtain between the beds and speaking in a calm, quiet manner.

EQUIPMENT PREPARATION FOR A FRIENDLIER ENVIRONMENT

Just the sight of needles, syringes, and a person in a white laboratory coat can be frightening to a child. Nurses and other health care providers working with children frequently wear bright, colorfully printed uniforms or smocks to create a child-friendly environment. Equipment, too, can be modified to appear less threatening. As an example, prepare the phlebotomy equipment and supplies prior to entering the child's room so that the child does not become even more anxious by watching the preparation. Use shorter needles if possible, and keep threatening-looking supplies (such as needles) covered and out of sight. If the hospital policy requires goggles or face shields for blood-exposure precautions, put this equipment on after greeting the child. Praise the child throughout the procedure. At the completion, reward the child with a colorful bandage, a sticker, an age-appropriate toy, or with parental permission, a lollipop. If no parent is present to assist in relieving the anxiety, you or the nurse may cuddle, rock, and offer a pacifier to an infant or gently stroke or talk softly to sooth a small child.

POSITIONS FOR RESTRAINING A CHILD

Holding the child may be required to ensure that the child does not move the limb during blood collection. Restraining techniques should be compassionate, safe, and performed quickly. A supportive parent who has been properly instructed can assist with restraining while providing comfort to the child.

Two preferred methods of restraining a child to immobilize the arm are the vertical position and the horizontal, or supine, position (Figures 12–2 ■ and 12–3 ■).[2,5] In both cases, the parent's face is in close proximity to the child's, thereby providing a comforting and secure feeling. The vertical technique, which works well for toddlers, requires the child to be held on the parent's lap. As the parent hugs and holds the child's body and the arm not being used, the health care worker can firmly hold the other arm to perform the procedure.

In the horizontal position, an older child lies supine, with the health care worker on one side of the bed and the parent on the opposite side. The parent gently but firmly leans over the child, restraining the near arm and the body while holding the opposite, extended arm securely for the health care worker.

Neonates and infants younger than 3 months usually do not require restraint and can be managed by the health care worker alone. Swaddling helps to control and comfort an upset newborn.

COMBATIVE PATIENTS

At times, a child will become uncooperative even after the proper steps have been followed to gain cooperation. Children may become combative—kicking and thrashing—if force is used. Because sharps are involved in blood collection, the health care worker must be certain that the procedure can be performed safely. Using force to the point of potential physical injury is unethical and unprofessional. Therefore, if the risk of injury to the child or the health care worker is likely, the blood collection attempt should be discontinued, and the

Figure 12–2. Supine (lying) Position for Restraining Child to Perform Blood Collection

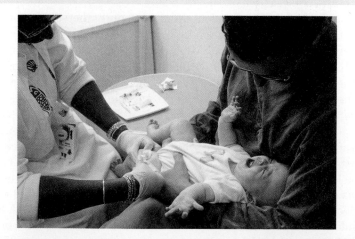

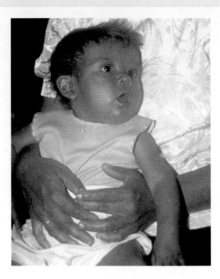

Figure 12–3. Vertical Position for Restraining a Child to Perform Blood Collection

nurse or the physician notified.[6] In such instances, alternative coping measures or pharmacological intervention may be necessary prior to the next attempt.

 ## INTERVENTIONS TO ALLEVIATE PAIN

The International Group for Neonatal Pain presented guidelines for preventing and managing pain during painful procedures. The guidelines encourage a combination of behavioral and pharmacological interventions to give an additive effect. These interventions may include EMLA, oral sucrose, a pacifier, and swaddling.[7,8]

Depending on the anticipated duration of the procedure, the severity of the child's illness, and the anxiety of the child, pharmacological intervention may be used to alleviate pain and anxiety. A topical anesthetic, EMLA, can be applied to intact skin by a nurse or physician. EMLA (eutectic mixture of local anesthetics) is an emulsion of lidocaine and prilocaine. This local anesthetic is ideal for use prior to venipuncture or starting intravenous (IV) therapy because it does not require a needle. EMLA penetrates both the epidermal and dermal layers, anesthetizing to a depth of 5 mm. It is applied to the skin as a patch or a cream that is then covered with a transparent occlusive dressing. Optimal anesthesia occurs after 60 minutes and may last as long as 2 to 3 hours. Drawbacks to the use of EMLA are cost, the need to apply it 60 minutes prior to the procedure, and having to know in advance the location of the vein to be used. Two separate locations may be anesthetized if the child has difficult venous access. EMLA has minimal side effects but may cause pallor at the application site or erythema due to the adhesive covering. EMLA should not be used if the child is allergic to local anesthetics.[2,7,8,9] Product information from Astra Pharmaceuticals indicates that EMLA can be used on neonates (minimum of 37 weeks gestation) and children weighing less than 20 kilograms. However, the area and duration of application should be limited.

ORAL SUCROSE

Studies have shown that 12 to 24 percent sucrose is effective in reducing pain during a painful procedure for an infant up to 6 months of age. A 24 percent solution of sucrose can be prepared by mixing 4 teaspoons of water with 1 teaspoon of sugar. The sucrose can be carefully administered by oral syringe, dropper, nipple, or on a pacifier. A sucrose nipple is given 2 minutes before heelsticks, and its action lasts about 5 minutes. Once the infant is crying vigorously and the heart and respiratory rates have increased, a pacifier alone has no significant effect on changing the rates but offers a degree of comfort.[10] Infants given pacifiers or sucrose have also been shown to be more alert following the procedure, to be less fussy, and to cry for a shorter duration.[7,11]

■■■■■ PREVENTION OF DISEASE TRANSMISSION— STANDARD PRECAUTIONS

If a child is in isolation, a sign posted on the door will describe the type of precautions to take and the personal protective equipment (PPE) to be worn. Isolation categories are based on the mode of transmission: contact, droplet, or airborne. All necessary supplies—a gown, gloves, and a mask—should be available at the room. If the child is on airborne precautions, a NIOSH-approved N-95 respirator must be used. Prior to using this respirator the health care worker must first complete a medical questionnaire and be fit tested. Check with the nurse in charge before entering the room[12,13] (See Chapter 5, Infection Control). Hands should be washed or disinfected with an alcohol hand rinse according to policy, before and after gloving. Usually, an anteroom is available before the isolation room, where you may sanitize your hands and put on the personal protective equipment.

To prevent transmission of bloodborne pathogens, Standard precautions should be followed throughout pediatric phlebotomy procedures. All children should be treated as if they could be potentially infectious. Standard precautions are used in addition to transmission based isolation precautions.[12,13] (See Chapter 5, "Infection Control," and Chapter 6, "Safety and First Aid").

PRECAUTIONS TO PROTECT THE CHILD

Premature babies, newborns, infants, and children who are chronically ill, immunocompromised, or have extensive burns are more likely to be susceptible to environmental microorganisms. To protect these children from these potentially harmful microorganisms, some hospitals may require protective precautions. In this instance, PPE—gowns, gloves, and masks—will be worn as indicated before entering the room. Remove the PPE according to policy and dispose of it in the appropriately marked container. Hands should be washed or sanitized according to policy. Alcohol-based waterless rubs, foams, or rinses are as effective as hand washing if the hands are not soiled.[14] Put on a clean gown and gloves before attending to the next infant or child.

▆▆▆▆ LATEX ALLERGY ALERT

Some children and health care workers may be allergic to latex. Usually, a sign posted on the door will note the child's allergy, or the child may wear a bracelet indicating a latex allergy or a latex alert. Several brands of nonlatex gloves should be available for use with children who have this allergy. Children with spina bifida and those with congenital urinary tract abnormalities or neurogenic bladders are particularly sensitive to latex. If a tourniquet is used it should also be latex-free.[15,16]

▆▆▆▆ PEDIATRIC PHLEBOTOMY PROCEDURES

Two methods are used to obtain blood from infants and children: microcapillary skin puncture and venipuncture. The previously described steps for preparing the child and the parent should be taken before the procedure is performed.

MICROCAPILLARY SKIN PUNCTURE

Skin punctures are useful for pediatric phlebotomy when only small amounts of blood are needed and can be adequately tested. It is particularly important to collect only the smallest amounts of blood necessary from neonates, infants, and children so that the effects of blood volume reduction are minimal. Overcollecting during phlebotomy may require packed cell transfusion in an infant. Studies have shown that patients lose 4 mg of iron for every 10 ml of blood collected.[17]

A 10 mL sample taken from a premature or newborn infant is equivalent to 5 to 10 percent of the infant's total blood volume. Calculation of blood volume is based on weight and can be calculated for any size person if the weight (in kilograms) of the individual is known. The total blood volume of a person is calculated by multiplying weight (kg) by the following blood volumes:

115 mL/kg	Premature infants
80–110 mL/kg	Newborns
75–100 mL/kg	Infants and children
70 mL/kg	Adults

Clinical Alert

Small infants can become anemic if too much blood is taken.

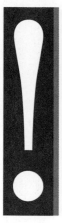

Clinical Alert

Puncturing deep veins in children may cause cardiac arrest, hemorrhage, venous thrombosis, damage to surrounding tissues, and infection.

When performing skin punctures, the phlebotomist collects the hematology specimens first to minimize platelet clumping, then for chemistry and blood bank specimens. Each laboratory has approved procedures for phlebotomy, including the volume of blood that is required for each test; these procedures should always be followed. Always record the amount of blood collected.

Skin Puncture Sites

- Lateral or medial plantar surface of the heel
- Palmar surface of the finger's distal phalanx

The heel is the most desirable site for skin puncture of the infant or neonate. The most medial or most lateral section of the plantar, or bottom, surface of the heel should be used (Figure 12–4 ■). The central area of the infant's heel should NOT be used for blood collection. For children older than 1 year, the palmar surface of the tip of the third or fourth finger is most frequently used, as the thumb has a pulse and the index finger may be more sensitive. The fifth finger is not used because the skin is too thin. (see Chapter 10, "Skin Puncture Procedures"). The plantar surface of the great toe is NOT recommended for skin

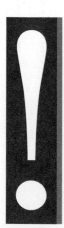

Clinical Alert

A 3 kg infant (approximately 6.6 pounds) will have a total blood volume of between 225 to 300 ml. It is important to monitor how much of this is withdrawn each day.[18] The table in Appendix 6 provides amounts of blood to be drawn from patients based on weight and maximum cumulative amount of blood to be drawn during a given hospital stay of 1 month or less.

Figure 12–4. Heel Sites for Capillary Puncture

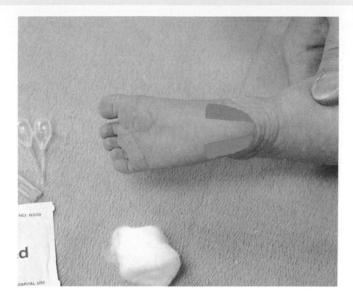

puncture. The skin-puncture device should be of proper pediatric size, making an incision that is less than 2.0 mm deep (see Figure 12–5 ■). Major blood vessels lie 0.3 to 1.6 mm beneath the skin at the dermal–subcutaneous junction in newborns.[19,20] If an incision goes deeper, the calcaneus or heel bone may be hit and may lead to osteomyelitis.[21,22]

Equipment for Microcapillary Sampling by Skin puncture

(See Chapter 8, "Blood Collection Equipment," for additional information.) The following equipment is necessary for pediatric skin puncture procedures:

1. Sterile, automatic, disposable pediatric skin-puncture safety devices in different manufacturers' incision depths (0.65–0.85 mm for premature neonates, 1.0 mm for larger infants)
2. Seventy percent isopropyl alcohol swabs
3. Sterile 2″ × 2″ gauze sponges.
4. Plastic capillary collection tubes and sealer
5. Microcollection containers, plastic capillary tubes, and BD Unopettes
6. Glass slides for smears
7. Puncture-resistant sharps container
8. Disposable gloves (nonlatex if child is allergic)
9. Compress (towel or washcloth) to warm heel if necessary
10. Marking pen
11. Laboratory request slips or labels

Figure 12–5. Performing a Heelstick on an Infant

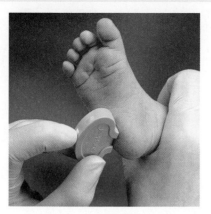

Courtesy of BD VACUTAINER Systems, *Preanalytical Solutions,* Franklin Lakes, NJ

Special Equipment for Capillary Blood Gas Collection

See Chapter 13, "Arterial, Intravenous (IV), and Special Collection Procedures," for details on capillary blood gas collection.

HEELSTICK

Specific guidelines for performing a heelstick include the following:

- Position the infant in the supine position (face up). Allow the foot to hang lower than the torso to improve blood flow.
- Warm the skin site prior to making the puncture
- Hold the infant's foot firmly but gently to prevent sudden movement. Holding the foot too tightly may cause bruising and restricts blood flow.
- Avoid excessive milking or squeezing, which causes hemolysis and dilutes the blood with interstitial and intracellular fluid.

Clinical Alert

Do not obtain blood by skin puncture from the central area of an infant's heel, as this may result in injury to nerves, tendons, and cartilage; fingers of infants less than 1 year old; or from previously punctured sites. If an infant has compromised circulation to the extremity, as in shock, or has edema, bruises, rashes, or infection at the heel, another site should be used.

1. Prepare and assemble supplies.
2. Introduce yourself to the parents, explain the procedure and use appropriate comfort techniques.
3. Identify the infant properly. If the infant is not wearing an identification bracelet, the floor nurse must identify the infant by name, address, and identification number and/or birth date and compare with laboratory test request form.
4. Wash or sanitize hands with an alcohol hand rinse, then put on gloves. If required, the health care worker should don a gown and a mask.
5. The selected area should be inspected and assessed for proper warmth. If it is cool or a blood gas specimen is to be collected, prewarm the foot with a warm, wet towel or a chemical heel-warming pack, according to policy. Wipe the heel dry after removing the warm towel.
6. The ideal posture for this procedure is with the baby in a supine position with the knee at open end of the bassinet. This position allows for the foot to hang lower than the torso, improving blood flow. When the baby is in an acceptable position for this procedure, clean the incision of the heel with an antiseptic swab. Allow the heel to air dry. Do not touch the incision site or allow the heel to come into contact with any nonsterile item or surface (Figure 12–6 ■).

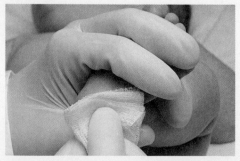

Figure 12–6 *Courtesy of ITC, Edison, NJ*

7. Remove the appropriate Tenderfoot device from its blister pack taking care not to rest the blade slot end on any nonsterile surface (Figure 12–7 ■).

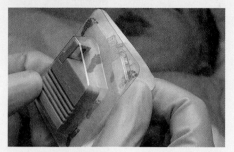

Figure 12–7 *Courtesy of ITC, Edison, NJ*

8. Remove the safety clip. Note: The safety clip may be replaced if the test is momentarily delayed; however, prolonged exposure of any Tenderfoot device to uncontrolled environmental conditions prior to use may affect its sterility. Once the safety clip is removed, DO NOT push the trigger or touch the blade slot (Figure 12–8 ■).

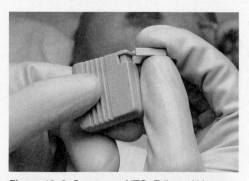

Figure 12–8 *Courtesy of ITC, Edison, NJ*

9. Raise the foot above the baby's heart level and carefully select a safe incision site (avoid any edematous area or site within 2.0 mm of a prior wound). Place the blade-slot surface of the device flush against the heel so that its center point is vertically aligned with the desired incision site (Figure 12–9 ■).

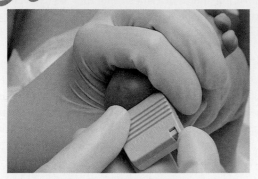

Figure 12-9 *Courtesy of ITC, Edison, NJ*

10. Ensure that both ends of the device have made light contact with the skin, and depress the trigger. After triggering, immediately remove the device from the infant's heel (Figure 12–10 ■).

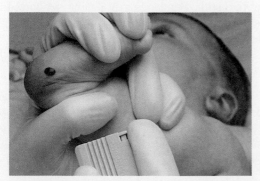

Figure 12-10 *Courtesy of ITC, Edison, NJ*

11. Using only a dry sterile gauze pad, gently wipe away the first droplet of blood that appears at the incision site (Figure 12–11 ■).

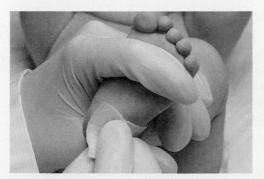

Figure 12-11 *Courtesy of ITC, Edison, NJ*

12. Taking care not to make direct wound contact with the collection container or capillary tube, fill to the desired specimen volume (Figure 12–12 ■).

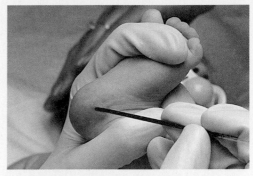

Figure 12-12 *Courtesy of ITC, Edison, NJ*

13. Following blood collection, gently press a dry sterile gauze pad to the incision site until bleeding has ceased. This step will help prevent a hematoma from forming (Figure 12–13 ■).

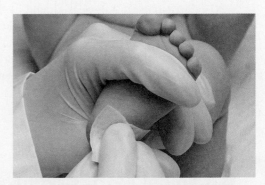

Figure 12-13 *Courtesy of ITC, Edison, NJ*

14. Label the specimen container and verify identification. Record time of collection.
15. Remove gloves and gown and mask if worn, and perform hand hygiene before proceeding to the next patient.

Heel Warming

The amount of blood that can be obtained from a single heelstick is limited, so to obtain an adequate sample, prewarming the heel may be indicated. Prewarming the heel increases blood flow and arterializes the specimen. This step is essential for drawing specimens for capillary blood gas analysis.

A warm, wet towel at a temperature no more than 42°C is wrapped around the infant's foot. If the temperature of the towel exceeds 44°C, it may burn the infant. Encase the wrap in a plastic bag to help retain heat and to keep the patient's bed dry. Prewarm the site for 3 to 5 minutes. Chemical heel-warming packs are also available commercially for this purpose.[23] Caution should be used if the towel is heated in a microwave oven because heating is uneven, and the towel may have hot spots. Depending on the institution's policy, the nurse may be called in advance to prewarm the infant's heel.

Care of the Heel after Collection

The heel should be elevated above the body, and a sterile gauze sponge pressed against the puncture site until the bleeding stops. This helps to prevent formation of a hematoma. Use of an adhesive bandage over skin-puncture sites is controversial on children less than 2 years old. Infants have delicate skin that may be irritated by the adhesive strip, and an older infant might remove it and put it in its mouth. Bandages can also be swallowed by older children. The primary care nurse should monitor the infant's heel site for the first hour following the puncture for late bleeding and inflammation.

Clean Up

Used skin-puncture devices should be disposed of in a sharps container with a biohazard label. The infant's bed must be checked for any equipment or trash left behind. Blood-soaked gauze sponges, grossly contaminated items, and gowns or gloves used in isolation rooms should be discarded in biohazardous waste containers. Gowns and gloves that are not from isolation rooms may be disposed in regular trash. Hands should be washed or sanitized after removing the gloves.

Clinical Alert: Complications from Heelstick

Some complications associated with neonatal heelsticks include celluitis, osteomyelitis of the calcaneus, abscess formation, tissue loss, scarring of the heel, and calcified nodules. Calcified nodules occur most commonly in infants who, as preemies (premature babies) or neonates, received multiple heelsticks. In neonates, these nodules appear as small depressions, which progress to firm nodular lesions that appear 4 to 12 months later, migrate to the skin surface, and disappear by 18 to 20 months.

NEONATAL SCREENING

In the United States, newborns are routinely screened for a variety of metabolic and genetic defects by analysis of blood collected on a special filter paper. Screening newborns is important for the early detection, diagnosis, and treatment of certain genetic, metabolic, and infectious diseases. The federal government has not set any national standards, so screening tests required for newborns vary widely from state to state.[24] Neonatal screening for phenylketonuria (PKU), congenital hypothyroidism, is mandated in all states and galactosemia (GAL) in all but one. Screening for sickle cell disease is mandated in all but three states. Most states test for maple syrup urine disease (MSUD), homocystinuria (HCY), biotinidase deficiency (BIO), and congenital adrenal hyperplasia (CAH). Two states test for toxoplasmosis, nine for cystic fibrosis, and only New York requires screening for HIV. Many of these diseases can result in severe abnormalities, including mental retardation, if not discovered and treated early.[25]

Tandem mass spectrometry screening (MS/MS) is a new technique that can detect blood components associated with over 30 inherited metabolic disorders in newborns in just one blood sample analysis collected on special filter paper. The U.S. National Screening Status Report contains up-to-date information on your state's specific requirements. In some states a neonate may be screened for only a few disorders while another may require screening for as many as 20. The National Newborn Screening Task Force recommends more education and standardization among states for newborn screening procedures and policies. The following websites should be reviewed for more specific information: Maternal and Child Health Bureau (MCHB) of the Health Resources and Services Administration (HRSA) at www.mchb.hrsa.gov and the American Academy of Pediatrics (AAP) at www.aap.org.

Blood spot testing for screening is performed before the newborn is 72 hours old. The American Academy of Pediatrics states that the optimal time for collection from a healthy newborn is as close to discharge as possible. If the blood specimen is collected before the newborn is 24 hours of age due to early discharge from the hospital, a second specimen for screening must be collected before 2 weeks of age. In classic galactosemia, symptoms occur within the first 2 weeks of life.[23] Filter specimens must be obtained from newborns prior to any transfusions for valid test results. Blood cells from transfusion provide normal enzymes that may invalidate screening results.

! Clinical Alert: Fingerstick

A fingerstick to obtain blood for routine laboratory analysis is usually preferred for children older than 1 year (Figure 12–14 ■). Also, a fingerstick may be necessary if a child has damaged veins from repeated venipuncture or if the veins are covered with bandages or casts. Do not perform a fingerstick if the extremity has compromised circulation, is edematous, or is infected.

Box 12-1

The heel of the neonate is the most frequently used site for collection of blood for screening.

- To prevent contamination, do not touch with hands or gloves any part of the filter paper circles before, during, or after collection. Do not allow the filter paper to come in contact with substances such as alcohol, formula, water, powder, antiseptic solutions, or lotion.
- Appropriate collection cards are kept in the hospital laboratory or the nursery. Circles are printed on the filter paper portion of the card.
- Wash hands well and put on gloves.
- Positively identify the newborn.
- Prepare the infant in the same manner as for a heelstick.
- Once the puncture is made wipe off the first drop of blood with sterile gauze. The initial drop contains tissue fluids that may dilute the sample.
- Allow another large blood drop to form.
- Lightly touch the printed side of the filter paper with the blood drop and fill each printed circle. Allow the blood to soak through and completely fill the circle with a single application to the large blood drop.
- If the circle does not fill entirely, the heel is wiped and another, larger drop is expressed to a different circle. Do not add a second drop of blood to a previously used circle.
- The filter paper must not touch the skin puncture site.
- Only one side of the filter paper should be used.
- Dry blood spots on a clean, dry flat nonabsorbent surface for a minimum of 4 hours.
- Direct application of blood from the heel to the card is the technique of choice; however, blood from a heparinized capillary tube may be applied if care is taken not to scratch or dent the filter paper. (See Figure 12–15 ■.)
- Correctly complete all the information on the screening card so that follow up can be done if the results are abnormal. The screening card should be placed in an appropriate envelope and sent to the laboratory within 24 hours.

Precautions

Use a pediatric safety skin-puncture device designed for the age and size of the child. An automatic skin-puncture device controls the puncture depth, which should not exceed 2.0 mm in small children. The distance from the skin surface to bone or cartilage in the middle, or third, finger is between 1.5 and 2.4 mm. Automatic puncture devices are available in sizes that incise to depths of 0.85 mm for preemies, 1.25 mm for infants and 1.75 mm for toddlers. For a detailed description of the blood collection procedure and supplies, refer to Chapter 10, "Procedures for Collecting Capillary Blood Specimens," and Chapter 8, "Blood Collection Equipment."

VENIPUNCTURE

Venipuncture in children is used when larger quantities of blood are needed for sampling. The veins of the antecubital fossa or the forearm (see Figure 12–16 ■) are the most accessible and are chosen for most toddlers and children. Dorsal hand veins are preferred sites for venous access in neonates and well infants.[26] If a venipuncture is done on a child younger than 2 years of age, the site should be limited to a superficial vein. Other sites used for venipuncture are the medial wrist, the dorsum of the foot, the scalp, and the medial ankle. Always check the policy at your facility before performing venipuncture on foot or ankle veins. If the neonate or child is receiving fluid or medication intravenously, the dis-

Figure 12–14. Collecting Blood via Fingerstick from a Toddler

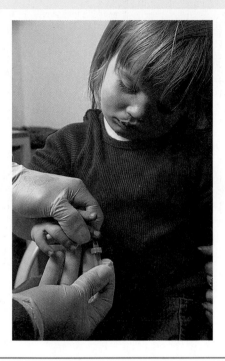

Figure 12–15. Collecting a Blood Sample from the Newborn for Neonatal Metabolic Screening

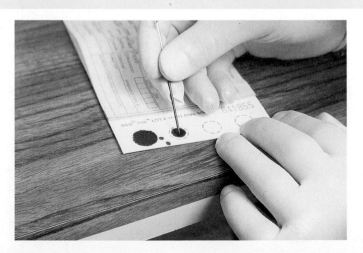

Figure 12–16. Veins in the Arm

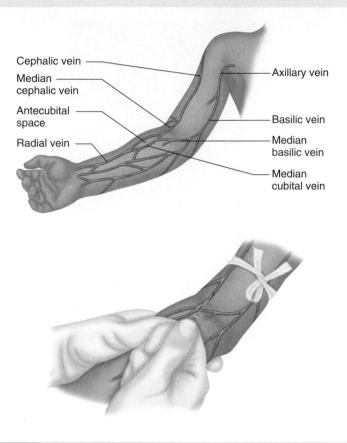

Cephalic vein

Median cephalic vein

Antecubital space

Radial vein

Axillary vein

Basilic vein

Median basilic vein

Median cubital vein

tal veins should be avoided for phlebotomy and preserved for IV therapy. Venipuncture is indicated for blood sampling for routine laboratory tests, erythrocyte sedimentation rate (ESR), blood cultures, cross-matching, coagulation studies, and drug and ammonia levels. Do not use veins in an extremity or area if there is edema or infection or if an IV line is present. Avoid deep veins in a child with hemophilia or other bleeding disorders.

Precautions

Remove the tourniquet before withdrawing the needle. Apply pressure with the gauze sponge for 3 minutes to prevent a hematoma. Do not use alcohol pads to apply pressure, as it will cause stinging and prevent hemostasis. Equipment of choice for venipuncture on a neonate is a small, winged safety (butterfly) needle. If feasible, use a winged safety needle for small children as well.

Equipment for Venipuncture

The equipment necessary for a pediatric venipuncture include the following:

1. Winged safety infusion (butterfly) needle, 23- or 25-gauge or transparent hub needle (21 gauge × 1 in. or 23 gauge × ¾ in.).
2. Syringes slightly larger than the volume of blood needed
3. Large-bore or 19-gauge needle
4. Seventy percent isopropyl alcohol swab in a sterile package
5. 2″ × 2″ gauze sponges
6. Appropriate specimen containers
7. Pediatric-size tourniquet (nonlatex if child is allergic)
8. Sterile disposable gloves (nonlatex if child is allergic)
9. For blood culture:
   a. Bottles, both aerobic and anaerobic. For smaller children use a special pediatric bottle. The required volumes are: for children 2 to 12, 2–4 ml; for infants under 2 years, 1 ml.
   b. Iodine swabs
   c. Chlorhexidine gluconate swabs (use for infants rather than iodine)
10. Paper tape and adhesive strip (for use only with older children)
11. Marking pens
12. Biohazardous waste container

Dorsal Hand Vein Technique

The dorsal hand vein technique is appropriate for neonates and infants who are younger than 2 years old.

Although the neonate may not need restraint, an older infant can be wrapped snuggly in a receiving blanket or restrained by an assistant to minimize movement.

Figure 12–17. Hand Veins

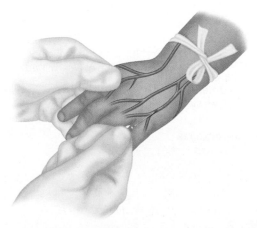

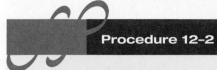

Procedure 12-2 Dorsal Hand Vein Procedure

1. Positively identify the infant.

2. Prepare and organize equipment. A 23-gauge butterfly safety needle attached to a 3–5 ml syringe is preferred.

3. Perform hand hygiene and put on gloves.

4. Select the hand that has easily visible veins. No tourniquet is necessary. Warm the site if the hand is cool.

5. The phlebotomist's middle and forefinger should encircle the infant's wrist and are used to apply pressure to distend the dorsal veins. The phlebotomist's thumb is placed against the infant's fingers to flex the infant's wrist downward as the dorsum of the hand is examined.

6. Be careful not to bend the wrist too much or the vein may collapse. Lightly palpate the back of the infant's hand to select the best vein and determine its direction.

7. Once the optimal vein has been chosen, the finger tourniquet should be released to allow blood to recirculate. If a vein cannot be seen or felt, do not attempt the venipuncture.

8. Disinfect the back of the infant's hand with the 70 percent alcohol swab. Allow the area to dry, then wipe with sterile gauze.

9. Select the appropriate needle according to the size of the vein.

10. Reposition infant's wrist, apply finger tourniquet and flex the infant's hand as described above.

11. Hold the needle with the wings of the butterfly needle bent together. The needle should be angled about 15 degrees to the skin, bevel up and parallel to the vein. The skin should be pierced 3–5 mm distal to the vein and advanced slowly and carefully until the vein is punctured.

12. As soon as blood appears in the tubing of the butterfly or hub of the needle, stop advancing and let the wings of the needle unbend. The blood may flow slowly, as venous pressure is very low. If no blood appears, it may be necessary to reposition the needle gently. It is not necessary to hold the needle, because the surrounding skin will hold it in place.

13. Pull the syringe plunger gently to fill with amount of blood required.

14. Microcollection tubes should be filled directly from the hub of the butterfly.

15. Release the finger tourniquet intermittently to allow the vein to refill. If the blood flow slows or stops, gently rotating the needle without advancing it may reestablish the flow.

16. Release fingers from the infant's wrist, quickly remove the needle, and apply pressure with a dry gauze sponge placed over the puncture site.

17. Direct pressure should be maintained for 2 to 3 minutes or until the bleeding stops. Adhesive strips should not be used on neonates, because their skin is fragile.

18. Engage safety device on butterfly. Disconnect the blood-filled syringe from the butterfly assembly.

19. Connect the syringe to transfer blood into vacuum tubes with a safety blood transfer device. Let the vacuum draw the blood into the tubes. Discard the syringe, safety blood transfer device, and needle in the sharps container.

20. Comfort the infant and offer a sucrose nipple, if permitted.

21. Discard remaining supplies, gloves, and gown, and wash hands.

22. Properly label the filled tubes.

Dorsal hand vein venipuncture has several advantages over skin puncture: it is less stressful for the infant and the health care worker; there is less dilution of the specimen with tissue fluids and less hemolysis; and fewer punctures are required.[27]

VENIPUNCTURE AT OTHER SITES

The procedure for performing venipuncture on children is similar to that for adults (see Chapter 9). The differences include the necessary preparation of the child and the parent, assistance in restraining the child, and the use of special pediatric-size needles or safety winged infusion sets. After the child is securely positioned, place the tourniquet proximal to the selected vein to distend it. If necessary, the limb may be lowered, rubbed gently, or warmed to promote dilation of the vein. Disinfect the site thoroughly. Allow the alcohol to dry completely. Then, hold the two wings of the infusion set together in the dominant hand as the other hand pulls taut the skin below the puncture site. After inserting the needle, and when blood appears in the tubing, release the wings of the infusion set. The skin will hold the needle in place, or paper tape can be used to secure it. Gently aspirate the syringe until the required amount of blood is withdrawn. Release the tourniquet and apply pressure over the puncture site with a gauze pad as the infusion set is quickly removed. Ask the parent or the nurse to hold pressure on the site until the bleeding stops. An adhesive strip may be used on an older child. Remove the syringe from the infusion set, attach it to a blood-transfer device for safe transfer of blood to the collecting tubes.

Scalp Vein Venipuncture

Scalp veins may be used on infants when access to other veins is difficult or undesirable. Figure 12–18 ■ shows the scalp veins used for peripheral vascular access. Additional equipment required for this procedure includes a disposable razor and a large, flat rubber band. A 23- or 25-gauge safety winged infusion set (butterfly needle) is used for the venipuncture.

Figure 12–18. Infant Scalp Veins

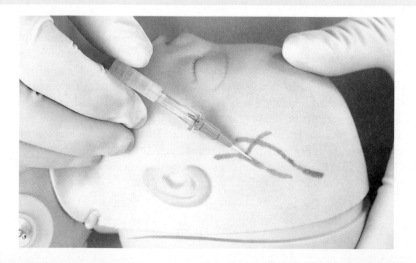

The appropriate procedures should be followed: hand washing and gloving, preparing the infant, and positioning with an assistant to provide restraint. If the scalp veins are not readily visible through the hair, a disposable razor may be used to shave the hair carefully in the frontal or parietal scalp area. A prominent vein may be occluded proximally with a finger as in the dorsal hand vein technique. Feel for a pulse to prevent hitting an artery. If a vein cannot be distended with the finger, a large, flat rubber band may be placed around the upper head as a tourniquet. (Placing a gauze pad under an area of the band helps in removing it after the procedure.) Disinfect the scalp with a povidone–iodine (Betadine) preparation or with alcohol, allow the scalp to dry, and then wipe it with sterile gauze. After the scalp is inspected for the desired vein, release the tourniquet to permit refilling of the veins. Reapply finger pressure or the rubber band. Hold the skin taut with the nondominant hand distal to the site to be punctured. Hold the infusion set with the two wings folded together and the bevel of the needle up. Position the needle at a 15-degree angle over the vein in the direction of the blood flow. Puncture the skin, and slowly advance the needle until blood begins to flow into the tubing of the needle set. Attach the syringe. Gently and slowly aspirate the blood to prevent hemolysis or occlusion by the vein wall. When sufficient blood is collected, release the finger tourniquet or rubber band. Place the sterile gauze pad over the puncture site, and apply pressure before quickly removing the needle. Apply additional pressure for several minutes to ensure that the bleeding has stopped. The remaining Betadine is removed with a sterile saline solution or water to prevent absorption. Fill the collecting tubes in the usual fashion. Comfort the infant by stroking softly, or by offering a pacifier with sucrose, if permitted. Be sure all used supplies are removed from the bed area.

COLLECTING BLOOD FROM IV LINES

Hospitalized children who are undergoing IV therapy (Figure 12–19 ■), whether for total parenteral nutrition (TPN), administration of an antibiotic, or chemotherapy, often have poor veins. They may have a heparin or saline lock or a central venous catheter (CVC) when long-term access is required. For more information on the types of central venous lines, see the following chapter. Some blood tests can be performed with blood drawn from these lines, but some hospitals limit the number of times a line can be accessed. Use 10 mL or larger syringe on any long term CVC to avoid overpressurizing and rupture of the catheter.[28,29] Confirm the amount of blood that can be drawn based on the child's weight (see table in Appendix 6). Check with the nurse in charge or the doctor to verify the policy.

In an effort to reduce sharps injuries as mandated by OSHA, latex or silicone membrane ports on CVCs are recommended. These ports allow penetration with a needleless access device and can be easily disinfected before each entry thereby reducing the risk of bacterial entry. When accessing a latex/silicone membrane port or a connector, the following are considered essential technique: 1) perform hand hygiene; 2) establish a sterile workspace using sterile gauze; and 3) prepare the access port with 70 percent alcohol, using sufficient friction and allowing the surface to dry[30,31] (Figure 12–20 ■).

Figure 12-19. Intravenous Line in Infant

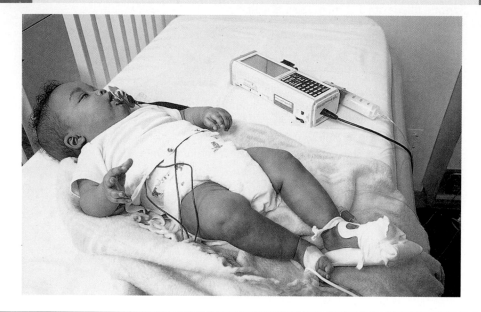

 Figure 12-20. Collecting Blood from an IV Line

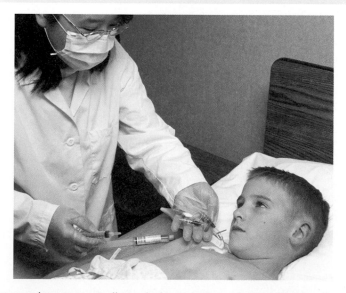

The health care worker uses sterile technique and carefully examines the central line to plan access from the correct port for blood collection.

Equipment

The equipment required for blood withdrawal from IV lines includes the following:

1. Syringe filled with 3–4 ml of normal saline
2. Syringe filled with 2–3 ml of heparinized flush solution; 100u/ml (1 ml for heparin lock)
3. 5-ml syringe for discard
4. 10-ml syringe for blood specimen
5. Small blood collection tubes
6. Transfer device for transferring blood to tubes
7. 19- to 25-gauge needles or needleless cannula for gaining access to heparin lock
8. Isopropyl alcohol or povidone–iodine (Betadine) swabs
9. Sterile double stopcock for central line
10. Sterile intermittent injection port or Luer-Lok catheter cap.
11. Sterile 4″ × 4″ gauze sponge
12. Mask
13. Gloves (nonlatex if child is allergic)

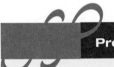

Procedure 12-3   Procedure for Heparin or Saline Lock

1. Perform hand hygiene.
2. Identify the patient using two identifiers.
3. Disinfect the catheter injection port with an alcohol or a povidone–iodine (Betadine) swab and let dry.
4. Check patency of the line by attaching syringe with normal saline and flushing with a small amount.
5. Attach a needle or needleless cannula to the discard syringe, and insert it into the cap of the lock.
6. Gently withdraw approximately 2 to 3 ml of fluid and blood, remove the syringe and needle, and discard in a sharps container.
7. Insert another needle/needleless device and syringe to collect the blood sample. When a sufficient amount of blood has been obtained, withdraw the needle and fill the collection tubes using a safety blood transfer device.
8. Clean the cap or injection port of the heparin lock with an alcohol swab, then insert the syringe with the heparinized flush solution, injecting slowly.

Procedure 12-4   Procedure for Central Venous Catheter

1. Identify the patient.
2. Assemble equipment.
3. Explain procedure to patient and parent in developmentally appropriate terms.
4. Stop all CVC intravenous fluids. Clamp all CVC access ports.
5. Perform hand hygiene and put on mask and gloves.
6. Open a sterile 4 × 4 inch gauze sponge, and place it under the catheter port to serve as a sterile field.
7. Option 1—Through injection port:
   a. Clean port with povidone–iodine swab. Allow iodine to dry then wipe with alcohol swab.
   b. Aseptically insert syringe with saline using needleless system. Unclamp catheter. Flush central line port with normal saline. Remove and discard syringe and needleless system access.
   c. Aseptically insert the next syringe using needleless system. Withdraw enough blood to clear the volume of the catheter. This amount will vary with different catheters. The manufacturers of the catheters specify a flush volume to determine the discard volume. Remove and discard syringe and needleless device in biohazardous waste container.
   d. Aseptically insert the next syringe using needleless system. Withdraw appropriate volume of blood for blood sample. Remove syringe and needleless system and insert blood sample into appropriate lab tubes.
8. Option 2—Catheter hub to syringe hub:
   a. If CVC is a triple lumen device, use the access port closest to the child. Clamp the catheter, then remove the intermittent injection cap after vigorously scrubbing connection with povidone–iodine or 70 percent alcohol for 30 seconds. Allow to dry.
   b. Disconnect IV tubing from catheter and cover with sterile capped needle.
   c. Aseptically connect the discard syringe and collection syringe to the sterile stopcock to ensuring a tight seal; attach to the port.
   d. Unclamp the catheter, open the stopcock to the discard syringe, and withdraw 3 to 5 ml of fluid based on catheter volume. Close that port, then open the stopcock port to the collection syringe and aspirate the required amount of blood. Close that port, and remove the syringe.
   e. Attach the syringe with the heparinized solution to the port. Gently aspirate to clear the stopcock of air, holding the syringe vertically to allow bubbles to rise. Tap the syringe to free any bubbles sticking to its side.
   f. Flush the catheter with 5 ml of saline, close that port, and then open the port to the heparinized solution and flush with 5 ml.
   g. Reclamp the catheter and remove the stopcocks.
   h. Clean the connection site of the catheter with a new alcohol pad, then attach a new Luer-Lok cap.
   i. Attach the safety blood transfer device to the syringe and fill the collection tubes.
9. Discard used items in the appropriate containers. Remove gloves and mask, and wash hands.

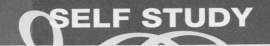
KEY TERMS

age-specific care considerations

blood volume

calcaneus

eutectic mixture of local anesthetics
   (EMLA)

heelstick

hemolysis

hypothyroidism

latex allergy

neonatal screening

neonates

osteomyelitis

parental involvement

pediatric phlebotomies

phenylketonuria (PKU)

premature Infant

sucrose nipple or pacifier

STUDY QUESTIONS

The following questions may have more than one correct answer.

1. Performing a phlebotomy on a child is challenging because:
   a. a child is less emotionally mature
      than an adult
   b. a child is small
   c. smaller equipment must be used
   d. a child's blood clots more quickly

2. Which of the following describes the behavior of an adolescent undergoing a
   painful procedure?
   a. fears separation from parent
   b. is embarrassed to show fear
   c. fears injury to body
   d. may not want parent present during
      the procedure

3. Which of the following are important steps in preparing the child and the parent for a
   phlebotomy?
   a. assess their past experience with
      blood drawing
   b. perform the phlebotomy as quickly
      as possible
   c. ask the parent to leave the room
   d. use a doll or puppet to demonstrate
      the procedure

4. Which is the *best* location for performing a phlebotomy on a hospitalized child?
   a. bedside in a chair
   b. playroom
   c. treatment room
   d. in his or her bed

5. The preferred technique(s) for restraining a child is/are:
   a. vertical with child sitting in parent's
      lap
   b. total sedation
   c. mechanical restraint
   d. supine with parent leaning over child

6. Which of the following are acceptable interventions to alleviate pain?
   a. xylocaine injection
   b. oral sucrose
   c. ice pack
   d. EMLA cream

7. Which is the preferred site for a heelstick?
   a. anteromedial aspect
   b. medial or lateral aspect
   c. posterior curve
   d. a previous puncture site

8. Warming the heel provides which of the following benefits?
   a. arterializes blood
   b. dramatically increases blood flow
   c. prevents hemolysis
   d. hastens hemostasis

9. Methods of distracting a child to alleviate anxiety include:
   a. counting
   b. blowing bubbles or a pinwheel
   c. music
   d. pinching an alternate site

10. The optimal lancet-device depth for a fingerstick on a child is:
    a. greater than 3.0 mm
    b. less than 2.0 mm
    c. less than 0.5 mm
    d. less than 0.25 mm

11. Strategies to prevent bloodborne disease transmission include:
    a. wearing gloves
    b. standard precautions
    c. safety sharps devices
    d. none are necessary, as children do not usually have bloodborne diseases

12. Neonatal blood screening is used to identify all of the following except:
    a. congenital hypothyroidism
    b. cystic fibrosis
    c. PKU (phenylketonuria)
    d. spina bifida

References

1. Mehne, C: Cultivating a tender touch. *MT Today,* September:12–16, 1992.
2. Schechter, N, et al.: Reducing the anxiety and pain of injections: A guide for managing the pediatric patient. Franklin Lakes, NJ: Becton Dickinson and Company 10/98.
3. London, ML, Ladewig, P, Ball, J, Bindler, R: *Maternal–Newborn and Child Nursing.* Upper Saddle River, NJ: Prentice Hall, 2002.
4. Joint Commission on Accreditation of Healthcare Organizations: 2004 National Patient Safety Goals for Ambulatory Care (online). Accessed July 18, 2003, http://www.jcaho.org.
5. Markenson, D, *Pediatric Prehospital Care.* Upper Saddle River, NJ: Prentice Hall, 2002.
6. Kelly, S: Pediatric blood collection made easy. *Lab Med,* 1993; 24(4): 247–248.
7. Mitchell, A, Waltman, PA. Oral sucrose and pain relief for preterm infants. *Pain Management Nursing* 4(2): 62–69, 2003.

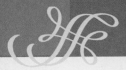

8. Gradin, M, et al.: Pain reduction at venipuncture in newborns: Oral glucose compared with local anesthetic cream. *Pediatrics,* Dec 2002; 110: 1053–7.

9. Lal, MK, McClelland, J, Phillips, J, Taub, NA, Beattie, RM: Comparison of EMLA cream versus placebo in children receiving distraction therapy for venipuncture. *Acta Paediatr,* Feb 2001; 90(2): 154–9.

10. Lindh, V, Wiklund, U, Hakanssom, S: Assessment of the effect of EMLA during venipuncture in newborn by analysis of heart rate variability. *Pain,* 2000; 86: 247–54.

11. Lindh, V, Wiklund, U, Blomquiat, HK, Hakansson, S: EMLA cream and oral glucose for immunization pain in 3-month-old infants. *Pain,* Jul 2003; 104 (1–2): 381–8.

12. National Committee for Clinical Laboratory Standards (NCCLS): Protection of Laboratory Workers from Occupationally Acquired Infections, Approved Guideline, 2nd ed. M29-A. Wayne, PA: NCCLS, December 2001.

13. Gardner, J, and Hospital Infection Control Practices Advisory Committee: Guideline for isolation precautions in hospitals. *American Journal of Infection Control* 1996; 24: 24–52.

14. CDC Guideline for Hand Hygiene in Health-Care Settings. *MMWR Recommendations and Reports,* October 25, 2002: 51 (RR-16).

15. Food and Drug Administration (FDA): Allergic reactions to latex-containing medical devices. *FDA Med Alert,* March 29, 1991.

16. Shriners Hospitals for Children: Patient Education, Latex Allergy in Children, http://shrinershq.org/patientedu/latex.html, accessed March 28, 2003.

17. Hicks, JM Q & A, Blood volumes needed for common tests. *Laboratory Medicine,* 2001; 4(2): 187.

18. National Committee for Clinical Laboratory Standards (NCCLS): Procedures and Devices for the Collection of Diagnostic Capillary Blood Specimens. 4-A5. Wayne, PA: NCCLS, 2004.

19. Reiner, CB, Meites, S, Hayes, JR: Optimal depths for skin puncture of infants and children as assessed from anatomical measurements. *Clinical Chemistry,* March 1990; 36(3): 547–9.

20. Jain, A, Rutter, N: Ultrasound study of heel to calcaneum depth in neonates. *Arch Dis Child Fetal Neonatal Ed,* May 1999; 80(3): F243–5.

21. Vertanen, H, Fellman, V, Brommels, M, Viinikka, L: An automatic incision device for obtaining blood samples from the heels of preterm infants causes less damage than a conventional manual lancet. *Arch Dis Child Fetal Neonatal Ed,* January 2001; 84: F53–F55.

22. Meites, S, Hamlin, CR, Hayes, JR. A study of experimental lancets for blood collection to avoid bone infection of infants. *Clinical Chemistry* 38: 908–910, 1992.

23. Ladeweg, P, London, M, Moberly, S, Olds, S: *Contemporary Maternal-Newborn Nursing Care,* 5th ed. Upper Saddle River, NJ: Prentice Hall, 2002.

24. American Academy of Pediatrics (AAP) Task Force on Newborn Screening: Newborn screening: A blueprint for the future—A call for a national agenda on state newborn screening programs. *Pediatrics,* August 2000; (106(2): 389–422.)

25. National Newborn Screening and Genetics Resource Center, US National Screening Status Report, http://genes-r-us.uthscsa.edu/resources/newborn/screenstatus.htm, updated February 06, 2004

26. Johnston, V: News and views: Venipuncture better for newborns? *Lab Med,* 1998; 29(6): 329.

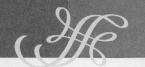

27. Clagg, ME: Venous sample collection from neonates using dorsal hand veins. *Lab Med,* 1989; 20(4): 248–250.

28. Keller, CA: Methods of drawing blood samples through central venous catheters in pediatric patients undergoing bone marrow transplant: Results of a national survey. *Oncology Nurses Forum,* June 1994; 21(5): 879–84.

29. Schallom, L, Bisch, A: Blood sampling techniques for patients with arterial or venous catheters. AACN Practice Resources; Ask the Experts, April 2001; 21(2).

30. Kilbride, H, Powers, R, Wirtschafter, D, et al.: Evaluation and development of potentially better practices to prevent neonatal nosocomial bacteremia. *Pediatrics,* April 2003; 111(4).

31. CDC Guidelines for the Prevention of Intravascular Catheter-Related Infections. *MMWR Recommendations and Reports,* August 9, 2002; 51(RR-10).

13

Arterial, Intravenous (IV), and Special Collection Procedures

CHAPTER OBJECTIVES

Upon completion of Chapter 13, the learner is responsible for the following:

1. Explain the special precautions and types of equipment needed to collect capillary or arterial blood gases.

2. Describe the equipment that is used to perform the bleeding-time test.

3. Discuss the requirements for the glucose and lactose tolerance tests.

4. Differentiate cannulas from fistulas.

5. List the steps and equipment in blood culture collections.

6. List the special requirements for collecting blood through intravenous (IV) catheters.

7. Differentiate therapeutic phlebotomy from autologous transfusion.

8. Describe the special precautions needed to collect blood in therapeutic drug monitoring (TDM) procedures.

9. List the types of patient specimens that are needed for trace metal analyses.

 MediaLINK

Access the accompanying CD-ROM to explore a wide variety of review questions and interactive activities for this chapter, including multiple choice, true/false, and video exercises.

Depending on the specific needs of individual clinical settings, health care workers may be required to perform a variety of special tests or procedures in addition to routine skin punctures and venipunctures. This chapter presents the basic techniques and precautions for various special tests. Extensive training sessions and supervision should accompany the student in these procedures, because they can harm the patient if performed incorrectly.

ARTERIAL BLOOD GASES

Arterial blood gases (ABGs) provide useful information about the respiratory status and the acid–base balance of patients with pulmonary (lung) disease or disorders. In addition, critically ill patients with other diseases, such as diabetes mellitus, benefit from ABG measurement, which is used to help manage their electrolyte and acid–base balance. Arterial blood is used rather than venous blood because arterial blood has the same composition throughout the body tissues, whereas venous blood has various compositions relative to metabolic activities in body tissues.

Arterial puncture to obtain arterial blood for blood gas evaluation requires skill and knowledge of technique. A health care provider must undergo extensive training on arterial punctures, including demonstration of the procedure, observation, and, under the supervision of a qualified instructor, several performances on patients.

RADIAL ARTERY PUNCTURE SITE

When an ABG analysis is ordered, the experienced health care worker, nurse, medical technologist, or physician should palpate the areas of the forearm where the artery is typically close to the surface. The radial artery, located on the thumb side of the wrist (as shown in Figure 13–1 ■) is the artery most frequently used for blood collection for ABG analysis.[1]

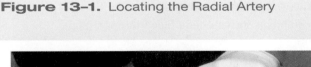

Figure 13–1. Locating the Radial Artery

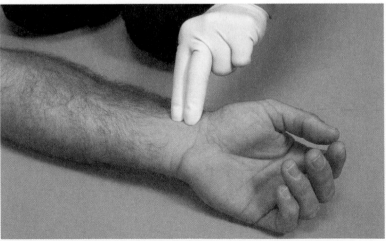

Source: Michal Heron/Pearson Education/PH College.

Using your index and middle fingers, the pulses from the radial artery should be palpated about 1 inch above the wrist (see Figure 13–1). This artery has widespread collateral flow, which means that the hand area is supplied with blood from more than one artery. Arterial blood flows into the hand from both the radial and the ulnar arteries. In addition, the radial artery lies over ligaments and bones of the wrist and can be easily compressed to lessen the chance of a hematoma during the procedure. A drawback to using the radial artery is its small size.

To use the radial artery for blood collection for ABG analysis, the health care provider must first perform the modified Allen test to make certain that the ulnar and radial arteries are providing collateral circulation (Figure 13–2 ■). The modified Allen test is performed as follows: (1) the health care provider compresses both arteries with the index and middle fingers, and the patient is asked to tightly clench his or her fist; (2) The patient is then asked to open his or her hand, and the health care provider releases the pressure on the ulnar artery; and (3) the hand should fill with blood within 5 to 10 seconds; if so, the Allen test is positive. If color returns to the hand after 5 to 10 seconds, the Allen test is negative. A negative Allen test indicates the inability of the ulnar artery to supply blood to the hand adequately and shows a lack of collateral circulation. Thus, the radial artery should not be used in a negative Allen test, since this artery might be accidentally damaged during puncture, resulting in total lack of blood flow to the hand.

BRACHIAL AND FEMORAL ARTERY PUNCTURE SITES

The brachial artery is an alternative site for blood collection for ABG analysis. The brachial artery is in the cubital fossa of the arm, as shown in Figure 13–3 ■.

Another choice, the femoral artery, is the largest artery used in ABG collections. It is located in the groin area of the leg, lateral to the femur bone, as shown in Figure 13–3. Even though the brachial and femoral arteries are larger than the radial artery, they are used less frequently because they lack collateral circulation. A four-year study on blood collections from the brachial artery has demonstrated that brachial artery puncture is an acceptably safe procedure and a very reasonable alternative to radial artery puncture.[2] The femoral artery is a site sometimes used on patients with cardiovascular disorders. The possibility of releasing plaque from the inner wall of the artery in geriatric patients, however, is a definite disadvantage of using the femoral artery as a puncture site. Usually, the femoral artery is the last choice for an arterial puncture site, and the health care provider must have expertise in obtaining blood from this artery.

PREPARATION OF SUPPLIES AND PATIENT

The necessary equipment and supplies, as listed in Table 13–1, should be gathered and organized for a successful arterial puncture. (See Procedure 13–1 on p. 367.)

- The patient must be properly identified and informed of the arterial puncture procedure.
- It should be determined that the patient has been in a stable state for at least the previous 30 minutes (i.e., no respiratory changes).
- The health care provider should attempt to calm the patient before collecting the specimen if the patient appears anxious. The anxiety can lead to hyperventilation, which will falsely alter the ABG levels.
- Before proceeding, the health care provider must also determine whether the patient is on anticoagulant therapy or is allergic to iodine or lidocaine, and must record the pa-

Figure 13-2. Modified Allen Test

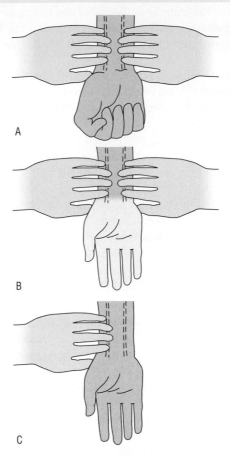

A. Using the index and middle fingers, the health care worker compresses the patient's ulner and radial arteries. The patient tightly clenches his or her fist. B. The patient opens the hand and the health care worker releases the pressure. C. If the patient's hand refills with blood (i.e., color returns) within 5 to 10 seconds, the test is positive, if not, the test is negative.

tient's temperature, oxygen concentration from the respirator (if applicable), and respiratory rate.

Arterial blood results for some analytes (e.g., ammonia, glucose, lactic acid, alcohol) may differ from venous blood results because of metabolic activities. Therefore, arterial blood samples should be collected for the blood gas measurements only when specifically requested by the attending physician. In such situations, the request slip must indicate that arterial blood was collected for the analytes.

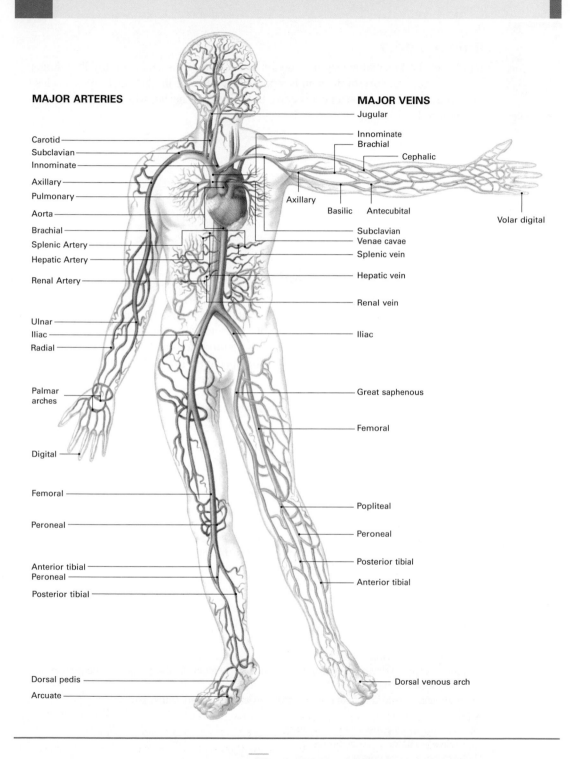

Figure 13-3. Arteries in the Arm and Leg for Puncture Sites

MAJOR ARTERIES

Carotid
Subclavian
Innominate
Axillary
Pulmonary
Aorta
Brachial
Splenic Artery
Hepatic Artery
Renal Artery
Ulnar
Iliac
Radial
Palmar arches
Digital
Femoral
Peroneal
Anterior tibial
Peroneal
Posterior tibial
Dorsal pedis
Arcuate

MAJOR VEINS

Jugular
Innominate
Brachial
Cephalic
Axillary
Basilic
Antecubital
Volar digital
Subclavian
Venae cavae
Splenic vein
Hepatic vein
Renal vein
Iliac
Great saphenous
Femoral
Popliteal
Peroneal
Posterior tibial
Anterior tibial
Dorsal venous arch

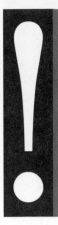

Clinical Alert

The pulse of the brachial artery may be felt at the fold of the elbow on the little finger side of the arm. Puncture of the vein is a possibility because the brachial artery is close to the veins. The brachial artery lies close to the median nerve, which can be accidentally punctured.

CAPILLARY BLOOD GASES

Arterial blood is the specimen of choice for testing the pH, oxygen (O_2) content, and carbon dioxide (CO_2) content of the blood. Skin puncture blood is less desirable as a specimen because it contains blood from capillaries, venules, and arterioles, and fluids from the surrounding tissue. In addition, common collection methods for capillary blood gas specimens employ an open collection system in which the specimen is temporarily exposed to room

TABLE 13–1.   Equipment and Supplies for an Arterial Puncture

Tincture of iodine solution or chlorhexidine gluconate
½ to 1 percent lidocaine to numb site
Prefilled heparinized safety syringe, 1 to 5 ml (especially designed plastic syringe for collections for ABG analysis)
Needles (20- to 22-gauge, for collections for ABG analysis)
Needles (25- to 26-gauge, for lidocaine administration)
Safety syringe for lidocaine administration (1- or 2-ml plastic syringe)
Gauze squares to be held on site after puncture
Plastic bag or cup with crushed ice and water
Patient identification label
Laboratory requisition slip
Waterproof ink pen
Alcohol pad
Adhesive bandage strip
Oxygen-measuring device to record on laboratory requisition slip the oxygen concentration on patient receiving oxygen
Thermometer to record patient's temperature on laboratory requisition slip
Mask
Gloves (nonlatex if patient has latex allergy)
Protective laboratory coat or smock
Biohazardous waste containers for sharps

Procedure 13-1   Radial ABG Procedure

1. The experienced phlebotomist, nurse, or physician should wash his or her hands, put on gloves, a facial mask, and a protective laboratory coat, and then palpate the radial artery in the forearm. The radial artery in the patient's nondominant hand is usually the best choice.

2. With the forefinger or first two fingers, the health care worker should press at these sites to find the artery (see Figure 13–1). The thumb should never be used for palpating because there is a pulse in the thumb that may be confused with the patient's pulse. Any site that has a hematoma or that was previously used for an arterial puncture should be avoided.

3. The patient's arm should be positioned with the wrist slightly extended and rotated. Check for adequate collateral circulation using the modified Allen test.

4. Once the radial artery site is chosen, the area should be cleaned well with tincture of iodine.

5. If a local anesthetic is desired by the patient, fill a 1-cc syringe with lidocaine and inject the lidocaine with the 25- to 26-gauge needle subcutaneously around the anticipated puncture site.

6. No tourniquet is required, because the artery has its own strong blood pressure. A prefilled heparinized safety syringe (1 to 5 ml) with a needle can be used to withdraw the sample.

7. The health care worker should pull the skin taut and pierce the pulsating artery at a high angle, usually no less than 45 degrees. Little or no suction is needed because the blood pulsates and flows quickly into the syringe under its own pressure.

8. When approximately 1 ml of blood is collected, the health care worker withdraws the needle carefully to avoid introducing bubbles into the syringe and applies gauze and direct manual pressure on the site for at least 5 minutes.

9. The safety syringe cover should be engaged to cover the needle exposure, then the blood in the syringe gently mixed with the heparin, and the syringe then labeled and immediately placed in ice water in an effort to prevent blood gases from escaping into the atmosphere.

10. Before leaving the patient, the health care worker should clean the puncture site with an alcohol pad to remove the excess iodine solution; a pressure bandage should be left on.

11. If bleeding from the site persists, the health care worker should apply more manual pressure and ring for assistance from the patient's primary nurse. The health care worker should never leave a patient who is bleeding, particularly after an arterial puncture.

12. The primary nurse should be notified after an arterial puncture is performed so that the area may be checked frequently for deep or superficial bleeding.

13. Ideally, the specimen should be analyzed within 10 minutes of collection. Therefore, the specimen should be transported immediately to the laboratory.

air, theoretically allowing for a brief exchange of gases (both O_2 and CO_2) before sealing the specimen from the air.

Blood for capillary blood gas analysis is often collected from small children and babies for whom arterial punctures can be too dangerous. They are collected from the same areas of the body as other capillary samples, such as the lateral posterior area of the heel, or the ball of the finger. (See Chapter 12, "Pediatric Procedures.")

When a capillary blood gas analysis is ordered, the health care worker first should choose a site. The puncture site should be cleaned and entered in the usual manner for skin punctures (as discussed in Chapter 10).

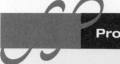

Procedure 13-2 | Collection for Capillary Blood Gas Testing

1. A heparinized safety plastic capillary tube (Figure 13–4 ■) should be used for the collection.

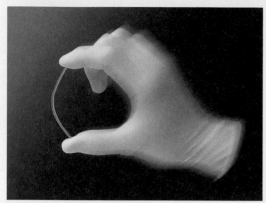

Figure 13–4 *SAFE-T-FILL Blood Gas Capillary Tube—100% Plastic for Safety*

Courtesy of Ram Scientific, Inc., Needham, MA

2. A minute metal filing (referred to as a "flea") may be inserted into the tube before collecting to help mix the specimen while it is entering the tube (see Figure 13–5 ■).

3. It is extremely important that the specimen be collected with no air bubbles, which can distort the values obtained from the specimen.

4. When the tube is full, the ends should be sealed with plastic caps, and a magnet should be used to draw the metal filing (flea) back and forth across the length of the tube to mix the specimen completely.

5. The tube should then be labeled and submerged in a slurry of ice water for transfer to the laboratory. The sample should be analyzed immediately in the laboratory; however, if the specimen is stored horizontally, capped, and in the slurry of ice water, it can be kept as long as 2 hours without serious degradation.

6. The skin puncture site should be pressed with a clean gauze sponge until the bleeding stops.

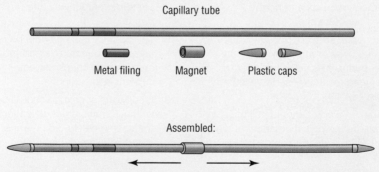

Figure 13–5 *Capillary Blood Gas Tube, Metal Filing (flea), and Plastic Caps*

BLEEDING-TIME TEST

The bleeding-time test is a useful tool for testing platelet plug formation in the capillaries. This diagnostic tool is most frequently used as a preoperative screening test.

The test is performed by making a minor standardized incision on the forearm and recording the length of time required for bleeding to cease. The duration of bleeding from

Figure 13–6. Surgicutt

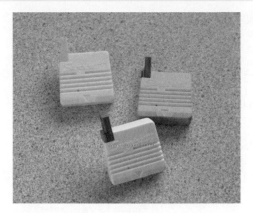

Courtesy of ITC, Edison, NJ.

a punctured capillary depends on the quantity and quality of platelets and the ability of the blood vessel wall to constrict.

Clinical research has led to the development of automated incision-making instruments for bleeding-time tests, such as the Surgicutt (Figure 13–6 ■).[3] It is a sterile, standardized, easy-to-use, disposable instrument that makes a uniform, surgical incision. This instrument is a spring-activated surgical steel blade housed in a self-containing plastic unit from which the blade protracts and retracts automatically, eliminating the variable of blade incision. See Procedure 13–3.

POSSIBLE INTERFERING FACTORS

A prolonged bleeding time may indicate the need for further testing (e.g., platelet count). In addition, the following items should be considered:

- The ingestion of aspirin-containing products up to 7 to 10 days prior to testing may affect results.
- Other drugs (e.g., dextran, streptokinase, streptodornase, ethyl alcohol, mithramycin) may cause a prolonged bleeding time.

There are other variations of this same procedure using different devices. For reproducible results, it is important to follow the manufacturer's instructions and to teach all health care workers in the same manner.

 BLOOD CULTURES

Blood cultures are often collected from patients who have fevers of unknown origin (FUO). Sometimes during the course of a bacterial infection in one location of the body, bacteremia or septicemia (presence of bacteria or toxins in the blood) may result and become the

Procedure 13–3   Surgicutt Bleeding Time Test[4]

1. Prior to beginning the procedure, patients should be advised that there is an occasional scarring problem inherent in the bleeding time test. Butterfly-type bandages can reduce the potential scarring by applying one to the incision area for a 24-hour period. If there is ooze from the incision, as may be encountered in severe primary hemostatic disorders, then a pressure-type dressing should be used in conjunction with the butterfly-type bandage. If the puncture site is still bleeding beyond 15 minutes, the test should be discontinued by applying pressure to the area. A physician should be notified. The patient can also be asked if he or she has taken aspirin or other salicylates within the previous 2 weeks; these drugs interfere with the test.

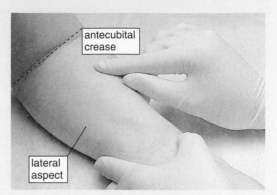

Figure 13–7a *Courtesy of International Technidyne Corp.*

2. Materials and supplies should be prepared before beginning the procedure. The following items are needed:

   • Surgicutt instrument. Each self-containing unit is sufficient for a single bleeding time determination. (NOTE: If package has been broken, do not use.)

   • Gloves

   • Antiseptic swab

   • Blood pressure cuff (sphygmomanometer)

   • Surgicutt Bleeding Time Blotting Paper Disk

   • Butterfly-type bandage

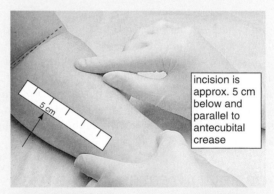

Figure 13–7b *Courtesy of International Technidyne Corp.*

3. Place the patient's arm on a steady support with the volar surface exposed. The incision is best performed over the lateral aspect (Figure 13–7a ■), volar surface of the forearm, approximately 5 cm below the antecubital crease (Figure 13–7b ■). Avoid surface veins, scars, bruises, and edematous areas. Lightly shave the area if body hair will interfere with the test.

4. Place the blood pressure cuff on the upper arm. Inflate the cuff to 40 mm/Hg for adults (Figure 13–8 ■). The time between inflation of the cuff and the incision should be 30 to 60 seconds. Hold at this exact pressure for the duration of the test.

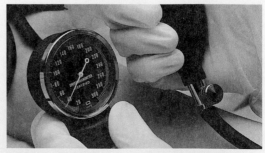

Figure 13–8 *Courtesy of International Technidyne Corp.*

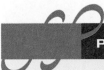

Procedure 13-3 *(continued)*

5. Cleanse the area (Figure 13–9 ■) with an antiseptic swab and allow to air dry. Remove the Surgicutt device from the package, being careful not to contaminate the instrument by touching or resting the blade-slot end on any unsterile surface.

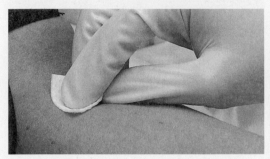

Figure 13–9 *Courtesy of International Technidyne Corp.*

6. Remove the safety clip (Figure 13–10 ■). (Safety clip may be replaced if the test is momentarily delayed; however, prolonged exposure of Surgicutt to uncontrolled environmental conditions prior to use may affect its sterility.) Once safety clip is removed, DO NOT push the trigger or touch the blade slot.

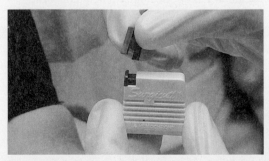

Figure 13–10 *Courtesy of International Technidyne Corp.*

7. Hold the device securely between the thumb and the middle finger (Figure 13–11 ■). Gently rest it on the patient's forearm and apply minimal pressure so that both ends of the instrument are lightly touching the skin. A horizontal incision parallel to the antecubital crease is the most sensitive technique for the bleeding time.

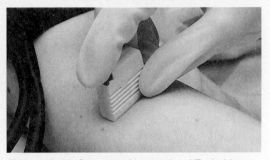

Figure 13–11 *Courtesy of International Technidyne Corp.*

8. Gently push the trigger, starting the stopwatch simultaneously. The blade will make an incision 5 mm long by 1 mm deep. Remove the device from the patient's forearm immediately after triggering (Figure 13–12 ■). After 30 seconds, wick the flow of blood with filter paper. Bring the Surgicutt blotting paper close to the incision, but DO NOT touch the paper directly to the incision, so as not to disturb the formation of a platelet plug.

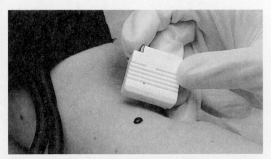

Figure 13–12 *Courtesy of International Technidyne Corp.*

Procedure 13-3 *(continued)*

9. Wick the blood every 30 seconds thereafter until blood no longer stains the paper (Figure 13–13 ■). Stop the timer. Bleeding time is determined to the nearest 30 seconds. Reference ranges vary from one health care facility to another. Most, however, are in the approximate range of 2.0 to 8.0 minutes.

10. Remove the blood pressure cuff and cleanse the incision site with an antiseptic swab. Apply the nonallergenic butterfly-type bandage for 24 hours.

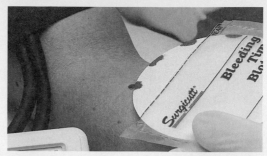

Figure 13–13 Courtesy of International Technidyne Corp.

dominant clinical feature. Septicemia is a major cause of death in the United States.[5] Blood cultures aid in identifying the specific bacterial organism causing the infections.

Prior to beginning the procedure, the health care provider should briefly explain the test to the patient.

SITE PREPARATION

Then, the following steps should be taken for blood culture collection:

1. The necessary equipment and supplies should be gathered and prepared next to the patient, as listed in Table 13–2.
2. After donning gloves (nonlatex if patient has latex allergy), locate the vein, loosen the tourniquet, scrub the site of the venipuncture with 70% alcohol for 60 seconds to rid the site of excess dirt, and then scrub with the iodine tincture (chlorhexidine gluconate for patients sensitive to iodine or for infants) for at least 30 seconds. The iodine swab

TABLE 13–2. Equipment and Supplies for Blood Culture Collections

Gloves (recommended sterile gloves for aseptic technique)
3 alcohol/acetone or alcohol preps
2 iodine-tincture scrub swabsticks or chlorhexidine gluconate swabsticks
2 blood culture vials (1 for anaerobic microorganisms and 1 for aerobic)
SPS evacuated tubes
Needles (22- or 20-gauge) or blood collection set
Safety syringe or evacuated safety tube assembly
Sterile gauze pads
Nonlatex bandages
Nonlatex tourniquet
Patient identification labels
Laboratory requisition slip and pen
Biohazard waste container

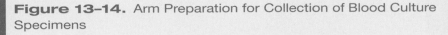

Figure 13–14. Arm Preparation for Collection of Blood Culture Specimens

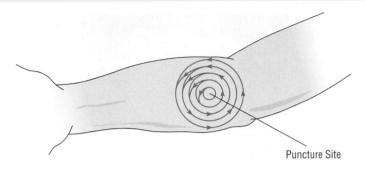

Puncture Site

should initially be placed at the site of needle insertion and then moved outward in concentric circles to a diameter of approximately 4 inches, as shown in Figure 13–14 ■.

3. Some health care facilities use a blood culture preparation kit that has a one-step application (e.g., ChloroPrep-Medi-Flex, Inc., Overland Park, Kansas). The application has chlorohexidine gluconate/isopropyl alcohol antiseptic combined for an effective 30-second cleansing of the venipuncture site (Figure 13–15 ■). The phlebotomist's gloved forefinger should also be cleaned in the same manner. Other blood culture preparation kits are also available commercially (Figure 13–16 ■). Through research, it was shown the blood culture collection sites prepared using iodine tincture instead of iodophor (e.g., povidone) were superior in combating contamination of sites where cultures were collected by "non-phlebotomy" personnel.[6]

Do not go back over any area that has been prepped. Allow the area to dry for 1 minute in order for the antiseptic to be effective against skin bacteria.

Figure 13–15. One-step 30-second Application for Blood Culture Venipuncture Preparation

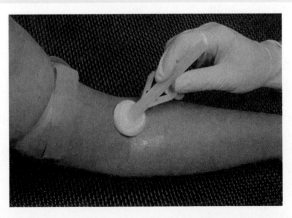

Courtesy of Medi-Flex Hospital Products, Inc., Overland Park, Kansas

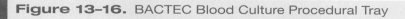

Figure 13–16. BACTEC Blood Culture Procedural Tray

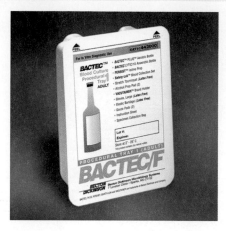

Courtesy of Becton Dickinson Microbiology Systems, Sparks, MD

4. As the venipuncture site dries, prep the tops of the blood culture vials or SPS evacuated tubes with a new iodine tincture swab stick, then wipe the tops of the vials with a new alcohol prep. This wipes the iodine away and decreases the likelihood of iodine entering with the blood into the vial. For some manufacturers of blood culture vials, it is recommended to clean the vial top with only alcohol after removing the cap from the vial. The prepping of the vials should occur IMMEDIATELY prior to the blood collection.

   Removal of the entire metal ring on some manufacturer's bottles introduces air into the vials and can cause contamination. Read the manufacturer's directions on blood culture vials before using them, because they may vary as to the size of blood sample needed and their preparation requirements.

The venipuncture procedure can be performed three different ways: by syringe, vacuum tube, and safety butterfly assembly.

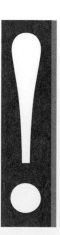

Clinical Alert

- For any of the blood collection procedures, the venipuncture site MUST NOT be repalpated after the venipuncture site is prepared for blood collection.
- Relocating the vein by repalpation after sterilization recontaminates the site.
- Make a mental note of the vein's location in relation to skin features such as a mole, crease, freckles, etc.
- If you must repalpate, do not palpate at the actual venipuncture site.

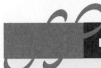

Procedure 13–4   Syringe Blood Culture Collection

Using a safety syringe, it is commonly recommended to do an adult collection of 20 ml and transfer the first 10 ml to the anaerobic vial and then 10 ml to the aerobic vial. The procedural steps include the following:

1. After the collection of the blood into the syringe, activate the safety needle cover and aseptically dispose of the needle into the sharps container without touching the needle.

2. Then, a blunt-tipped cannula (connector) should be placed on the syringe and the blunt-tipped connector attached to the direct-draw holder/adapter (Figure 13–17 ■).

3. Starting with the anaerobic microbiology vial (Figure 8–3) in an upright position, place the direct-draw holder/adapter on the vial, fill to the desired amount, and remove the syringe with the direct-draw holder/adapter from this vial. Then place the syringe with the holder/adapter over the upright aerobic bottle and fill this bottle to desired amount (10 ml). NEVER push on the syringe plunger. Allow the vacuum in the microbiology vials to pull the blood into the vials.

4. If the blood collector can only collect 3 ml or less, the entire amount should be placed in the aerobic vial.

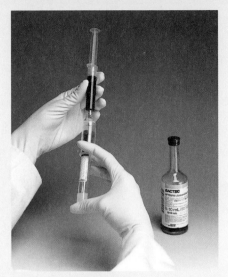

Figure 13–17 Courtesy of Becton Dickinson Microbiology Systems, Sparks, MD

5. For pediatric patients younger than 10 years old: it is recommended to collect for the blood culture workup 1 ml of blood for each year of life.[7]

POSSIBLE INTERFERING FACTORS

- If blood culture collections are ordered with other laboratory tests, blood culture specimens must be collected first. If an evacuated blood collection tube is used prior to the blood culture vials or SPS evacuated tubes, the needle can become contaminated.
- When entering the needle into the venipuncture site, do not scrape the needle across the skin, since this can contaminate the needle and, thus, blood cultures.
- The anaerobic blood culture vial must be inoculated first in all procedures except the butterfly assembly method, because injection of air into the anaerobic bottle can cause the death of some anaerobic microorganisms and result in a false-negative culture.

Box 13–1   Vacuum Tube Blood Culture Collections

As in other venipuncture collections (see Chapter 9), a safety holder/needle apparatus can be used to collect blood for blood cultures in the yellow-topped evacuated tubes containing sodium polyanethole sulfonate (SPS), or in vials (bottles), such as the BACTEC culture collection kit, that are shaped to fit into the barrel apparatus just as an evacuated tube would, thereby eliminating one step (see Figure 13–18).

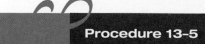

Procedure 13–5   Safety Butterfly Assembly Blood Culture Collection

1. A safety butterfly assembly (safety blood collection set) (Figure 8–11) is used for insertion of the butterfly needle into the venipuncture site after the appropriate skin preparation.

2. A strip of tape is then placed over the butterfly wings to keep the needle in place as the blood culture vials are filled with the blood.

3. The blood is transferred to the microbiology vials via a direct draw adapter that fits directly over the blood culture vial (Figure 13–18 ■).

4. Using this method, blood is transferred to the aerobic vial first, since the assembly tubing contains air.

5. The safety butterfly set should never be used without a direct draw adapter for transfer of the blood to the vials. If the needle is not concealed in this transfer of blood, the needle poses a risk of accidental needlestick as it is pushed into the microbiology vial.

6. Also, it is important to check with the manufacturers of blood collection safety-holder/needle devices before attempting blood culture collections, since some of these devices do not accommodate the blood transfer to blood culture bottles.

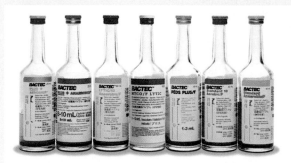

Figure 13–18 *BACTEC Direct Draw Culture Vials*
Courtesy of BD-Becton-Dickinson and Company, Sparks, MD

- Some culture vials contain resin beads that neutralize antibiotics in the patient's blood specimen. If these vials are not gently mixed to neutralize the antibiotics in the blood, the antibiotics can inhibit bacterial growth and cause false-negative results.

After collecting the blood, remove the iodine from the patient's skin with an alcohol prep. The health care provider must initial the patient identification labels, indicate the time and date of collection on the labels, and attach a label to each vial or tube.

Changing needles should not occur after collecting blood for culture, because it can lead to a needlestick injury to the phlebotomist. Careful skin cleansing has been shown to be the important factor in minimizing the specimen contamination rate.

◼◼◼◼ GLUCOSE TOLERANCE TEST (GTT)

For patients who have symptoms suggesting problems in carbohydrate metabolism, such as diabetes mellitus, the glucose tolerance test can be an effective diagnostic tool. When a

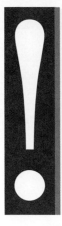

Clinical Alert

Note: Microbiology culture bottles MUST be held upright during the venipuncture collection to avoid reflux of culture media into the patient.

glucose tolerance test is to be performed, the patient should be given complete instructions about the procedure so that his or her cooperation can be ensured (Box 13–2).

For best results, the patient should:

1. Eat normal, balanced meals for at least 3 days prior to the test
2. Fast 12 hours prior to the beginning of the test
3. Drink water
4. Not drink unsweetened tea, coffee, or any other beverage during fasting or during the procedure
5. Not smoke, chew tobacco, or chew gum (including sugarless gum) during the fasting time or during the procedure. (Note: If a patient is chewing gum prior to this procedure or during, note this on the requisition form since gum may interfere in the test results.)

The test is performed by first obtaining a fasting blood specimen. The fasting blood specimen should be taken to the laboratory for test results. If the result is normal, then the patient can be given a standard load of glucose (e.g., Glucola), and subsequent blood and urine samples can be obtained at intervals, usually during a 2- to 3-hour period. If the fasting specimen is abnormal, the physician must be notified before giving the load of glucose. Each specimen is then analyzed for its glucose content. In general, glucose levels should return to normal within 2 hours after ingestion of the glucose. During the test, the patient drinks a standard dose of glucose: 75 grams for adults or approximately 1 gram per kilogram of body weight for children and small adults. A dose of 50 gram or 75 gram is recommended for diagnosis of gestational diabetes.[8] Gestational diabetes occurs during pregnancy, usually the second or third trimester. (See Postprandial Glucose Test.) Commercial preparations are available as flavored drinks to make the glucose more palatable. The patient must start and finish the drink within 5 minutes. Water intake is encouraged throughout the procedure. If the patient should vomit at any point in the procedure, the physician should be notified immediately to decide whether the test should be continued or stopped.[9]

When the patient finishes drinking the solution, the time is noted, and 30-, 60-, 120-, and 180-minute blood specimens are obtained.

Box 13-2	Sample Patient Information Card

PATIENT INFORMATION CARD GLUCOSE TOLERANCE TEST

Introduction

A glucose tolerance test (GTT) has been ordered by your physician. The purpose of a GTT is to test the efficiency of your body's insulin-releasing mechanism and glucose-disposing system.

You must prepare your body for the GTT by changing your eating and medication routines slightly for 3 days before the test. It is very important that you follow the instructions below in order for accurate results to be obtained.

Basically, you will need to follow these three guidelines to prepare for your GTT test:

1. Your carbohydrate intake must be at least 150 g per day for 3 days prior to the GTT.

2. Do not eat anything for 12 hours before the GTT, but do not fast for more than 14 hours before the test.

3. Do not exercise for 12 hours before the GTT.

Preparation: Medication

Before proceeding with the GTT, you must tell your physician if you are currently using any of the following medications, because they may interfere with test results:

- Alcohol
- Anticonvulsants (seizure medication)
- Blood pressure medication
- Clofibrate
- Corticosteroids
- Diuretics (fluid pills)
- Estrogens (birth control pills or estrogen replacement pills)
- Salicylates (aspirin, pain killers)—only if taken in high doses, such as for rheumatoid arthritis

Preparation: Diet and Exercise

Remember that for 3 days prior to your test, your diet must contain at least 150 g of carbohydrates per day. The following is a list of high-carbohydrate foods:

- **Milk and milk products**—12 g of carbohydrates per serving. One serving is equal to 8 oz. of milk (whole, skim, or buttermilk), 4 oz. of evaporated milk, or 1 cup of plain yogurt.
- **Vegetables**—5 g of carbohydrates per serving. One serving is equal to ½ cup of any vegetable, excluding starches (e.g., potatoes, corn, or peas).
- **Fruits and fruit juices**—10 g of carbohydrates per serving. One serving is equal to ½ cup of juice, 1 small piece of fresh fruit, or ½ cup of unsweetened canned fruit, with the following exceptions:

Apple juice	⅓ cup
Grape juice	¼ cup
Raisins	2 tbsp.
Watermelon	1 cup
Prunes	2 medium
Banana	½ small
Dates	2
Cantaloupe	¼ 6-inch melon
Honeydew melon	⅛ 7-inch melon

(continued)

Box 13-2   (continued)

- **Breads and starches**—15 g of carbohydrates per serving. One serving is equal to 1 slice of bread or 1 small roll. Other one-serving sizes are:

Bagel/english muffin	½
Tortilla	1
Cooked cereal	½ cup
Dry cereal	¾ cup
Cooked rice, noodles, pasta	½ cup
White potatoes, dried beans, and peas	½ cup
Yams	¼ cup
Corn	⅓ cup
Crackers	5 to 6

- **Meats, cheeses, and fats**—These foods contain few or no carbohydrates.
- **Miscellaneous**

Ice cream	½ cup	15 g of carbohydrates
Sherbet	½ cup	30 g of carbohydrates
Gelatin	½ cup	30 g of carbohydrates
Jams, jellies	1 tbsp.	15 g of carbohydrates
Sugar	1 tsp.	4 g of carbohydrates
Carbonated beverage	6 oz.	20 g of carbohydrates
Hard candy	2 pcs.	10 g of carbohydrates
Fruit pie	⅙ pie	60 g of carbohydrates
Cream pie	⅙ pie	50 g of carbohydrates
Plain cake	¹⁄₁₀ cake	30 g of carbohydrates
Frosted cake	¹⁄₁₀ cake	38 g of carbohydrates

Preparation: General Health

The following physical conditions should be reported to your doctor because they too may affect the results of your test:

Acute pancreatitis

Adrenal insufficiency

Diabetes mellitus

Hyperinsulinism (excess insulin secretion, resulting in hypoglycemia)

Hyperthyroidism

Hypopituitarism (decreased function of pituitary gland)

Pregnancy

Stress

If you have any difficulty making the necessary alterations in your diet or medication schedule, please inform your doctor. For accurate test results, the instructions on this card must be followed.

Courtesy of Division of Laboratory Medicine, University of Texas M.D. Anderson Cancer Center, Houston, TX.

Figure 13–19. Graph of Glucose Tolerance Test Results

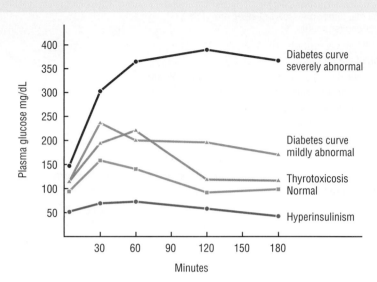

Examples of timed blood collections for GTT are as follows:

- Fasting specimen obtained and sent to laboratory (lab result okay to proceed with GTT)
- Glucose load given (i.e., Glucola) at 7:00a
- ½ hour specimen at 7:30a
- 1 hour specimen at 8:00a
- 2 hour specimen at 9:00a

The tubes should be labeled with the time (Figure 13–19 ∎) as well as "30 minutes," "1st hour," and so on. Upon collection, each specimen should be sent to the laboratory for immediate testing. Venous blood is the preferred specimen for glucose tolerance tests because glucose normal values are determined on venous blood. If serum samples are collected, the serum separator tube should be used. The grey-topped tubes have a preservative and can also be used for this procedure.

∎ POSTPRANDIAL GLUCOSE TEST

The 2-hour postprandial glucose test can be used to screen patients for diabetes, (including gestational diabetes) because glucose levels in serum specimens drawn 2 hours after a meal are rarely elevated in normal patients. In contrast, diabetic patients usually have increased values 2 hours after a meal.

For this test, the patient should be placed on a high-carbohydrate diet 2 to 3 days before the test. The day of the test, the patient should eat a breakfast of orange juice, cereal with sugar, toast, and milk to provide an approximate equivalent of 100 g of glucose. A blood specimen is taken 2 hours after the patient finishes eating breakfast. The glucose level of this specimen is then determined, and the physician can decide whether further carbohydrate metabolism tests (such as a glucose tolerance test) are needed.

LACTOSE TOLERANCE TEST

Some otherwise healthy adults experience difficulty in digesting lactose, a milk sugar. They appear to lack a mucosal lactase enzyme that breaks down the lactose into the simple sugars glucose and galactose. Instead, gastrointestinal discomfort may result, followed by diarrhea. These patients usually show no further symptoms if milk is removed from their diet.

To determine if a patient suffers from lactose intolerance, a physician may order a lactose tolerance test. In this procedure, a solution containing 50 grams of lactose is given to the patient. The standard procedure includes the collection of a baseline specimen and 5-, 10-, 30-, 60-, 90-, and 120-minute specimens for plasma glucose measurements. When the results are graphed, the curve should be similar to that obtained from the glucose tolerance test, if the patient has the mucosal lactase enzyme and digests the sugar properly. If the patient is intolerant to lactose, his or her blood glucose level will increase by no more than 20 mg/dl from the fasting sample level.

The health care worker should be sure that a bathroom is located near the patient testing area because patients who are lactose intolerant may experience severe discomfort during the testing.

THERAPEUTIC DRUG MONITORING (TDM)

Therapeutic drug monitoring (TDM) is used to monitor the serum concentration of certain drugs. It is an important laboratory assessment tool in the following circumstances:

- If the drug is highly toxic.
- When underdosing or overdosing can have serious consequences.
- If use of multiple drugs may alter the action of the drug being measured.

Box 13-3

Laboratory personnel must acquire and document additional information when performing TDM. A health care worker may be asked to acquire the following information:

- Patient's name
- Patient's identification number
- Patient's location
- Test ordered
- Requesting physician
- Collection time and date
- Mode of collection (e.g., venipuncture, central venous catheter collection)
- Whether the order is for a peak level, a trough level, or a continuous-infusion random level determination
- Time and date of last dose
- Time and date of next dose
- A unit nurse's verification that the dose was administered

Specific specimen guidelines for each drug should be established by pharmacy and laboratory staff and strictly adhered to.

- If individual patients metabolize drugs at different rates.
- If the effectiveness of the drug is questionable.

TDM is often used for patients taking anticonvulsant drugs, tricyclic antidepressants, digoxin, theophylline, lithium, chemotherapeutic agents such as methotrexate, or antibiotics such as gentamicin.

Laboratory drug monitoring of therapeutic agents is a complex endeavor that requires much coordination among laboratory, nursing, and pharmacy personnel. A basic understanding of the variables, information needed, and definitions of terms is important to obtain accurate laboratory results. For most drugs, either plasma, serum, or whole blood is used to determine circulating levels of the drug.[10]

To adequately evaluate the appropriate dosage levels of many drugs, the collection and evaluation of specimens for trough and peak levels are necessary. The trough level is the lowest concentration in the patient's serum; that is, the specimen should be collected immediately prior to administration of the drug to ensure that the medication level stays within the therapeutic (effective dosage) range. The peak level is the highest concentration of a drug in the patient's serum (Figure 13–20 ■). The time required to reach the highest concentration varies with the mode of administration (intramuscular injection versus IV infusion) and the rate at which the drug is infused. In addition, random levels may be appropriate for monitoring the drug dosage if the drug is administered by continuous infusion and if enough time has elapsed for the drug to reach equilibrium.

Blood specimens for TDM should be maintained in an upright position during transportation. In addition, because falsely low levels of lidocaine, phenytoin, and pentobarbital have occurred with the use of gel serum separator tubes, this type of evacuated blood collection tube should be evaluated and determined not to cause interferences.[11,12]

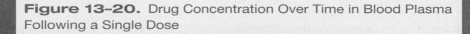

Figure 13–20. Drug Concentration Over Time in Blood Plasma Following a Single Dose

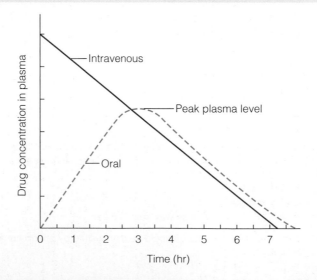

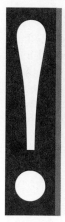

Clinical Alert

The time of collection is much more critical for drugs with shorter half-lives (e.g., gentamicin, tobramycin, and procainamide) than for those with longer half-lives (e.g., phenobarbital and digoxin). In addition, certain drug levels (e.g., aminoglycosides) in the blood can be falsely altered if collected through a central venous catheter. Also, blood should not be taken from the arm into which drugs or other fluids are being infused.

Most TDM assays should be performed on clotted blood. The National Committee for Clinical Laboratory Standards (NCCLS) has devised toxicology and drug-monitoring requirements for blood collection containers; these requirements can be helpful to the pharmacy and laboratory personnel who are responsible for establishing specific specimen guidelines for each drug.

COLLECTION FOR TRACE METALS (ELEMENTS)

Testing for trace metals involves the use of specially prepared trace-metal-free evacuated blood collection tubes. Also, special acid-washed plastic syringes are usually suitable for trace metal testing. For aluminum level determinations, a needle that is free of aluminum must be used. For lead level determinations, lead-free heparinized evacuated blood tubes equipped with sterilized stainless steel needles should be used for blood collection. Specific specimen collection guidelines should be established as part of the clinical laboratory's technical procedures for trace metal testing. The NCCLS guidelines entitled Control of Preanalytical Variation in Trace Element Determinations are very helpful in the preparation of procedures to collect trace elements.[13]

GENETIC MOLECULAR TESTS

The proper collection of a blood specimen for genetic molecular tests is critical to obtain accurate results. To collect for molecular testing requires special informed consent forms to be signed by the patient and collection of the specimen in acid-citrate-dextrose (ACD) or EDTA, depending on laboratory protocol. In addition to the blood specimen, the patient's correct demographics (i.e., vital statistics such as age, place of birth, parents' ethnicity/race, etc.) must be obtained, which is more essential for genetic laboratory tests than for other types of assays. The genetic material (e.g., RNA) is only viable for approximately 6 to 24 hours, and thus the specimens must be sent to the laboratory immediately. This new type of testing will become increasingly popular and expansive in genetic assays. Thus the health care worker needs to stay up-to-date on the necessary blood collection protocols for genetic molecular tests.

◼◼◼◼ IV LINE COLLECTIONS

Drawing blood specimens through intravenous (IV) or central venous catheter (CVC) lines requires special techniques, training, and experience. A CVC, also called a central intravenous line, is one of numerous vascular access devices (VADs). The CVC is usually inserted into the (1) subclavian vein, which is in the chest area below the clavicle; (2) jugular vein; or (3) superior vena cava (Figure 13–3). A dressing covers the tubing that extends above the skin. Another type of VAD is a peripherally inserted central catheter (PICC), which is inserted into the arm or hand veins (Figure 13–21 ◼). The PICC is usually only used for blood collection when it is first inserted, because it can become easily infected around the area.

COLLECTING BLOOD THROUGH A CVC

Usually, managers of health care facilities require nursing or laboratory personnel to take specialized training courses prior to allowing them to collect blood from a central venous line (See Procedure 13–6).[14]

The following equipment and supplies should be prepared prior to the procedure:

- Laboratory requisition forms
- Tubes and labels for the specimen
- Sterile gloves
- 10-ml disposable syringe with needleless cannula (transfer connector from syringe to vacuum tubes)

Figure 13–21. Inserting the Peripherally Inserted Central Catheter (PICC)

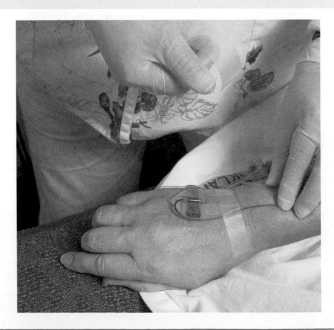

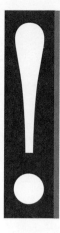

Clinical Alert

The IV line is a direct pathway into the patient's bloodstream. Each time the IV system is entered, the possibility of contamination and infection exists.

- One 10-ml syringe with needleless cannula filled with injectable heparinized saline (used for flushing the catheter)
- 4 × 4-inch piece of sterile gauze
- Linen protector to provide a clean work area
- A plastic or paper container for wastes or soiled items
- Adhesive tape
- Alcohol wipes
- VACUTAINER safety needle/holder set

 ## CANNULAS AND FISTULAS

A cannula is a tubular instrument that is used in patients with kidney disease to gain access to venous blood for dialysis or blood collection. Blood should be drawn from the cannula of these patients only by specially trained personnel because the procedure requires special techniques and experience.

A fistula is an artificial shunt in which the vein and artery have been fused through surgery. It is a permanent connection tube located in the arm of the patients undergoing kidney dialysis. Only specialized personnel can collect blood from a fistula. The health care worker should use extreme caution when collecting a blood specimen from these patients and avoid using the arm with the fistula as the site for venipuncture. If no other location can be found for the venipuncture site, the patient's arm must be cleaned thoroughly prior to blood collection. If the venipuncture site in this arm becomes infected, the inflammation in the blood vessels of the arm may shut down all the veins, requiring surgery to place a new shunt in the patient.

 ## DONOR ROOM COLLECTIONS

Properly trained health care providers may be employed in a regional blood center or a hospital blood donor center to screen and collect blood from donors. This section summarizes the procedure outlined by the American Association of Blood Banks (AABB).[15] Only an experienced, properly trained health care worker or technologist should be considered for this function because a physical, emotional, or traumatic experience may keep a donor from volunteering in the future.

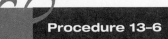

Procedure 13-6 Collecting Blood through a CVC

The procedure may involve the following steps but is subject to differences among hospitals and must be performed by authorized personnel only and under institutional guidelines.[14,15]

1. Check patient's chart for physician's order to draw blood through CVC.

2. Obtain laboratory requisitions and labels that reflect patient location and tests for which blood is needed.

3. Check labels against slips and patient's identification bracelet as described in Chapter 9.

4. Assemble equipment, wash hands, and put sterile gloves on.

5. Aseptically draw up to 10 ml injectable normal saline in syringe.

Note: Take only tubes for the patient, no others.

6. Identify patient by armband ID, noting full name and hospital number. Check against preprinted labels.

7. Explain procedure to patient.

8. Provide adequate room and light for procedure.

9. Position patient by elevating the bed to a comfortable working level and making the bed flat, and have catheter hub at or below the level of the patient's heart.

10. After placing linen protector on the bed, place tray of supplies on protector. Place sterile 4 × 4-inch gauze under connection site.

11. Shut off IV fluids infusing through line and unclamp most proximal lumen of multilumen catheter. Stop infusion for 3 minutes prior to blood collection (Figure 13–22 ■). Swab cap and hub with tincture of iodine for 30 seconds and allow to dry. Note: for blood culture collection, disinfect cap and hub with 70 percent alcohol and allow to dry. Then repeat disinfection of cap and hub with tincture of iodine.

12. Aseptically insert needleless cannula of 10-ml syringe into cap and unclamp catheter (see Figure 13–23 ■).

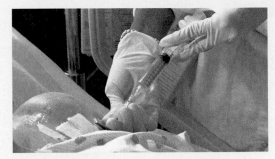

Figure 13–23

13. Aspirate (slowly and steadily) the following amount of blood for discard (Figure 13–24 ■):

   • Pediatrics—2 ml

   • Adults—5 to 7 ml

   • Coagulation studies—withdraw 20 ml of blood (13 ml may be used for testing after discarding 7 ml); collect 3 ml in a separate syringe. This process is only required when the CVC has been used to infuse heparin.

Close clamp, remove syringe with blood, and place in tray in order to discard later.

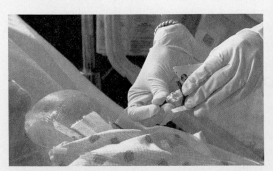

Figure 13–22

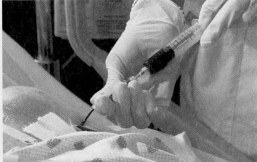

Figure 13–24

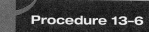

Procedure 13-6 *(continued)*

14. Swab cap again and aseptically insert Vacutainer holder as shown in Figure 13–25 ■.

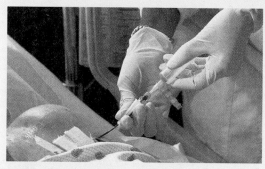

Figure 13–25

15. As shown in Figure 13–26 ■, insert partial draw or pediatric vacuum collection tube (for slower, gentle blood flow to avoid hemolysis) and withdraw required amount of blood for laboratory tests. Fill tube until blood flow into tube ceases.

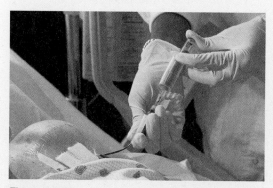

Figure 13–26

16. As shown in Figure 13–27 ■, remove vacuum tube from holder and insert next tube (again, use partial or pediatric vacuum tube) into holder to obtain required blood. Gently mix tubes with blood as described in Chapter 9.

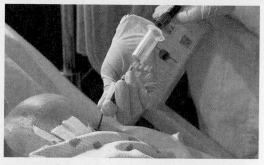

Figure 13–27

17. If blood culture vials are to be collected, these tubes MUST BE collected prior to other vacuum collection tubes. The "order of draw" as described in Chapter 9 should be followed.

18. Close catheter and withdraw VACUTAINER holder as shown in Figure 13–28 ■.

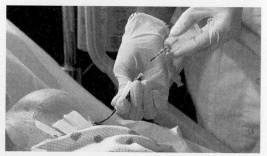

Figure 13–28

19. As shown in Figure 13–29 ■, the cap needs to be swabbed to aseptically clean it.

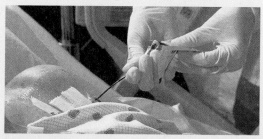

Figure 13–29

Procedure 13-6   *(continued)*

20. Complete irrigation of catheter with remaining 10 ml saline flush to avoid possibility of occlusion (Figure 13–30 ■). Some institutions require flushing also with a heparin solution.

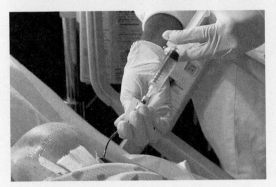

Figure 13–30

21. Determine that IV fluids are infusing properly at rate set by unit nurse. Note: If pump is being used, make certain pump is ON and alarm is ON. If the rate of IV flow appears altered, the unit nurse should be notified immediately.

22. Make sure the patient is in a safe and comfortable position, with the bed down, siderails up, and bedside table and call light accessible to patient. Place used equipment and supplies in appropriate discard containers. (Figure 13–31 ■).

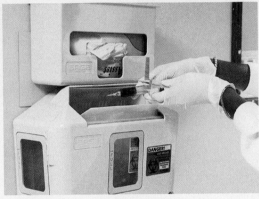

Figure 13–31

23. Always immediately label the blood specimens and indicate that these specimens were collected by a line draw. Dispatch to laboratory in usual manner.

24. Document completion of procedure and any problems in the patient's medical record.

DONOR INTERVIEW AND SELECTION

Not everyone who wants to donate blood is eligible, so the interviewer must determine the eligibility of each potential donor. Carefully determining donor eligibility not only helps prevent the spread of disease to blood product recipients but also prevents untoward effects on the potential donor.

The following information on every donor should be kept on file indefinitely and is initially obtained from every prospective donor, regardless of the acceptability of his or her donation:[15]

1. Date and time of donation
2. Last name, first name, and middle initial
3. Address
4. Telephone number
5. Gender
6. Age and birth date (Donors should be at least 17 years of age; however, minors may be accepted if written consent is obtained in accordance with applicable state law. Elderly prospective donors may be accepted at the discretion of the blood bank physician.)

7. Written consent form signed by the donor (1) allowing the donor to defer from being a donor if he or she has risk factors for HIV, the causative agent of acquired immunodeficiency syndrome (AIDS), or (2) authorizing the blood bank to take and use his or her blood

8. A record of reasons for deferrals, if any

9. Social security number or driver's license number (may be used for additional identification but is not mandatory)

10. Name of patient or group to be credited, if a credit system is used

11. Race (not mandatory, but this information can be useful in screening patients for a specific phenotype [chromosomal makeup])

12. Unique characteristics about a donor's blood (Donated blood that is negative for cytomegalovirus or that is Rh-negative group-O blood is used for neonatal patients.)

To help minimize the incidence of dizziness, fainting, or other reactions to blood loss, donors are encouraged to eat within 4 to 6 hours of donating blood. Eating a light snack just before the phlebotomy may help prevent these reactions, but a donor should not be required to eat if he or she does not want to do so.

Blood bank records must link each component of a donor unit (red blood cells [RBCs], white blood cells [WBCs], platelets, etc.) to its disposition. If the donation is a "replacement for credit" for a particular patient, the donor must supply the patient's name or the group name that is to be credited.

A brief physical examination is required to determine whether the donor is in generally good condition on the day that he or she is to donate blood. The physical examination entails a few simple procedures easily mastered by the health care worker:

1. Weight. Donors must weigh at least 110 lb (50 kg); if the weight is less, the volume of blood donated must be carefully monitored and care taken that not too much blood is collected. Also, the anticoagulant in the bag must be modified for the lesser donation. Most blood banks will not routinely accept donors who weigh less than 110 lb.

2. Temperature. The donor's oral temperature must not exceed 37.5°C (99.5°F).

3. Pulse. The donor's pulse should be regular and strong, between 50 and 100 beats per minute. The pulse should be taken for at least 15 seconds.

4. Blood pressure. The systolic blood pressure should measure no higher than 180 mm Hg, and the diastolic blood pressure should be no higher than 100 mm Hg. People with blood pressure outside these limits should be deferred as donors and referred to their physicians for evaluation of a possible health problem.

5. Skin lesions. Both arms should be examined for signs of drug abuse, such as needle marks or sclerotic veins. The presence of mild skin disorders, such as a poison ivy rash, does not necessarily prohibit an individual from donating unless the lesions are in the antecubital area or the rash is particularly extensive. The skin at the site of the venipuncture must be free of lesions.

6. General appearance. If the donor looks ill, excessively nervous, or under the influence of alcohol or drugs, he or she should be deferred.

7. Hematocrit or hemoglobin values. The hematocrit value must be no less than 38 percent for donors. The hemoglobin value must be no less than 12.5 g/dl. A finger stick is commonly used to draw blood for such determinations. The health care worker may either collect blood in a plastic hematocrit tube for centrifuging and reading, measure hemoglobin spectrophotometrically, or use the copper sulfate method, in which the

hemoglobin is qualitatively determined. (For further details on the copper sulfate method, please refer to the AABB technical manual.[15])

8. An extensive medical history must be taken on all potential donors, regardless of the number of previous donations on record. Most blood bank donor rooms have a simple card listing all the questions to be asked and "yes" or "no" columns that are used to indicate the donor's responses. The health care provider should refer to the protocol of the donor room at the institution's blood bank or the AABB technical manual, which sets guidelines for donor screening and acceptance.

COLLECTION OF DONOR'S BLOOD

The health care worker in a donor room must operate under the supervision of a qualified, licensed physician. Blood should be collected by using aseptic technique; a sterile, closed system; and a single venipuncture. If a second venipuncture is needed, an entirely new, sterile donor set is necessary; the first is discarded according to the contaminated material disposal protocol of the institution.

A donor should never be left alone either during or immediately after blood collection. The health care worker should be well versed in donor reactions, equipment safety precautions, first-aid techniques, and location of first-aid equipment in case it is needed in the course of donation. See Appendix 7 for comprehensive standard operating procedures for donor phlebotomy.

THERAPEUTIC PHLEBOTOMY

Therepeutic phlebotomy is the intentional removal of blood for therapeutic reasons (Figure 13–32 ■). It is used in the treatment of some myeloproliferative diseases, such as polycythemia, or other conditions in which there is an excessive production of blood cells. Records in the blood bank should indicate the patient's diagnosis, the physician's request

Figure 13–32. Therapeutic Phlebotomy Collection

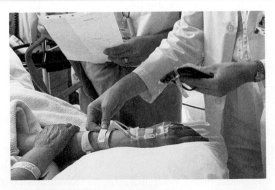

As in other donor collections, health care workers must be experienced and properly trained to collect blood from these patients.

for the phlebotomy, and the amount of blood to be taken. The medical director of the blood bank must decide whether the patient is to be bled in the donor room or in a private section of the blood bank. Some patients are visibly ill and weak, and their presence may have an adverse psychological effect on the healthy donors in the donor room. When a patient is obviously ill, his or her physician or the medical director of the blood bank should be present during the phlebotomy. Generally, the patient should be bled more slowly than a healthy donor, and the resting period should be extended.

The blood obtained through therapeutic bleeding may be used for homologous transfusion if the unit is deemed suitable by the director of the blood bank. If it is to be used, the recipient's physician must agree to use the blood from his or her patient, and a record of the agreement should be kept. The unit is then labeled and processed in the usual manner. The label must indicate that the blood is the result of a therapeutic bleed and must include the patient's diagnosis. If the unit is unsuitable for transfusion, the entire unit is disposed of in the usual manner for contaminated wastes.

AUTOLOGOUS TRANSFUSION

A practice that is frequently used is autologous transfusion: the patient donates his or her own blood before anticipated surgery. The reason for this type of transfusion is that the safest blood a recipient can receive is his or her own blood. The autologous transfusion prevents transfusion-transmitted infectious diseases (e.g., HIV, hepatitis) and eliminates the formation of antibodies in the transfused patient.

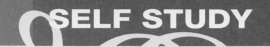

KEY TERMS

Allen test
arterial blood gases (ABGs)
autologous transfusion
bacteremia
bleeding-time test
blood cultures
brachial artery
cannula
capillary blood gas analysis
central intravenous line
femoral artery
fevers of unknown origin (FUO)
fistula
glucose tolerance test

heparin or saline lock
implanted port
intravenous (IV) catheter
lactose tolerance test
peripherally inserted central catheter
   (PICC)
postprandial glucose test
radial artery
septicemia
sodium polyanethole sulfonate (SPS)
therapeutic drug monitoring (TDM)
therapeutic phlebotomy
trace metals
vascular access devices (VADs)

■ STUDY QUESTIONS

For the following, choose the one best answer.

1. What is a cannula?
   a. the fusion of a vein and an artery
   b. a good source of arterial blood
   c. a tubular instrument used to gain access to venous blood
   d. an artificial shunt that provides access to arterial blood

2. Which of the following is a milk sugar that sometimes cannot be digested by healthy individuals?
   a. glucose
   b. glucagon
   c. lactose
   d. lactate

3. Which of the following is the preferred site for blood collection for ABG analysis?
   a. subclavian artery
   b. femoral artery
   c. ulnar artery
   d. radial artery

4. Which of the following supplies is not needed during an arterial puncture for an ABG determination?
   a. tourniquet
   b. heparin
   c. lidocaine
   d. syringe

5. What is the reason for performing the modified Allen test?
   a. to obtain the oxygen concentration of the patient
   b. to determine whether the patient's blood pressure is elevated
   c. to test for the possibility of a hematoma
   d. to determine that the ulnar and radial arteries are providing collateral circulation

6. When blood is drawn from the radial artery for an ABG determination, the needle should be inserted at an angle of no less than
   a. 20 degrees
   b. 30 degrees
   c. 45 degrees
   d. 65 degrees

7. Which of the following evacuated tubes is preferred for the collection of a blood culture specimen?
   a. yellow-topped evacuated tube
   b. green-topped evacuated tube
   c. light-blue-topped evacuated tube
   d. red-topped evacuated tube

8. During a glucose tolerance test, which procedure is acceptable?
   a. a standard amount of glucose drink is given to the patient, then a fasting blood collection is performed
   b. the patient should be encouraged to drink water throughout the procedure
   c. the patient is allowed to chew sugarless gum
   d. all the patient's specimens are timed from the fasting collection

9. The bleeding-time test is used for what purpose?
   a. check for vascular abnormalities
   b. diagnose diabetes mellitus
   c. determine whether the patient's blood pressure is low
   d. assess liver glycogen stores

10. Autologous transfusion is to prevent which of the following possibilities?
    a. transfused patient developing diabetes mellitus
    b. antibodies forming in the transfused patient
    c. antigens forming in the transfused patient
    d. polycythemia developing in the transfused patient

References

1. Chang, DW, Elstun, LR, Jones, AP: *The Multiskilled Respiratory Therapist.* Philadelphia: FA Davis Co, 2000, 68–88.

2. Okeson, GC, Wulbrecht, PH: The safety of brachial artery puncture for arterial blood sampling. *Chest,* 1998; 114: 748–751.

3. Smith, C: Surgicutt: A device for modified template bleeding times. *J Med Technol,* 1986:3(4).

4. International Technidyne Corporation: *Surgicutt: Package Insert of Procedure.* Edison, NJ: International Technidyne Corporation, 2003.

5. Ruge, D, Sandin, R, Siegelski, S, Greene, J, Johnson, N: Reduction in blood culture contamination rates by establishment of policy for central intravenous catheters. *Lab Med,* 2002; 33(10): 797–800.

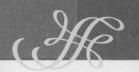

6. Schifman, R, Pindur, A: The effect of skin disinfection material on reducing blood culture contamination. *Am J Clin Pathol,* 1993; 99: 536–538.

7. Koneman, E, Allen, S, Janda, W, et al. (eds): *Color Atlas and Textbook of Diagnostic Microbiology,* 5th ed. Philadelphia: Lippincott, 1997.

8. American Diabetes Association: Gestational Diabetes Mellitus-Position Statement: Diabetes Care, 2000; 23(Suppl.1): 1–6. http://journal.diabetes.org.

9. Report of the Expert Committee on the Diagnosis and Classification of Diabetes Mellitus: Diabetes Care, 2000; 23(suppl. 1). http://journal.diabetes.org.

10. Kaplan, LA, Pesce, AJ, and Kazmierczak (eds): Therapeutic drug monitoring. In *Clinical Chemistry: Theory, Analysis Correlation,* 4th ed. St. Louis: Mosby, 2003, 1073–1084.

11. Quattrocchi, F, Karnes, H, Robinson, J, et al.: Effect of serum separator blood collection tubes on drug concentration. *Ther Drug Monit,* 1983; 5: 359–362.

12. Dasgupta, A, Dean, R, Saldora, S, et al.: Absorption in therapeutic drugs by barrier gels in separator blood collection tubes. *Am J Clin Pathol,* 1994; 101: 456–461.

13. National Committee for Clinical Laboratory Standards: Control of Preanalytical Variation in Trace Element Determinations: Approved Guidelines. Document C38-A. Wayne, PA: NCCLS, 1997.

14. Becan-McBride, K, Baranowski, L: *BD Pre-Analytix Training Program: Interactive Education Program for Health Professionals.* Franklin Lakes, NJ: Becton-Dickinson & Co, 2000.

15. Vengelen-Tyler, V (ed): *Technical Manual of the American Association of Blood Banks,* 14th ed. Bethesda, MD: 2002.

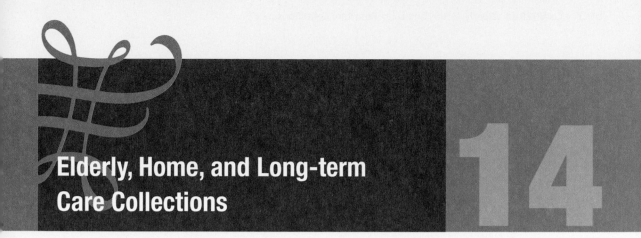

Elderly, Home, and Long-term Care Collections

14

CHAPTER OBJECTIVES

Upon completion of Chapter 14, the learner is responsible for the following:

1. List two other terms that are synonymous with point-of-care testing.

2. Define five physical and/or emotional changes that are associated with the aging process.

3. Describe how a health care worker should react to physical and emotional changes associated with the elderly.

4. Identify four analytes whose levels can be determined through point-of-care testing.

5. Describe the most widely used application of point-of-care testing.

6. Define quality assurance and its requirements.

 MediaLINK

Access the accompanying CD-ROM to explore a wide variety of review questions and interactive activities for this chapter, including multiple choice, true/false, and video exercises.

With new emerging technology, laboratory testing services and results delivery have expanded beyond the laboratory to the hospital bedside, the home, the nursing home, and any other direct-contact patient setting.[1]

Box 14–1

The terms used for these direct laboratory services include:

- decentralized laboratory testing
- on-site testing
- alternate-site testing
- near-patient testing
- patient-focused testing
- point-of-care testing
- bedside testing

With the increasing health care requirements of the growing U.S. elderly population, nurses, laboratorians, and other health care providers will increasingly perform additional on-site laboratory testing to obtain various types of laboratory test results. The demand for point-of-care testing is increasing because rapid turnaround of laboratory test results is necessary for prompt medical decision making.

■■■■■ CONSIDERATIONS FOR THE ELDERLY

The elderly, or geriatric, population comprises about 15 percent of the U.S. population and uses 31 percent of the nation's health care services (Figure 14–1 ■). In 25 years, the geriatric population will have reached 20 percent of the total U.S. population.[2] Physical condi-

Figure 14–1. Increasing Geriatric Population in the United States

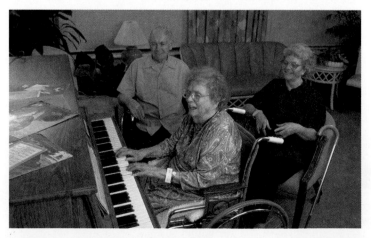

The number of elderly citizens is rapidly increasing due to the advancing age of the Baby Boomer generation. (Source: Michal Heron/Pearson Education/PH College.)

tions, such as arthritis, Parkinson's disease (a disease causing tremors), and other debilitating diseases in the elderly will continue to increase point-of-care testing by skin puncture due to the difficulty of obtaining blood by venipuncture. In addition, this patient population will increasingly need point-of-care testing and other health care services in their homes, nursing homes, rehabilitation centers, and other long-term care facilities (i.e., where the length of stay is over 30 days).

The process of aging presents physical and emotional problems that can be challenging for health care workers. Whatever the case, elderly individuals should be treated with the utmost respect and dignity. Physical problems that are common in older individuals include the following:

- Hearing loss may cause embarrassment and frustration. Repeating instructions or adjusting one's position to speak in the "good" ear may be necessary for the patient to truly understand a procedure.
- Failing eyesight is common, so the health care worker should take care to guide the elderly individual to the appropriate seat for blood collection or to the bathroom for urine collections.
- Loss of taste, smell, and feeling can accompany the aging process. Elderly people may lack an appetite, which may lead to malnourishment. They may tend to drop things or not be able to make a fist due to muscle weakness. The health care worker should make a note of these clues, particularly if the patient is homebound without a caregiver.
- Memory loss can affect the patient's ability to take medications or to remember the last time he or she ate. These factors may interfere with the interpretation of laboratory results.
- Skin tissue becomes thinner, thereby making venipuncture more difficult. The phlebotomist must hold the skin extra taut so that the vein does not "roll." Also, the arm should not be "slapped" when trying to locate the vein. This causes bruising. Use of heated compresses can be helpful.
- Muscles become smaller, so the angle of penetration of a venipuncture needle may need to be more shallow.
- Increased susceptibility to accidental hypothermia (a subnormal drop in body temperature) can make the elderly patient feel cold. Thus, specimen collection may require warming of the site.
- Increased sensitivities and allergies. Therefore patients should be asked if they are allergic to anything.

Emotional problems that are associated with aging include the possible loss of career, spouse, close friends, or relatives and can be reflected by depression or anger at life in general. Health care workers should remember to address the elderly with dignity and respect by using "Mr./ Mrs./ Miss," etc. Respect for privacy should also be considered.

▆▆▆▆ GLUCOSE MONITORING

One of the most widely used applications of point-of-care testing is blood glucose monitoring, in which commercially available instruments, such as the one shown in Procedure 14–1, are used to determine blood glucose levels. Such determinations allow the physician to choose appropriate treatment regimens for patients with diabetes mellitus, a chronic disease in which the pancreas cannot produce enough insulin or cannot use the insulin that it

Box 14–2	Considerations in Home Care

Factors related to the physical setting can also affect a phlebotomist's work. If specimens are to be collected in homes, all procedures are similar except that extra care must be taken for the following:

- Extra supplies and equipment, including biohazard containers for disposables and a specimen transport container, should be taken into the home.
- The patient should be positively identified if possible. If not possible, then procedures of the health care organization should be developed and followed.
- The patient should be placed in a comfortable, preferably reclining, position in case of fainting.
- The phlebotomist should transport a hand disinfectant with other supplies and equipment and use the disinfectant on his/her hands before the collection of blood occurs.
- The health care worker should carefully inspect the area after the procedure to assure that all trash and used supplies have been properly discarded.
- Specimens should be carefully labeled and placed in leakproof containers with the biohazard sign on the container. Appropriate temperatures for transport should be checked.
- Health care workers who are working in high-crime areas should take security precautions, travel with a mobile phone, and carry maps of the area to avoid getting lost on the way to or from the patient's home.
- Delays in returning specimens to the laboratory should be carefully documented.

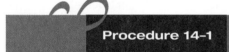

Procedure 14–1	Obtaining Blood Specimen for Glucose Testing (Skin Puncture)

Preparation

1. Gather equipment-safety automatic lancet
2. Cleanse your hands
3. Don gloves

Procedure

1. Choose and wash patients' fingertip (especially side of finger (Fig 14–2A).

2. Cleanse skin with alcohol wipe (Fig 14–2B) and allow skin to dry.

3. Gently massage the finger five or six times from base to tip to aid blood flow (Fig 14–2C).

4. Decide which side of the finger to make the incision (Fig 14–2D).

5. Remove the safety lancet from the protective paper without touching the tip and as you hold the patient's finger firmly with one hand, make a swift, deep puncture with the retractable safety puncture device (Fig 14–2E).

6. Wipe the first three drops of blood away with clean gauze (Figure 14–2F).

7. Gently massage the finger from base to tip to obtain the needed drop of blood (Fig 14–2G).

8. Apply the Hemocue® microcuvette to the drop of blood. The correct volume is drawn into the cuvette by capillary action (capillary, venous, or arterial blood can be used) (Fig 14–2H).

9. Wipe off any excess blood from sides of cuvette (Fig 14–2I).

10. Place the microcuvette into the cuvette holder and insert it into the photometer (Fig 14–2J).

11. The laboratory test result is displayed automatically (Fig 14–2K).

continued

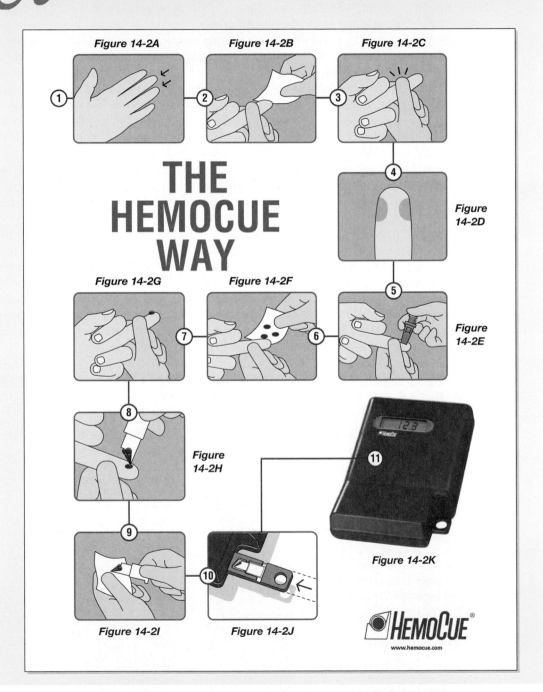

Figure 14-2A

Figure 14-2B

Figure 14-2C

Figure 14-2D

Figure 14-2E

Figure 14-2F

Figure 14-2G

Figure 14-2H

Figure 14-2I

Figure 14-2J

Figure 14-2K

THE HEMOCUE WAY

HEMOCUE®
www.hemocue.com

does produce. Insulin is a chemical that is released into the bloodstream by the pancreas when glucose levels in the blood increase after meals. Insulin causes the glucose to be absorbed from the blood into the body tissues, where it is used for energy. Because of the lack of insulin in patients with diabetes mellitus, glucose is not properly absorbed by the tissues, and the glucose levels within the blood increase.

During the past decade, small glucose-monitoring instruments, such as those shown in Figure 14–2 and described in Table 14–1, became commonplace in the home, in the nursing home, and at the hospital bedside. These "rapid" methods (Figure 14–3 ■) require whole blood samples collected by skin puncture from the finger, heel (for infants), or a flushed heparin line. As for any blood collection procedure, appropriate safety protocols must be followed (e.g., wearing gloves), and disposal of potentially contaminated waste must be part of the quality control and safety guidelines (see Chapters 5 and 6). These bedside procedures are handy for quick screening in a hospital or outpatient setting. Extreme caution must be taken, however, to provide a rigid, up-to-date, quality control and training program for personnel before they begin to implement such procedures. Not following the written instructions about product storage or procedural steps can lead to errors in the test results.[3,4]

To perform the blood glucose determinations, health care providers need to gather the appropriate supplies (Figure 14–2) and must be aware of the total quality assurance procedures that are required to obtain accurate and precise results. The timing of the reaction is critical, and most of these instruments call the time to the attention of the operator by buzzing, sounding an alarm, or digitally displaying the glucose result. Also, the health care provider needs to know what type of blood—blood from a fingerstick and/or blood from venipuncture—can be used to perform glucose determination with the point-of-care instrument and the patient age group that the blood instrument can be used for.

TABLE 14–1.   Blood Glucose Monitors

INSTRUMENT (MANUFACTURER)	FEATURES	TEST TIME	VOLUME
Accu-Chek Active (Roche Diagnostics Corp.) www.accu-chek.com	Photo-reflectance assay; 200 tests	5 sec	1 μL
Medisense Soft-Tact (Abbott Laboratories) www.medisense.com	Electrochemical assay; 450 tests	20 sec	3 μL
Ascensia Glucometer DEX2 (Bayer Diagnostics) www.bayercarediabetes.com	Electrochemical assay; 100 tests	30 sec	3–4 μL
One Touch Ultra (Life Scan) www.lifescan.com	Electrochemical assay; 150 tests	5 sec	1 μL
FreeStyle (TheraSense) www.therasense.com	Electrochemical assay; 250 tests	15 sec	0.3 μL

Figure 14-3. Use of Glucose Meters

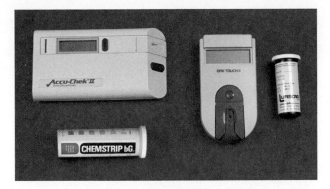

Many types of glucose meters are available today.

As an example, the HemoCue β-Glucose Analyzer (Figure 14–4 ■) is an instrument that can obtain test results from capillary, venous, or arterial whole blood. It uses a microcuvette rather than a test strip and does not require blotting. Also, it can be used to monitor blood glucose in neonates as well as adults and children.

QUALITY IN POINT-OF-CARE TESTING (POCT)

Some glucose-monitoring instruments should be calibrated with glucose standards (calibrators). The glucose values must be monitored daily with quality control material and whenever a battery is changed or the meter is cleaned. This control material should be similar to the patient's specimen in order to determine if the analytic system is working properly. For example, the glucose control material should be based on the use of whole blood because this type of body fluid is used for measurements with bedside glucose-monitoring instruments.

In addition, some instruments have automatic control, or "electronic quality control" (EQC). The purpose of EQC is to test the electronics: the internal and analyte circuits of the instrument. Both the liquid and electronic QC should be performed.

For each day the glucose assay or other point-of-care test is performed on patients' blood specimens, control material should be analyzed so that the mean and standard deviation

Box 14-3	Proper Technique for Accurate Point-of-Care Testing

- Carefully read the package insert and user manual
- Watch an experienced laboratory professional, doctor or nurse perform the test
- Strictly follow daily quality control procedures
- Carefully record the results, including the date, time, and health care worker identification, as well as verification that the results are from the bedside (or patient's home) rather than the clinical laboratory. (In some health care facilities, bedside test results are recorded on special bedside-testing written or computer forms or in a separate section of the patient's medical record.)

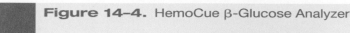

Figure 14–4. HemoCue β-Glucose Analyzer

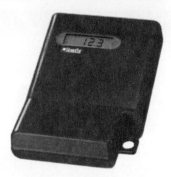

Courtesy of HemoCue, Inc., Lake Forest, CA

can be calculated. The calculations usually occur on 20 to 30 control values.[5] The control value obtained each day is plotted on a chart under the appropriate date, and the daily plots are joined with a straight line (Figure 14–5 ■). Interpretation of this chart is based on the fact that, for a normal distribution, 95 percent of the values about the mean, or average ($\bar{x}$), should be within plus or minus 2 standard deviations (SD) of the mean (average), and the fact that, for a normal distribution, 99 percent of the values are within plus or minus 3 SD of the mean. Tolerance limits are determined by pooling the data obtained during a 30-day test period and referring to the mean plus or minus 2 SD. If a daily control value exceeds the tolerance limits, corrective action must occur according to the manufacturer's directions and be documented for future reference.

Another quality control measure that can be taken when point-of-care monitoring instruments are used is purchasing the reagent strips and controls in quantities that enable health care workers to use constant pools of the same lot number. This leads to reproducibility of the results. Required preventive maintenance of each point-of-care instrument is critical for accurate results.

Some point-of-care testing instruments can store and download calibrators, controls, and patients' results and can, thus, provide a complete instrument log for quality assurance interpretation. Table 14–2 provides a list that will help lead to quality results through avoidance of these problems.

◼◼◼◼ BLOOD GAS AND ELECTROLYTE ANALYSIS

Blood gas analysis for critical patient care needs can also be accomplished through patient-focused testing using instrumentation such as the Nova Biomedical Stat Profile pHOx analyzer (Figure 14–6 ■). Blood gas analysis involves measurement of the partial pressure of oxygen (pO_2), partial pressure of carbon dioxide (pCO_2), and pH. The pO_2 and pCO_2 are analyzed whenever a patient has a heart or lung disorder. The blood pH determines whether the blood is too acidic or too alkaline. All of these analytes must be closely monitored in emergency care situations, critical care units, cardiac intensive care units, and other units requiring immediate patient diagnosis and treatment.

Figure 14–5. Quality Control Record

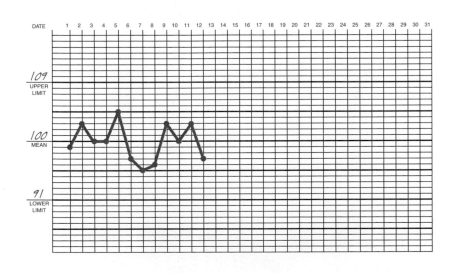

Glucose Monitor

QUALITY CONTROL RECORD

PRACTICE NAME
Med Mobile Clinic

INSTRUMENT *Glucose Monitor - Mobile Clinic*
CONTROL LOT# *54539*   EXPIRATION DATE *03/05/05*
DIRECTOR SIGNATURE/DATE:

NAME/LEVEL
Accu Glucose/Normal

TEST *Glucose *Glucose Monitor*   UNITS *mg/dl*

LOWER LIMIT *91*   MEAN *100*   UPPER LIMIT *109*

DATE	NO.	VALUE	TECH	COMMENT	DATE	NO.	VALUE	TECH	COMMENT
2/8/04	1	99	KBM			17			
2/9/04	2	103	KBM	prev. maintenance		18			
2/10/04	3	100	KBM			19			
2/11/04	4	100	KBM			20			
2/12/04	5	105	KBM			21			
2/15/04	6	97	KBM			22			
2/16/04	7	95	KBM			23			
2/17/04	8	96	KBM	new battery		24			
2/18/04	9	103	KBM			25			
2/19/04	10	100	KBM			26			
2/20/04	11	103	KBM			27			
2/21/04	12	97	KBM			28			
	13					29			
	14					30			
	15					31			
	16								

DATE   1 2 3 4 5 6 7 8 9 10 11 12 13 14 15 16 17 18 19 20 21 22 23 24 25 26 27 28 29 30 31

109 UPPER LIMIT

100 MEAN

91 LOWER LIMIT

TABLE 14–2. Problems to Avoid in Point-of-Care Testing

Specimen is inappropriately stored.

Contamination of the blood with alcohol. (After alcohol is used to cleanse the skin puncture site, the skin must dry completely before puncturing the site.)

Wrong volume of specimen is collected.

Instrument blotting/wiping technique is not performed according to manufacturer's directions.

Instrument is not clean.

Reagents are outdated.

Timing of the analytic procedure is incorrect.

Reagents are not stored at the proper temperature, leading them to deterioration.

Patient has not dieted properly for procedure.

Patient's result/time/date/etc. is mislabeled.

Recording of result is incorrect.

Battery for instrument is weak or dead.

Calibrators and/or controls are not properly used and/or recorded.

Results are not sent to appropriate individuals in timely manner.

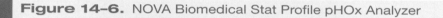

Figure 14–6. NOVA Biomedical Stat Profile pHOx Analyzer

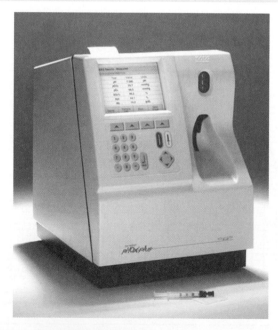

Courtesy of Nova Biomedical, Waltham, MA

In addition to monitoring blood gases, point-of-care instruments such as the Nova Stat Profile pHOx Plus can measure blood electrolyte levels—sodium (Na^+), potassium (K^+), chloride (Cl^-) or calcium (Ca^{++})—plus glucose, calculate bicarbonate (HCO_3^-) and total carbon dioxide (TCO_2) levels. These electrolyte measurements, as well as blood gas analysis, are needed immediately in critical care situations.

These instruments require preventive maintenance and quality control similar to the glucose-monitoring instruments; however, these instruments measure more than one analyte and thus have more complex operational, quality control, and maintenance needs than the glucose monitors. Consequently, as a health care professional involved in collecting blood and determining the analytes' results with these instruments, it is extremely important to be thoroughly trained in their use prior to actually testing patients' blood.

POINT-OF-CARE TESTING FOR ACUTE HEART DAMAGE

Another cardiac point-of-care test is the CARDIA STATus (Figure 14–7 ■) from Spectral Diagnostics for the measurement of troponin T, myoglobin, and creatine kinase–MB (CK-MB). These assays use whole blood, plasma, or serum. A positive test result is indicated by an observable purple-colored line, which identifies an increase in troponin T, myoglobin, and CK-MB as a result of cardiac damage. Another POC assay for the measurement of troponin to detect heart damage is the TROPT sensitive rapid assay from Roche Diagnostics.

Figure 14–7. Spectral CardiaSTATus

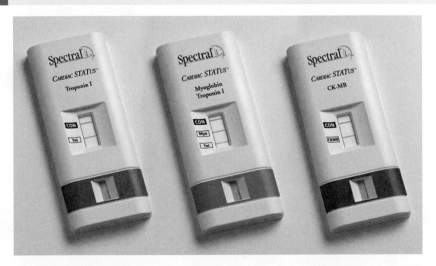

Courtesy of Spectral Diagnostics, Inc., Toronto, Ontario, Canada

■■■ ■ BLOOD COAGULATION MONITORING

Similar to glucose monitoring, monitoring blood coagulation through point-of-care testing provides immediate results that can be used in controlling bleeding or clotting disorders in patients.[6] A blood coagulation instrument, such as the CoaguChek System from Roche Diagnostics Corp., is a handheld instrument that can measure prothrombin time (PT) from an unmeasured drop of whole blood, providing results in 2 minutes (Figure 14–8 ■). The CoaguChek System can be used by home health care providers or other outpatient clinic providers to monitor long-term anticoagulation therapy in patients. The immediate test results allow rapid dose adjustments. Again, the health care provider using these instruments must be trained appropriately in the preventive maintenance and quality control parameters in order to obtain accurate results. Also, reading the manufacturer's directions is essential. For example, the CoaguChek System is calibrated to use the first drop of blood in skin puncture. The ProTime International Technidyne Corp., measures prothrombin time, using one or two drops from a finger stick. The blood is collected directly into the disposable cuvette.

Other point-of-care coagulation systems are the Actalyke Activated Clotting Time Test (ACT) System (Figure 14–9 ■), the Hemochron Jr. Instrument, the Rapidpoint Coag analyzer, and the INRatio Meter (Figure 14–10 ■). These instruments are designed for use at the patient's point of care (i.e., home, intensive care unit, physician's office) to monitor anticoagulation therapy such as heparin or warfarin sodium (Coumadin). The INRatio Meter

Figure 14–8. CoaguChek System

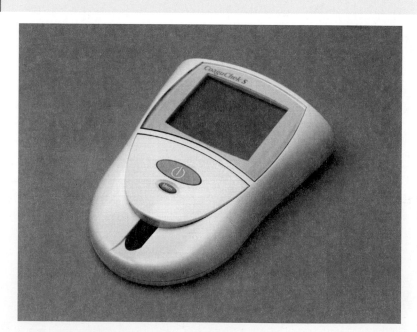

Courtesy of Roche Diagnostics Corp., Indianapolis, IN.

Figure 14–9. Actalyke Activated Clotting Time Test (ACT) System

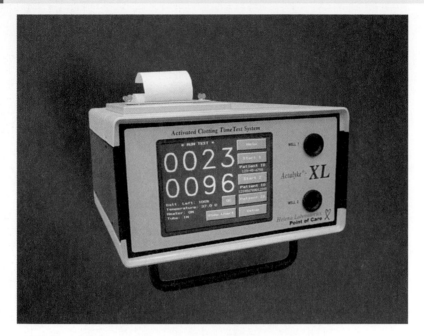

Courtesy of Helena Laboratories, Beaumont, TX.

provides prothrombin time (PT) and International Normalized Ratio (INR) results within 2 minutes.

 HEMATOCRIT, HEMOGLOBIN, AND OTHER HEMATOLOGY PARAMETERS

The hematocrit (Hct, packed cell volume [PCV], Crit) represents the volume of circulating blood that is occupied by red blood cells (RBCs). It is expressed as a percentage; thus, a hematocrit value of 38 percent indicates that 38 ml of each 100 ml of peripheral blood is composed of RBCs. Hematocrit values are obtained to aid in the diagnosis and evaluation of anemia, a less than normal number of erythrocytes, and may be used to evaluate blood volume and total RBC mass. Blood collection usually occurs by skin puncture. For accurate test results, remember not to squeeze the tissue to obtain capillary blood because doing so will dilute the sample with tissue fluid. It is very important to follow the healthcare facility's procedure. Plastic microcapillary tubes must be used to avoid the possibility of bloodborne pathogen exposure from a broken tube.

Determining a patient's hemoglobin level is another test to aid in the diagnosis and evaluation of anemia and other blood abnormalities. The hemoglobin test has been determined by the American Medical Association (AMA) to be more accurate than the hematocrit test in diagnosis and treatment. Also, the hemoglobin procedure is a safer method to detect

Figure 14–10. INRatio Meter

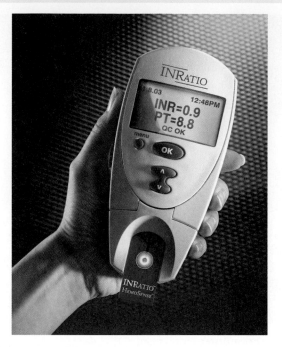

Courtesy of HemoSense, Milpitas, CA

anemia. A point-of-care analyzer that can be used to measure hemoglobin is the HemoCue β-Hemoglobin System (HemoCue, Inc., Mission Viejo, CA) (Fig. 14–11 ■). A patient's venous, capillary, or arterial whole blood sample placed in the microcuvette and inserted into this instrument provides the patient's hemoglobin value.

The Ichor automated cell counter (Helena Laboratories, Beaumont, TX) is an instrument for hematology analysis in acute (i.e., ICU) adult and pediatric patient management (Figure 14–12 ■). This system is used to determine the hematology parameters that include platelet count, hemoglobin, hematocrit, WBC count, RBC count, and platelet aggregation results. The results are available in about 1 minute.

■■■■■ CHOLESTEROL SCREENING

Another laboratory testing procedure that health care providers are performing through point-of-care testing is cholesterol screening. Using a finger stick drop of blood, total cholesterol (TC) values can be obtained.

The AccuTrend GC/Accu-Chek InstantPlus (Roche Diagnostics, Indianapolis, IN) provides blood total cholesterol and blood glucose with a fingerstick drop of blood in 3 minutes.

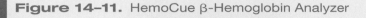

Figure 14–11. HemoCue β-Hemoglobin Analyzer

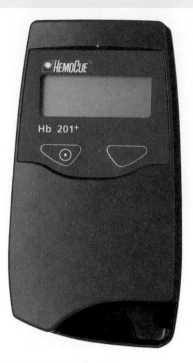

Courtesy of HemoCue, Inc., Lake Forests, CA

■■■■■ FUTURE TRENDS

Additional point-of-care testing procedures that have evolved include the hemoglobin A1c procedure to test for maintenance of blood glucose levels using the Bayer Diagnostics DCA 2000+ Analyzer; the handheld BiliCheck from Respironics, Inc., which noninvasively measures the concentration of bilirubin in the forehead skin of newborns; and a rapid HIV point-of-care test—the OraQuick Assay (see Chapter 2, "Legal and Regulatory Issues") manufactured by Abbott Diagnostics.

More point-of-care testing procedures are evolving that will inevitably involve phlebotomists, nurses, patient care technicians, and others who are providing care at the hospital bedside, nursing home, and/or home. For each new procedure, the health care worker must make a point of learning in detail the blood collection requirements, preventive maintenance, quality control, ethical and legal implications of doing such a test (e.g., HIV testing), record keeping, and calibration requirements in order to provide accurate and precise test results.

Figure 14–12. Ichor Automated Cell Counter

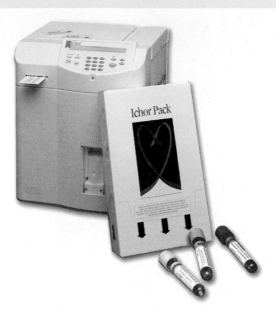

Courtesy of Helena Laboratories, Beaumont, TX

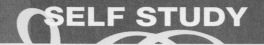

SELF STUDY

KEY TERMS

blood gas analysis

diabetes mellitus

insulin

Parkinson's disease

patient-focused testing

point-of-care testing

quality control material

troponin T

STUDY QUESTIONS

For the following, choose the one best answer.

1. Insulin is released into the bloodstream in which of these circumstances?
   a. blood cholesterol levels decrease
   b. blood glucose levels decrease
   c. blood glucose levels increase
   d. blood cholesterol levels increase

2. Diabetes mellitus is caused by the inability of the pancreas to make or to use which substance?
   a. glucose
   b. cholesterol
   c. sodium
   d. insulin

3. In which of the following organs is insulin produced?
   a. gallbladder
   b. pancreas
   c. liver
   d. kidney

4. What is the next step after the skin is punctured to obtain blood for glucose monitoring?
   a. use the first drop of blood for the glucose test
   b. use an alcohol pad to remove the first drop of blood
   c. use a dry, sterile gauze pad to remove the first drop of blood
   d. squeeze the patient's finger to make a big first drop of blood for the monitor

5. What should the blood collector do prior to using reagent strips and/or controls in point-of-care testing?
   a. check the date when the bottle was opened
   b. check the expiration date
   c. verify that they were stored at the appropriate temperature
   d. all of the above

6. How can a phlebotomist increase the blood flow from the skin puncture site for patient testing?
   a. squeeze the punctured finger
   b. massage the area
   c. puncture another site adjacent to the first puncture site
   d. none of the above

7. What do blood gas analyses measure?
   a. Na^+ and K^+
   b. pCO_2, pO_2, and pH
   c. Cl^- and HCO_3^-
   d. pCO_2, Na^+, and Cl^-

8. Which tests are measured through blood coagulation monitoring by point-of-care testing?

    a. PT and INR

    b. PT and pCO_2

    c. pO_2 and pCO_2

    d. PT, APTT, and pH

9. Which of the following is a blood glucose monitor?

    a. One Touch Ultra

    b. HemoSense INRatio Meter

    c. CoaguChek System

    d. TROPT Sensitive rapid assay

10. Which tests can be measured by electrolyte monitoring through point-of-care testing?

    a. Na^+, K^+, PT, and APTT

    b. pCO_2, pO_2, and Na^+

    c. Na^+, K^+, Cl^-, and HCO_3^-

    d. pCO_2, Cl^-, HCO_3^-, and pO_2

References

1. Kost, GJ: *Principles and Practice of Point-of-Care Testing.* Philadelphia, PA: Lippincott Williams & Wilkins, 2002.

2. Nixon, RG: *BRADY Geriatric Prehospital Care.* Upper Saddle River, NJ: Prentice Hall, 2003.

3. US Food and Drug Administration: Center for Devices and Radiological Health, Current Lab Safety Tips, http://www.fda.gov/cdrh/oivd/laboratory.html 5/21/2003.

4. Jacobs, E: Chapter 17: Point-of-Care (Near-Patient) Testing, In *Clinical Chemistry: Theory, Analysis, Correlation,* edited by Kaplan, LA, Pesce, AJ, and Kazmierczak. St. Louis: Mosby Publishers, 2003.

5. Westgard, J, Qia, E, Barry, T: *Basic QC Practices—Training in Statistical Quality Control for Healthcare Laboratories,* Westgard Quality Corp., www.westgard.com, 1998.

6. Despotis, GJ, Sontoro, SA, Spritznagel, E, et al.: Prospective evaluation and clinical utility of on-site monitoring of coagulation in patients undergoing cardiac operation. *J Thorac Cardiovasc Surg,* 1994; 107(1): 271–279.

Urinalysis, Body Fluids, and Other Specimens

15

CHAPTER OBJECTIVES

Upon completion of Chapter 15, the learner is responsible for the following:

1. Identify body fluid specimens, other than blood, that are analyzed in the clinical laboratory, and the correct procedures for collecting and/or transporting these specimens to the laboratory.

2. Identify specimens collected for microbiological, throat, and nasopharyngeal cultures and the protocol that must be followed when transporting these specimens.

3. List the types of patient specimens that are needed for gastric and sweat chloride analyses.

4. List three types of urine specimen collections and differentiate the uses of the urine specimens obtained from these collections.

 MediaLINK

Access the accompanying CD-ROM to explore a wide variety of review questions and interactive activities for this chapter, including multiple choice, true/false, and video exercises.

In addition to collecting and transporting blood specimens, health care workers usually are involved in the collection and/or transportation of urine and other body fluid specimens. The health care worker should be careful when transporting body fluids because they are difficult to obtain and because the quality of the clinical laboratory test result is only as good as the specimen that is collected and transported to the testing site. Also, because such specimens may be biohazardous, the health care worker must adhere to standard precautions (see Chapter 5, "Infection Control") during collection and transportation of these specimens. Just as for blood collections, the laboratory request slip must accompany the specimen, which must be properly labeled with the patient's name, the patient's identification number, the date, the time of collection, the type of specimen, and the attending physician's name. The label should be affixed on the container, NOT the lid as shown in Figure 15–1 ■. If different patients' urine specimens are in the same location for testing and the labeled lids are taken off the unlabeled containers for testing each urine specimen, it is highly likely that mismatching of the tests' results to the patients will occur.

■ URINE COLLECTION

Routine urinalysis (UA) is one of the most frequently requested laboratory procedures because it can provide a useful indication of body health. It can be performed on a "first morning" or "random" urine specimen. Various diseases and disorders, such as those listed in Table 15–1, can be detected through a routine UA. Some of the more common types of

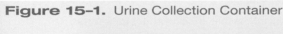

Figure 15–1. Urine Collection Container

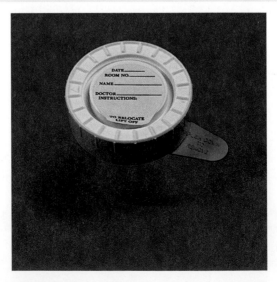

The label with necessary patient's information should be affixed to the container, NOT the lid.

TABLE 15–1.   Abnormal Urine Test Results and Associated Conditions

ABNORMAL URINE TEST RESULT	ASSOCIATED CONDITION
Presence of protein in urine (proteinuria)	Kidney disease
	Prolonged exercise
	Chemical poisoning
Presence of hemoglobin in urine (indicates blood destruction)	Kidney disease
	Malaria
	Severe burns
	Chemical poisoning
Presence of bilirubin in urine	Liver disease
	Obstructive jaundice
Presence of glucose in urine (glycosuria)	Diabetes mellitus
Presence of leukocytes in urine (white blood cells)	Infection of the kidney
	Infection of the urinary bladder
	Infection of the urethra
Presence of ketone bodies in urine (ketosis)	Diabetes mellitus
	Starvation

urine specimen collections and their uses are provided in Table 15–2. The routine UA includes a physical, chemical, and sometimes microscopic analysis of the urine sample. The physical properties include the following: color, transparency vs. cloudiness, odor, and concentration as detected through a specific gravity measurement.

TABLE 15–2.   Types of Urine Specimen Collections and Their Uses

SPECIMEN TYPE	REASON FOR COLLECTION	USE
Random	This type of specimen is most convenient to obtain.	Routine urinalysis (UA)
		Quantitative and qualitative
First urine of the morning	This urine excretion is the most concentrated.	Protein, nitrate, microscopic analysis
		Routine urinalysis (UA)
Fasting	Metabolic abnormalities are suspected	Glucose level determinations for diabetes mellitus testing
Clean-catch midstream	The specimen is free of contamination.	Culture for bacteria and/or microscopic analysis
Timed (e.g., 2 hour, 4 hour, 24 hour)	The excretion rate of the analyte can be determined.	Creatinine clearance test, urobilinogen determinations, hormone studies
Tolerance test	Timed blood and urine specimens are obtained to detect metabolic abnormalities.	Glucose tolerance test (GTT) and other tolerance tests

The chemical analysis for abnormal constituents is determined by using plastic reagent strips impregnated with color-reacting substances that test for the presence of glucose, protein, blood (red blood cells [RBCs] and hemoglobin), white blood cells (WBCs), ketones, bacteria, bilirubin, and other constituents (Figure 15–2 ■). The plastic reagent strip, which has a separate reagent pad for each chemical test, is dipped into the urine briefly (Figure 15–3 ■). The color of each reagent pad is compared to a color chart usually shown on the outer label of the reagent strip container. The results are reported according to the reagent label specifications (e.g., trace, 1+, 2+, and so on for a positive result, or negative when no reaction occurs). The strip is discarded after it is used one time. As for all types of point-of-care testing, quality control monitoring must be used to ensure accurate results. Other tests that can be performed on urine specimens are the pregnancy, myoglobin, and porphyrin tests. Urine is also the specimen of choice for drug abuse testing. Other laboratory procedures associated with the urinary system include the creatinine clearance test to determine the ability of the kidneys to remove creatinine from the blood and the blood urea nitrogen (BUN) test to measure the amount of urea in the blood.

SINGLE-SPECIMEN COLLECTION

The preferred urine specimen for most analyses is the first voided urine of the morning (Figure 15–4 ■), when urine is the most concentrated. The urine collection containers must be clean and dry prior to the collection process. For routine UA procedures, appropriate containers include plastic disposable cups or bags (for infants) with a capacity of 50 ml. The containers must be properly labeled (label on container, not the lid), free of interfering chemicals, able to be tightly capped, and leakproof (Figure 15–5 ■).

The specimen should be transported to the UA section promptly for analysis within 2 hours after the patient voids. If transportation or analysis cannot occur within this time period, the urine should be refrigerated.

Another type of single-specimen urine test is the urine culture and sensitivity (C&S). This specimen requires a clean-catch midstream urine collection. The patient is instructed to void approximately one half of the urine into the toilet, collect a portion in a readily available sterile container, and allow the rest to pass into the toilet.[1]

If asked, "What is a clean-catch urine specimen?" the procedure should be described, stating that this type of specimen is used to detect the presence or absence of infecting organisms. The specimen must be free of contaminating matter that may be present on the external genital areas. Thus, the steps in Box 15–1 should be explained to a female patient who is to obtain a clean-catch midstream urine specimen. For a male patient, the procedure in Box 15–2 should be adhered to for obtaining a clean-catch midstream urine specimen.[2]

The urine specimen must be transported to the microbiology section promptly. If it cannot be taken to the area for microbiological culturing within 1 hour of collection, the specimen should be refrigerated to prevent an overgrowth of contaminate bacteria.

TIMED COLLECTIONS

For some laboratory assays, such as the creatinine clearance test, urobilinogen determinations, and hormone studies, 24-hour (or other timed period) urine specimens must be obtained. Incorrect collection and improper preservation of this type of specimen are two

Figure 15–2. Keo-Diastix Strip

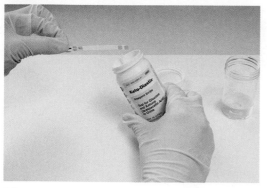

(a)

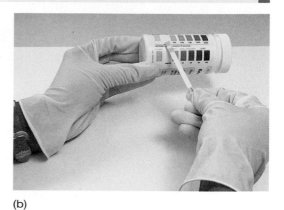

(b)

(a) The Keo-Diastix strip is used to check urine for ketone bodies. (b) The Keo-Diastix strip is checked against the chart found on the bottle after dipping the strip in the urine.

Figure 15–3. Dipping the Plastic Urinalysis Strip into the Urine for Chemical Analysis

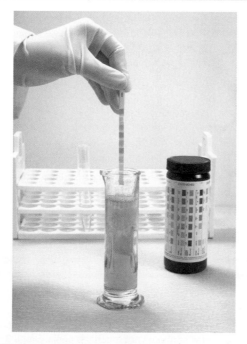

Source: Michal Heron/Pearson Education/PH College.

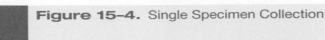

Figure 15–4. Single Specimen Collection

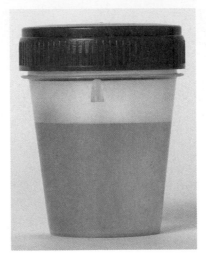

Urine is most concentrated in the morning. (Source: Dorling Kindersley Media Library)

Box 15–1   Clean-Catch Midstream Urine Collection Instructions for Women

1. After washing her hands, the woman should separate the skin folds around the urinary opening and clean this area with mild antiseptic soap and water or special towelettes.

2. Holding the skin folds apart with one hand and after urinating into the toilet, the patient should urinate into a sterile container. The container should not touch the genital area. It must be covered with the lid provided after urination. It is extremely important not to touch the inside or lip of the container with the hands or other parts of the body.

3. The health care worker or, sometimes, the patient will label the container with her name and the time of collection and deliver it to the requested location.

4. Health care personnel should refrigerate the urine specimen immediately.

Box 15–2   Clean-Catch Midstream Urine Collection Instructions for Men

1. The man should wash his hands and the end of his penis with soapy water or special tow-elettes and then let dry.

2. After allowing some urine to pass into the toilet, the patient should collect the urine in the sterile container. The container should not touch the penis. Steps 3 and 4 are the same as those for a woman (Box 15–1).

Figure 15–5. Patient's Labeled Urine Specimen Given to Health Care Worker

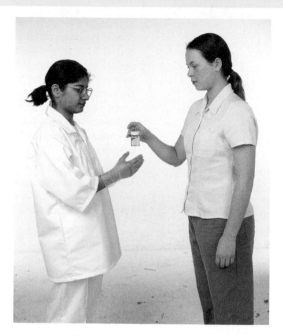

Source: Dorling Kindersley Media Library.

frequent errors affecting timed collections. Thus, the health care worker should be aware of the protocol for collecting a 24-hour urine specimen so that he or she can assist other health care professionals and the patient in preventing collection errors. The steps in Procedure 15–1 should be followed for a 24-hour urine collection.[3]

CEREBROSPINAL FLUID

Cerebrospinal fluid (CSF) is obtained by a physician through a spinal tap or lumbar puncture. The fluid is usually collected in three sterile containers numbered in the order in which they were collected. The first tube is usually contaminated with blood or tissue debris. Thus, the first tube is usually transported to the clinical chemistry or serological testing area of the laboratory. The second tube is used for clinical microbiology testing, and the third tube is usually used for cytological and microscopic analysis. Tests commonly performed on CSF include total protein level, glucose level, cell count, microbiological, chloride level, and cryptococcal antigen determinations. Wearing gloves, CSF must be immediately transported at room temperature to the clinical laboratory for STAT analysis. Transportation can occur to a reference laboratory if the CSF is maintained in an ice slurry;[4] however, it should not be frozen.

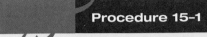

Procedure 15-1   Collecting a 24-Hour Urine Specimen

Equipment

Wide-mouthed, 3- to 4- liter container with lid

Preservative, if required

Label for specimen

Requisition slip

Container with ice, if required

Note: To obtain accurate test results, the laboratory needs the ENTIRE 24-hour urine specimen.

1. Explain the whole procedure to the patient and also provide written directions. Instructions should be in the patient's native language. Explain the importance of hand washing for the urine collection.

2. The patient should be given the container and lid. The laboratory personnel should add any required preservatives to the container prior to giving it to the patient. The preservative and any precautions should be written on the collection container label. The label should be placed on the container, not on the lid. Other information on the label should include the following:

   - Patient's name
   - Patient's identification number
   - Starting collection date and time
   - Ending collection date and time
   - Name of the requested laboratory test

   Other information may be required by the facility.

3. The patient should be instructed verbally that the collection of the 24-hour urine specimen begins with emptying the bladder and discarding the first urine passed. This first step in the collection process should start between 6 and 8 A.M., and the exact time should be written on the container label.

4. Except for the first urine discarded, all urine should be collected during the next 24-hour period. The patient should be reminded to urinate at the end of the collection period and to include this urine in the 24-hour collection. The patient should be told to urinate before having a bowel movement because fecal material in the urine specimen will make the specimen unacceptable for collection.

5. The patient should be instructed to refrigerate the entire specimen after adding each collection during the 24-hour period, except in the case of urate testing.

6. Some preservatives for 24-hour urine collection are corrosive if accidentally spilled or if the patient comes in contact with them during collection. Thus, the patient should be warned of any preservatives in the container.

7. The patient should be informed not to add anything except urine to the container and not to discard any urine during the collection period.

8. A normal intake of fluids during the collection period is desirable unless otherwise indicated by the physician.

9. Some laboratory assays require special dietary restrictions; these instructions should be given to the patient.

10. If possible, medications should be discontinued for 48 to 72 hours preceding the urine collection as a precaution against interference in the laboratory assays.

11. The 24-hour urine specimen should be transported to the clinical laboratory as soon as possible. The specimen should be placed in an insulated bag or a portable cooler to maintain their cool temperature.

▰▰▰▰ FECAL SPECIMENS

Stool (fecal) specimens are commonly collected in order to detect parasites (e.g., ova and parasites [O&P]), enteric disease organisms (e.g., Salmonella, Shigella, Staphylococcus aureus), and viruses. The specimen is collected in a wide-mouthed plastic or waxed cardboard container with a tight-fitting lid. If the patient is to collect the stool specimen at home, he or she should be given a collecting container and instructed to avoid urinating in the container because urine can kill the microorganisms in the collected stool specimen. For children, the container can be placed under the toilet seat so that the child can sit on the toilet. The patient should be instructed to wash the outside of the specimen container after collection and to wash his or her hands thoroughly. The specimen container must be properly sealed to prevent leakage and contamination, because fecal material from patients with infectious intestinal diseases is extremely hazardous. The specimen must be transported to the laboratory immediately and maintained at body temperature (37°C) for detection of parasitic infections.

In addition to the collection of stool specimens for microorganism detection, feces are collected to detect invisible (occult) quantities of blood that do not alter the appearance of the stool. Laboratory determination of occult blood assists in the confirmation of the presence of blood in black stools and can be helpful in detecting gastrointestinal (GI) tract lesions and colorectal cancer. Feces for occult blood tests are often collected by the patient using special test cards, such as ColoScreen-ES (Figure 15–6 ■). The card can be mailed or brought to the health care facility after collection. Manufacturers have also developed occult blood tests that can be performed at home without collecting a stool specimen. A chemically impregnated pad is dropped into the toilet by the patient after he or she has a bowel movement. The patient watches for a color change that he or she reports to the physician via a special test result card supplied with each patient kit. The health care workers involved in specimen collection and transportation should be aware of the procedural steps for these occult blood tests to instruct the patient for proper collections.[5] Many factors can contribute to false-negative or false-positive test results (e.g., patient's ingestion of aspirin, corticosteroids, ibuprofen, anticoagulants, and/or rare meats).

▰▰▰▰ SEMINAL FLUID

Semen is examined in the clinical laboratory to (1) determine the effectiveness of a vasectomy, (2) investigate the possibility of sexual criminal charges, and (3) assess fertility. Before collection of a semen specimen, the patient should be given clear instructions for proper specimen collection. Semen must be collected in containers that are clean and free of trace detergents. Condoms can be used but must be washed free of spermicidal substances prior to use. Specimens must not be exposed to extremes of temperature or light prior to being submitted to the clinical laboratory and should be transported within 2 hours of collection.

▰▰▰▰ AMNIOTIC FLUID

Fluid that bathes the fetus within the amniotic sac is called amniotic fluid. It may be collected by a physician when the pregnant patient is at approximately 16 weeks' gestation so that fetal abnormalities can be detected through chromosomal analysis and chemical tests,

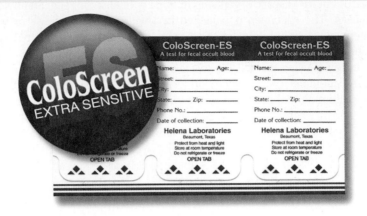

Figure 15–6. ColoScreen Take-Home Packs to Test for Occult Blood

Courtesy of Helena Laboratories, Beaumont, TX

such as the alpha-fetoprotein (AFP) assay. Occasionally, amniotic fluid is obtained in the last trimester of pregnancy to determine the lung maturity of the fetus. In addition to wearing gloves when transporting amniotic fluid to the laboratory, the specimen must be protected from light and transported immediately.

OTHER BODY FLUIDS

In addition to the fluids just discussed, other types of body fluids that sometimes must be transported to the laboratory include synovial fluid, which is extracted aseptically from joint cavities, and fluid aspirated from body cavities (e.g., pleural fluid obtained from the lung cavity, pericardial fluid from the heart cavity, peritoneal fluid from the abdominal cavity). Other specimens for forensic and toxicology studies are mentioned in Chapter 16.

Upon receiving any type of body fluid for transportation, it is important to verify that the container is properly labeled with the patient's name, the patient's identification number, the date, the time of collection, and the type of body fluid collected. If the containers holding any type of body fluids are contaminated on the outside, it is extremely important to wear gloves when transporting them.

CULTURE SPECIMENS

Other specimens that the health care worker may be requested to transport to the clinical laboratory include sputum (fluid from the lungs containing pus) (Figure 15–7 ■), throat and sinus drainage cultures, wound cultures, ear or eye cultures, and skin cultures. The health care worker should be extremely careful while transporting each type of specimen because the specimens can easily become contaminated and may be biohazardous. For safety, the health care worker needs to wear gloves when handling and transporting these specimens in their containers.

OTHER NONBLOOD PROCEDURES

THROAT AND NASOPHARYNGEAL CULTURE COLLECTIONS

Nasopharyngeal cultures are often performed to detect carrier states of *Neisseria meningitidis, Corynebacterium diphtheriae, Streptococcus pyogenes, Haemophilus influenzae,* and *Staphylococcus aureus.* For infants and children, from whom significant sputum cultures are difficult to obtain, nasopharyngeal cultures may be used to diagnose whooping cough, croup, and pneumonia. Throat cultures are most commonly obtained to determine the presence of streptococcal infections. Because coughing may force organisms from the lower respiratory tract into the nasopharynx, it may be best to perform a throat culture on a child or an infant and stimulate coughing in order to obtain a more significant nasopharyngeal culture. Health care workers should be thoroughly taught the correct procedures before they are allowed to acquire specimens from patients.

When a throat culture is ordered, the patient should be instructed to open the mouth wide (Figure 15–8 ■), as if to yawn. A light source should be directed into the mouth and throat so that areas of inflammation, ulceration, exudation, or capsule formation can be readily seen. A tongue blade or spoon is used to depress the tongue and to prevent contamination with organisms from the oral cavity. A sterile cotton swab should be used to swab the tonsil area from side to side, including any inflamed areas.[6]

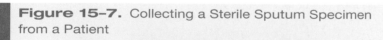

Figure 15–7. Collecting a Sterile Sputum Specimen from a Patient

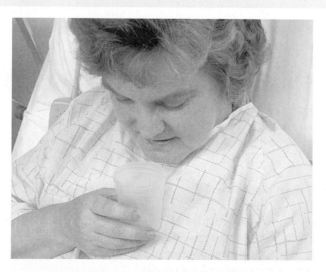

Figure 15-8. Obtaining a Throat Culture

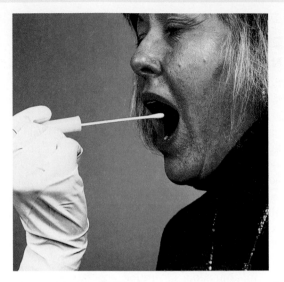

After swabbing throat from side to side, remove the applicator swab being careful to not touch any part of the mouth.

The swab can then be placed in a special transport medium (Figure 15–9 ■), or the fluid on the swab can be inoculated directly onto agar in a petri dish by rolling the swab across a small area of the medium. The specimen can then be transported to the laboratory, where it may be spread out, or "streaked," for distribution of the microorganisms. A Gram-stained smear is often useful to provide preliminary indications of infection and should be made with the swab by rolling it across a sterile slide before placing it in a transport medium or inoculating plate agar. The slide, the swab, and any inoculating media should be taken to the laboratory and processed as soon as possible after collection. The culture should be placed under optimal growth conditions for suspected pathogens (i.e., the culture should be incubated). Timely processing of the specimen helps prevent overgrowth of normal flora, which can inhibit or mask any pathogenic organisms present.

Nasopharyngeal specimens should be obtained with a Dacron- or cotton-tipped flexible wire that can be easily sterilized prior to use. Commercially packaged sterilized swabs are also available. The swab is passed gently through the nose and into the nasopharynx, where it is rotated. Then the swab is carefully removed and placed in a transport medium, or the fluid on the swab is inoculated onto a medium for isolation. Again, the timely processing of all specimens is crucial for best results.

Figure 15–9. Specimen Tube for Swab

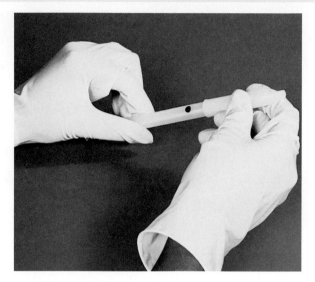

The applicator swab is being placed in specimen tube with caution to avoid contaminating the swab.

SKIN TESTS

On occasion, a nurse or other health care worker may be asked to perform a skin test. The health care worker should check the policies of the health care facility prior to performing the procedure. Skin tests are simple and relatively inexpensive. They determine whether a patient has ever had contact with a particular antigen and has produced antibodies to that antigen. A wide range of disease states stimulate antibody responses in individuals. Tests range from detection of ragweed and milk allergies in hypersensitive individuals, to detection of tuberculosis (TB) and fungal infections in persons who have had contact with these organisms. The allergy skin test is performed on the patient's forearm (Figure 15–10 ■) or back using a common procedure called the prick technique.

The TB skin test can be administered using an automatic device or by pulling 0.1 ml of diluted antigen into a tuberculin syringe. All air bubbles should be expelled by holding the syringe vertically and tapping the sides of the barrel. The volar surface of the patient's forearm should be cleaned with alcohol and prepared in the same manner as for a venipuncture (see Chapter 9). The area should be devoid of scars, skin eruptions, and excessive hair. Holding the syringe at a slight angle (approximately 20 degrees), the needle should be slipped just under the skin. The plunger should be pulled back to ensure that a blood vessel has not been entered. The fluid may be slowly expelled into the site. The needle should be promptly removed, and only slight pressure applied, with gauze, over the site. Care should be taken that the fluid does not leak onto the gauze or run out of the in-

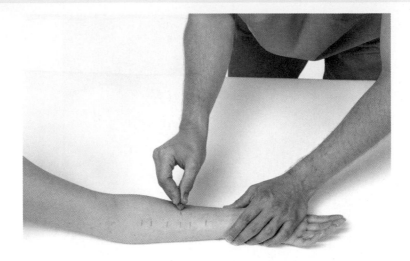

Figure 15–10. Allergy Skin Testing

Source: Andy Crawford/Dorling Kindersley Media Library.

jection site. The patient should hold the arm in an extended position until the site has time to close and retain the fluid. A bandage should not be used over the site because it may absorb some of the fluid and distort the results of the skin test by causing skin irritation from the adhesive.

The patient should report any reaction, no matter how slight, to the physician. Also, a return visit for proper interpretation of the skin reaction should be scheduled with the physician. At some health care agencies, the patient is asked to note the exact size of the reaction site or to compare their reaction with pictures on a prelabeled card that can be mailed back to the institution. When this is the case, patients should be fully informed about how to read positive and negative reactions.

GASTRIC ANALYSIS

Gastric analysis determines how much acid is produced in an individual's stomach. The stomach (gastric) contents are emptied through a gastric tube. Then histamine (a stimulant) is injected into the patient. Five minutes later, the stomach contents are emptied and tested for acidity. The procedure may be repeated several times. The test involves passing a tube through the patient's nose (intubating) and into the stomach (Figure 15–11 ■). The health care worker may be asked to assist and collect specimens as required. The responsibility for properly intubating the patient (using fluoroscopic examination) and administering the histamine intravenously usually rests with the physician or the nurse. The health care worker can be present to assist in patient care and to draw any required

Figure 15–11. Aspirating Gastric Contents from the Patient

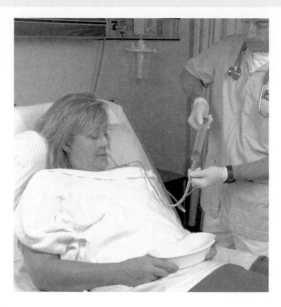

blood specimens, but under no circumstances should be expected to carry out the procedure unless properly trained. Improper placement of the tube poses a high risk to the patient and could result in a punctured lung if the tube enters the bronchial system instead of the esophagus. The health care worker can and should be responsible for proper labeling of gastric and blood samples when he or she is present and assisting during the procedure.

BREATH ANALYSIS FOR PEPTIC ULCERS

Helicobacter pylori is a bacteria that damages the stomach lining and causes peptic ulcers. A positive H-pylori test, antibody, antigen, or breath test indicates that the patient has been infected with this organism. The health care worker should be aware of the procedural steps to assist the patient.

SWEAT CHLORIDE BY IONTOPHORESIS

The sweat chloride test is used in the diagnosis of cystic fibrosis.[7,8] Cystic fibrosis is a disorder of the exocrine glands, generally thought to be enzymatic in nature, that causes changes in mucus-producing glands in the body. Primarily affected are the lungs, upper respiratory tract, liver, and pancreas. Patients with cystic fibrosis produce chloride in their sweat at two to five times the level produced by healthy individuals.

For the laboratory evaluation, pilocarpine hydrochloric acid (HCl) is iontophoresed into the skin of the patient to stimulate sweat production. The sweat is absorbed onto preweighed gauze pads, then the weight of the sweat is determined. The pad is then diluted with deionized water, and the chloride is generally read by titration with a chloridometer.

When a health care provider receives an order to perform a sweat chloride test on a patient, he or she should properly prepare for the procedure under the supervision of a clinical laboratory scientist. Four cups and lids should be preweighed with two 2-inch square gauze pads in each cup. Only two cups are normally used, but the other two can be used as backups, if needed. The patient needs to be appropriately dressed for the climate and drinking fluids to be well hydrated.

Choosing a site with the largest surface area (in children and infants, the leg is best suited), the health care worker should wipe the surface of the skin with an alcohol prep and then with a gauze pad soaked in deionized water. Tap water must not be used. Next, the area is wiped dry with a sterile gauze pad. Another 2-inch-square, eight-ply gauze pad is soaked in 0.07 moles/liter sodium bicarbonate and placed on the cleaned area. The negative electrode is placed on the gauze and taped securely to the skin. The electrode should not come into direct contact with the skin at any time when the current is on.

Another gauze square is soaked in 0.33 percent pilocarpine HCl and placed on the skin next to the sodium bicarbonate square but not touching it. The positive electrode should be placed on this piece of gauze and taped securely in place. Again, care should be taken that the electrode does not come into direct contact with the skin at any time during the procedure. Before the current is turned on, the area between and around the secured gauze squares should be wiped dry.

Next, the current is turned on and very slowly increased to 1 mA. The current must be incremented slowly because a sudden increase may electrically shock the patient. After 10 minutes, the current is decreased to zero. The switch is turned off, and the electrodes and gauze squares are removed and discarded. Reagent-grade water is used to wipe off the pilocarpine HCl area, which is then wiped dry.

A 2 × 2-inch square of thin waxed film, such as Parafilm, should be cut out and handled with clean forceps. Using the forceps, place the film against the cleaned area and taped securely onto the skin on adjacent sides. Still using the forceps, remove two gauze pads from a preweighed cup and place between the Parafilm and the skin. The remaining side can be taped securely. Tape may also be applied across the top of the Parafilm to prevent it from tearing. A timer set at 1 hour should be started. During that period, the procedure should be repeated on the other arm or leg.

After 1 hour, the tape should be carefully removed, and then the gauze sponges removed with forceps and returned to the original cup. The lid must be placed tightly on the cup, and the cup weighed again. After weighing, 200 ml of deionized water should be added to the cup. The lid should be replaced and wrapped securely with Parafilm. The gauze sponges should equilibrate 2 to 3 hours or overnight. The cups and a record of the weights measured during the procedure should be taken to the laboratory, where a clinical laboratory scientist will determine the chloride and calculate the results.

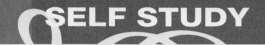

KEY TERMS

amniotic fluid

blood urea nitrogen (BUN)

cerebrospinal fluid (CSF)

clean-catch midstream

creatinine clearance test

culture and sensitivity (C&S)

gastric analysis

occult blood

ova and parasites (O&P)

pericardial fluid

peritoneal fluid

pleural fluid

random urine sample

skin test

sputum

sweat chloride test

synovial fluid

STUDY QUESTIONS

For the following, choose the one best answer.

1. What type of urine specimen is needed to detect an infection?
   a. random
   b. clean-catch
   c. routine
   d. 24-hour

2. Which of the following types of specimens is most frequently collected for analysis?
   a. amniotic fluid
   b. urine
   c. CSF
   d. pericardial fluid

3. Which of the following body fluids is extracted from joint cavities?
   a. pleural fluid
   b. peritoneal fluid
   c. synovial fluid
   d. pericardial fluid

4. The O&P analysis is requested on what type of specimen?
   a. CSF
   b. amniotic fluid
   c. fecal
   d. synovial fluid

5. Fetal abnormalities are detected through analysis of which fluid?
   a. pleural
   b. peritoneal
   c. amniotic
   d. CSF

6. The occult blood analysis is frequently requested on what type of specimen?
   a. CSF
   b. fecal
   c. throat culture
   d. seminal fluid

7. Ketosis is frequently detected with which of the following conditions?
   a. liver disease
   b. diabetes mellitus
   c. chemical poisoning
   d. infection

8. Which of the following body fluids is obtained from the abdominal cavity?

    a. synovial fluid   c. peritoneal fluid

    b. pericardial fluid   d. CSF

9. Which of the following can be used in children and infants to diagnose whooping cough?

    a. CSF culture   c. amniotic fluid culture

    b. nasopharyngeal culture   d. pericardial fluid culture

10. What is the specimen of choice for drug abuse testing?

    a. CSF   c. synovial fluid

    b. urine   d. gastric fluid

References

1. Garza, D: Urine collection and preservation. In Ross, DL, Neely, AE (eds), *Textbook of Urinalysis and Body Fluids.* New York: Appleton-Century-Crofts, 1983, p. 61.

2. Free, AH, Free, HM: *Urinalysis in Clinical Laboratory Practice.* Cleveland: CRC Press, 1975.

3. National Committee for Clinical Laboratory Standards (NCCLS): Urinalysis and Collection, Transportation, and Preservation of Urine Specimens, Approved Guideline, 2nd ed. NCCLS Document GP16-A2. Wayne, PA: NCCLS, 2001.

4. Guder, WG, Narayanan, S, Wisser, H, Zawta, B: *Samples: From the Patient to the Laboratory.* Darmstadt, Germany: Git Verlag Pub, 1996.

5. American College of Physicians: Suggested technique for fecal occult blood testing and interpretation in colorectal cancer screening. *Ann Intern Med* 1997; 126: 808.

6. Becan-McBride, K, Ross, D: *Essentials for the Small Laboratory and Physician's Office.* Chicago: Mosby-Year Book, 1988.

7. National Committee for Clinical Laboratory Standards (NCCLS): Sweat Testing: Sample Collection and Quantitative Analysis. NCCLS Document C34-A2. Wayne, PA: NCCLS, 2000.

8. Cystic Fibrosis Foundation: Clinical Practice Guidelines for Cystic Fibrosis. Bethesda, MD: April 2001, http://www.cff.org/living-withcf/sweat_testing.cfm.

Forensic Toxicology, Workplace Testing, Sports Medicine, and Related Areas

16

CHAPTER OBJECTIVES

Upon completion of Chapter 16, the learner is responsible for the following:

1. Define toxicology and forensic toxicology.
2. Give five examples of specimens that can be used for forensic analysis.
3. Describe the role of the health care worker, or "collector," in federal drug-testing programs.
4. Describe the function of a chain of custody, and of the Custody and Control Form.
5. Give examples of situations where drug testing might be valuable.
6. Describe how to detect adulteration of urine specimens.

 MediaLINK

Access the accompanying CD-ROM to explore a wide variety of review questions and interactive activities for this chapter, including multiple choice, true/false, and video exercises.

■■■■ OVERVIEW AND PREVALENCE OF DRUG USE

The use of illicit drugs (e.g., marijuana, cocaine, heroine, hallucinogens, inhalants, and the nonmedical use of prescription-type pain relievers, tranquilizers, stimulants, and sedatives) was monitored by a survey conducted by the Office of Applied Studies, Substance Abuse and Mental Health Services Administration (SAMHSA) in 2001. Approximately 15.9 million Americans (7.1 percent of the population age 12 or older) had used an illicit drug within the past month of the survey.[1] Box 16–1 describes additional facts about substance abuse. Alcohol is the most commonly used substance, and teenagers use alcohol and tobacco more than any other drugs; they are often referred to as "gateway drugs" because substance abuse problems tend to begin with alcohol and cigarettes. Among clients at adolescent substance abuse treatment facilities, 73 percent were treated for both alcohol and drug abuse problems, while 8 percent were treated for alcohol abuse alone.[2]

The development of modern collection devices, screening techniques, clinical laboratory automation, molecular advances, and computer technology have increased the variety of laboratory testing options available for the diagnosis and treatment of drugs of abuse and analysis of specimens in remote locations or from crime scenes. The following sections will provide basic guidelines and resources for further information.

Box 16–1   Facts about Substance Abuse

- Marijuana is the most commonly used illicit drug (used by 76 percent of the current illicit drug users)
- The states with the highest rates of illicit drug use for ages over 12 were Massachusetts, Vermont, Maine, Rhode Island, and New Hampshire. Utah and Idaho had the lowest rates.
- In 2002 about 11 million people aged 12 or older reported driving under the influence of illegal drugs, i.e., "drugged driving," during the past year. This represents 31 percent of the illicit drug users.
- 21 year olds were more likely than any other age group to drive under the influence of illegal drugs.
- Among adults aged 26 to 49, those who were unemployed were more likely than full- or part-time workers to report driving under the influence of illegal drugs.
- Related to workplace substance abuse and violence, in 1990 more than 1 million arrests were made for drug offenses (selling, manufacturing, or possession) and more than 3 million for alcohol offenses (driving under the influence (DUI), liquor law violations, drunkenness, or disorderly conduct).
- At least half of individuals arrested for major crimes including homicide, theft, and assault were under the influence of illicit drugs around the time of their arrest.
- Drug- and alcohol-related problems are among the top reasons for the rise in workplace violence.
- In 1997 drug abuse cost corporate America $85 billion; over 6 million employees were threatened in the workplace; and drugs accounted for up to 80 percent of losses due to theft in the workplace.
- One out of 4 substance abusers in treatment admitted stealing from their employer.
- The leading cause of death among people between 15 and 24 years of age is violence, including accidents, homicides, and suicides. Often these deaths are attributed to the use of drugs and alcohol.
- Among pregnant women approximately 25 percent use nicotine, and 5 to 8 percent are at risk for alcohol-related prenatal problems.
- It is estimated that 500,000 to 750,000 newborns are exposed to illicit drugs annually.
- Approximately 11 percent of women in a 36-hospital study had taken illicit drugs during pregnancy.[1,2,3,4,5,6]

The health care worker who is responsible for collecting the specimen plays a key role in ensuring the integrity of the specimen, especially in federal workplace drug-testing programs. The major responsibilities for the specimen collector include:

- Identification of both the donor and the specimen
- Prevention of specimen adulteration or substitution
- Tamper-proofing the collected specimen
- Initiation and accountability for the chain-of-custody
- Accurate and comprehensive documentation

████ FORENSIC TOXICOLOGY SPECIMENS

Toxicology is the scientific study of poisons (including drugs), how they are detected, their actions in the human body, and the treatment of the conditions they produce. Forensic specimens are those involved in civil or criminal legal cases. Forensic toxicology usually involves testing specimens for drugs of abuse in legal cases.

In toxicologic analysis, very small amounts of analytes are usually found in the blood, urine, or other specimens obtained for analysis. Thus, the type of specimen (e.g., venous blood, arterial blood, urine, hair, meconium), materials, and equipment used for collecting specimens for toxicologic analysis can greatly affect analytic results. The type of glass or plastic composing the collection tube, cover, or both may contain materials that will contaminate and/or react with or absorb the analytes. Even oils or bacteria from dirty fingers that handle specimens may cause contamination. Thus, for toxicologic specimens, the health care worker must strictly adhere to the facility's laboratory guidelines for collection of these types of specimens.

Extensive training, experience, and supervision are required for collecting specimens for forensic analyses. Box 16–2 includes types of specimens that may be used for forensic toxicology studies or other medical applications of a criminal investigation.

Box 16–2   Forensic Specimens

Specimens that may be used in forensic analyses:

- Anorectal swabs
- Arterial blood
- Bones
- Capillary blood
- Clothing
- Dried blood stains
- Hair
- Nails: nail scrapings or clippings
- Saliva
- Skin
- Sperm: semen residue
- Sweat
- Teeth: oral swabs
- Urine
- Venous blood
- Vaginal swabs[8,9,10,11]

Forensic laboratory analysis is completely different from other types of laboratory analyses in the following ways:[7,9]

- Specimens are very diverse, ranging from vaginal swabs in rape cases to contact lenses found on a sofa at a crime scene.
- Specimens may be exposed to the elements (rain, mud, mixed blood from multiple individuals).
- Specimens may be available in only trace amounts (a single hair or one smudge of blood).
- Forensic scientists must perform analyses in all types of environments, and their results must be able to stand up to the most intense judicial scrutiny.

Crime laboratories are involved in analyzing trace evidence (evidence found at the scene of the crime or on a person—fingerprints, shoe impressions, hairs, fibers, paint chips, glass fragments, soil samples); firearms and toolmarks (to analyze bullets and tool markings); drug chemistry (identification of drugs); toxicology (carbon monoxide, poisonings, drugs); arson and fire debris; biology and serology (semen stains, vaginal swabs from sexual assaults, crime scene specimens, DNA analysis); documents (paper, ink, type of printing, gum marks, etc.); and computers.[7]

DNA testing has become particularly helpful because of its accuracy in identification. Many highly publicized trials hinge on the outcome of DNA testing, and recently there have been reports of inmates released because of a wrongful conviction proven by DNA testing. In sexual assault cases, only 20 percent to 45 percent of the victims show signs of bodily injuries; therefore, laboratory evidence is vital to support the victim's claims. In general, DNA analysis is useful for the following reasons:[8,9]

- It is the same in all cells of the body (except eggs and sperm cells, which contain one-half of the DNA).
- It stays the same throughout life.
- It is present in all cells.
- It differs from one person to another except in the case of identical twins.

All specimens must be labeled using permanent markers with the victim's name, sample, site, and if possible an identification number for reference. The evidence must pass directly from the medical examiner to the individuals who will process specimens, using a chain-of-custody signature procedure. This provides a complete documentation system of all individuals who handle the specimen.

■■■■■ CHAIN OF CUSTODY

The chain of custody is a process for maintaining control of and accountability for each specimen from the time it is collected to the time of disposal. This process documents the identity of each individual that handles the specimen and each time a specimen is transferred in the chain. A chain-of-custody form is also required, which indicates specific identification of the patient or subject, the individual who obtained and processed the specimen, the date, the location, and the signature of the subject documenting that the specimen in the container is the one that was obtained from the person identified on the label. The specimen must be placed in a specimen transfer bag that is permanently sealed until it is opened for analysis. The seal ensures the "tamper-evident" transfer of contents until they reach their destination for analysis.[10]

FEDERAL WORKPLACE DRUG TESTING

Workplace drug-testing programs initially began when the Department of Health and Human Services (HHS) established guidelines for federal drug-testing programs, as well as standards for certification of laboratories engaged in urine drug testing for federal agencies such as the U.S. Department of Transportation (DOT), Department of Defense (DOD), Nuclear Regulatory Commission (NRC), and the Department of Energy (DOE). The standards relate to testing of specimens, quality assurance and quality control, the chain-of-custody form called the Custody and Control Form (CCF), personnel, and results reporting. Box 16–3, "Facts about Drug Testing in the Workplace," summarizes the rationale and procedures associated with drug-testing programs in the workplace.

Table 16–1 indicates the classes of drugs that are tested and the DHHS cut-off levels. These levels developed by the Department of Health and Human Services determine

---

Box 16–3   Facts About Drug Testing in the Workplace

- Workplace drug-testing programs are used for one or more of the following reasons:
  - To comply with federal regulations (DOT, DOD, NRC, DOE)
  - To comply with customer or contract requirements and insurance carrier requirements
  - To minimize the chances of hiring employees who are drug users/abusers
  - To reinforce the policy of "no drug use"
  - To identify users and refer them for assistance
  - To establish reasons for disciplinary actions
  - To improve safety, improve the health of employees, and reduce addiction
- Situations where drug testing is appropriate or necessary include:
  - **Preemployment testing**—Job offers made only after a negative drug test
  - **Prepromotion tests**—Employees testing prior to getting a promotion
  - **Annual physical tests**—To identify users/abusers so they can be referred for assistance and/or disciplinary action
  - **Reasonable suspicion/for-cause tests**—For employees who show signs of being impaired or have documented patterns of unsafe work practices
  - **Random tests**—Commonly used in safety- or security-sensitive jobs, involves testing at unpredictable times
  - **Postaccident tests**—Used to determine if drugs or alcohol were a factor in an employee being involved in an incident and/or accident
  - **Treatment follow-up or clearance to return to work**—Periodic testing for employees after participating in a rehabilitation program
- The consequences of testing positive involve the following:
  - Employers with workplace testing programs have guidelines in place that should explain procedures for what actions are taken after a positive test (paid or unpaid leave, referral to an employee assistance program, automatic discharge, disciplinary actions, and/or appeals procedures)
- Testing procedures:
  - Institutional procedures for drug testing are normally a part of the workplace drug-testing program.
  - Information may include where samples will be collected and tested, how results will be reported, the chain of custody, the drugs and cut-off levels used to determine if a test is positive or negative, and the confirmatory tests used if the initial test is positive.
  - The time to detect drugs is dependent on metabolic rate, dose of the drug, how it was taken, and the cut-off concentrations used by each laboratory. Generally drugs are detectable for several days.
  - Employees should be aware of the procedures.[12]

TABLE 16–1. Department of Health and Human Services Drugs and Cut-Off Levels

	CUT-OFF LEVELS INITIAL TESTS (NG/ML)	CUT-OFF LEVELS CONFIRMATORY TESTS (NG/ML)
Cocaine	300	150
Phencyclidine	25	25
Opiates	300	300
Amphetamines	1000	500
Cannabinoids	100	15

whether a test is positive or negative and have been proven accurate, reliable, and defensible in court.[12] These types of laboratory tests are considered "qualitative" because they detect presence or absence of the drug at a pre-determined cut-off level. Whereas "quantitative" tests determine the actual measurement or concentration of the substance being tested.

The Substance Abuse and Mental Health Services Administration (SAMHSA) has published a useful handbook for urine collection procedures in federal workplace drug-testing programs.[10] It provides guidance to health care workers responsible for collecting urine specimens for these programs.

The "collector" is the key to the success of a drug-testing program and is the one individual with whom all donors will have direct, face-to-face contact. "A collector is a trained individual who instructs and assists a donor at a collection site, receives and makes an initial

---

Box 16–4   Guidelines for Federal Drug Testing Custody and Control Form

The Office of Management and Budget (OMB) approved Federal Drug Testing Custody and Control Form (CCF; see Figure 16–1) must be used to document handling and storage of specimens from the time a donor gives the specimen to the collector to the final disposition of the specimen. The CCF is depicted below; it is a five part form and is usually obtained from the laboratory performing the testing. The CCF (OMB No. 0930-0158) is available on the SAMHSA Web site (www.health.org/workpl.htm), and collectors must be familiar with following the federal guidelines including:

1. Identification processes—including names, identifications, and contact information of the employer, the Medical Review Officer (MRO), and the donor, the reason for the test (e.g., random, pre-employment), and tests to be performed.

2. Giving the donor instructions about specimen collection and handling—including sealing the specimen after recording the temperature of the specimen as "acceptable" or "unacceptable," whether it is a split or single specimen, whether it was an "observed" collection and why, and if no collection was obtained and why (e.g., unable to urinate, or "shy bladder," etc).

3. Monitoring and documenting all circumstances that might indicate adulteration or substitution of the specimen.

4. Assuring that all 5 copies of the CCF go to the correct destinations (Laboratory copy, Medical Review Officer copy, Collector copy, Employer copy, and Donor copy).

inspection of the urine specimen provided by a donor, and initiates and completes the Federal Drug Testing Custody and Control Form (CCF)."[10] If the collector does not ensure the integrity of the specimen and adhere to the collection process, the specimen may not be considered a valid piece of evidence. If a specimen is reported positive for a drug or metabolite, the entire collection process must be able to withstand the closest scrutiny and all challenges to its integrity.[10] Figure 16–1 ■ indicates the format of the CCF.

▮▮▮▮▮ TAMPERING WITH SPECIMENS

Drug users have become very imaginative in ways to avoid a positive drug test result. Adulteration is a means of tampering with the specimen, usually urine, to make the specimen test negatively for drugs. It occurs in two ways: when substances are ingested by the patient to alter his/her own urine, and when substances are added or substituted for urine at the time of collection. Water is the most common substance added to the specimen or ingested to dilute the urine so that the drug concentrations are below the detection limit. Other substances that have been added to urine are liquid soap, bleach, salt, ammonia, vinegar, baking soda, UrinAid (glutaraldehyde), Klear (potassium nitrite), lemon juice, cologne, and other fluids.[13]

Detecting and deterring adulterants in urine can occur by:

- Sensory examination (odor and color) of the urine—For example bleach odor, foaming, or turbidity can be a sign of a liquid soap additive.
- Taking urine temperature—Temperature should be taken within 4 minutes after the donor provides the specimen. The acceptable temperature range is 32 to 38 degrees centigrade. Urine samples for drug testing contain a temperature strip affixed to the container.
- Simple tests such as specific gravity (it should not be less than 1.003 or greater than 1.025), and urine creatinine (less than 20 mg/dl) and electrolytes (to determine values outside the physiologic range). Klear can be detected as a strong positive nitrite in a urine specimen with no bacteria present.
- Working with the Substance Abuse and Mental Health Services Administration (SAMHSA) to seal off the water supply in the collection area, adding bluing to the toilet water, and preventing the patient from taking unneeded items into the collection stall.

If tampering is suspected or observed, the health care worker may conduct another collection procedure under "direct observation." Federal guidelines are very strict about the circumstances for this measure; however, there are situations when it is required.[10]

▮▮▮▮▮ DRUG TESTING IN THE PRIVATE SECTOR

Many private-sector employers, including hospitals and clinics, also choose to have workplace drug testing procedures in place, and the testing guidelines may vary slightly from the federal standards. However, private industries often elect to use laboratories that comply with the federal standards, so for purposes of this review the federal guidelines are discussed. Employees may be tested without prior notice; therefore, the collection procedure, processing, analysis, and reporting are very strict and well defined. Also, private employers may request that the certified laboratory test for several drugs or drug classes other than

Figure 16–1. Federal Drug Testing Custody and Control Form[10]

FEDERAL DRUG TESTING CUSTODY AND CONTROL FORM

SPECIMEN ID NO.   **1234567**   LAB ACCESSION NO.

OMB No. 0930-0158

STEP 1: COMPLETED BY COLLECTOR OR EMPLOYER REPRESENTATIVE

A. Employer Name, Address, I.D. No.   B. MRO Name, Address, Phone and Fax No.

C. Donor SSN or Employee I.D. No. _____

D. Reason for Test: ☐ Pre-employment ☐ Random ☐ Reasonable Suspicion/Cause ☐ Post Accident
                     ☐ Return to Duty ☐ Follow-up ☐ Other (specify)_____

E. Drug Tests to be Performed: ☐ THC, COC, PCP, OPI, AMP   ☐ THC & COC Only   ☐ Other (specify)_____

F. Collection Site Address:

Collector Phone No. _____

Collector Fax No. _____

STEP 2: COMPLETED BY COLLECTOR

| Read specimen temperature within 4 minutes. Is temperature between 90° and 100° F? ☐ Yes ☐ No, Enter Remark | Specimen Collection: ☐ Split ☐ Single ☐ None Provided (Enter Remark) ☐ Observed (Enter Remark) |

REMARKS

PRESS HARD - YOU ARE MAKING MULTIPLE COPIES

STEP 3: Collector affixes bottle seal(s) to bottle(s). Collector dates seal(s). Donor initials seal(s). Donor completes STEP 5 on Copy 2 (MRO Copy)

STEP 4: CHAIN OF CUSTODY - INITIATED BY COLLECTOR AND COMPLETED BY LABORATORY

I certify that the specimen given to me by the donor identified in the certification section on Copy 2 of this form was collected, labeled, sealed and released to the Delivery Service noted in accordance with applicable Federal requirements.

X _____   AM / PM

Signature of Collector   Time of Collection

_____   / /

(PRINT) Collector's Name (First, MI, Last)   Date (Mo./Day/Yr.)

SPECIMEN BOTTLE(S) RELEASED TO:

_____
Name of Delivery Service Transferring Specimen to Lab

RECEIVED AT LAB:

X _____
Signature of Accessioner

_____   / /
(PRINT) Accessioner's Name (First, MI, Last)   Date (Mo./Day/Yr.)

Primary Specimen Bottle Seal Intact
☐ Yes
☐ No, Enter Remark Below

SPECIMEN BOTTLE(S) RELEASED TO:

STEP 5a: PRIMARY SPECIMEN TEST RESULTS - COMPLETED BY PRIMARY LABORATORY

☐ NEGATIVE   ☐ POSITIVE for: ☐ MARIJUANA METABOLITE ☐ CODEINE ☐ AMPHETAMINE ☐ ADULTERATED
  ☐ DILUTE   ☐ COCAINE METABOLITE ☐ MORPHINE ☐ METHAMPHETAMINE ☐ SUBSTITUTED
  ☐ REJECTED FOR TESTING ☐ PCP ☐ 6-ACETYLMORPHINE ☐ INVALID RESULT

REMARKS _____

TEST LAB (if different from above) _____

I certify that the specimen identified on this form was examined upon receipt, handled using chain of custody procedures, analyzed, and reported in accordance with applicable Federal requirements.

X _____   _____   / /
Signature of Certifying Scientist   (PRINT) Certifying Scientist's Name (First, MI, Last)   Date (Mo./Day/Yr.)

STEP 5b: SPLIT SPECIMEN TEST RESULTS - (IF TESTED) COMPLETED BY SECONDARY LABORATORY

| Laboratory Name | ☐ RECONFIRMED ☐ FAILED TO RECONFIRM - REASON_____ |

I certify that the split specimen identified on this form was examined upon receipt, handled using chain of custody procedures, analyzed, and reported in accordance with applicable Federal requirements.

Laboratory Address

X _____   _____   / /
Signature of Certifying Scientist   (PRINT) Certifying Scientist's Name (First, MI, Last)   Date (Mo./Day/Yr.)

PEEL

1234567   A
SPECIMEN ID NO.

PLACE OVER CAP

1234567
SPECIMEN BOTTLE SEAL

/ /
Date (Mo. Day Yr.)

_____
Donor's Initials

PEEL

1234567   B (SPLIT)
SPECIMEN ID NO.

PLACE OVER CAP

1234567
SPECIMEN BOTTLE SEAL

/ /
Date (Mo. Day Yr.)

_____
Donor's Initials

COPY 1 - LABORATORY

Box 16–5	Blood Doping and Use of Erythropoietin (EPO)

The NCAA prohibits the practice of "blood doping," whereby whole blood, packed red blood cells, or blood substitutes are injected intravenously in athletes who try to increase their endurance by overloading their system with erythrocytes or drugs such as EPO. EPO increases the body's production of RBCs, thereby increasing the oxygen-carrying capacity. It can lead to performance advantages in endurance sports such as cycling. However, it has also been associated with cardiovascular problems, strokes, and deaths. While EPO is hard to detect, recent advances in blood and urine testing are becoming strong deterrents.[15,16,17]

those required by the federal agencies (Table 16–1), or they may use different testing levels for initial or confirmatory tests.

DRUG USE IN SPORTS

Using drugs and performance-enhancing substances in sports has become more prevalent and highly publicized in recent years. At many levels of competitive sports, including collegiate (e.g., National Collegiate Athletic Association [NCAA]) and professional (e.g., National Basketball Association [NBA], the National Football League [NFL], and the Olympics), drug use may be evident. The NCAA Drug-Testing Program tests more than 10,000 student athletes annually.

"The program involves urine collection on specific occasions and laboratory analyses for substances on a list of banned-drug classes developed by the NCAA Executive Committee. This list consists of substances generally purported to be performance enhancing and/or potentially harmful to the health and safety of the student-athlete." The drug classes are listed in the NCAA website and specifically include stimulants (such as amphetamines; caffeine or guarana if the urine concentration is greaterthan 15 micrograms/ml; ephedra; and cocaine), street drugs (such as heroin and marijuana), anabolic steroids, peptide hormones and analogues (such as human chorionic gonadotrophin, growth hormone, erythropoietin), and other drugs.[14]

PREFERRED SPECIMENS FOR DRUG TESTS

Even though blood is the best specimen for alcohol and EPO testing, urine remains the preferred specimen in sports drug testing for the following reasons:[16,17]

- Drugs and their metabolites are present in higher concentrations in urine than in blood
- Large specimen volumes are easily obtainable
- There is no pain or discomfort to the athlete when collecting the specimen
- The process of collection is noninvasive

As mentioned previously, the downside of using urine specimens for drug testing is that it is easily adulterated, or altered, by the donor. Urine drug detection times are also limited from about 12 hours to 2 or 3 weeks, with most drugs being undetectable in 2 to 5 days. Detection times for drugs in human hair are longer, ranging from weeks to months; however, detection is costly, and infrequent drug use will not likely be detected.

▮▮▮▮ BREATH TESTING FOR ALCOHOL

Breath is a useful specimen when alcohol use/abuse is suspected. Breath tests for alcohol are used instead of blood alcohol levels in situations outside of health care facilities because the procedure does not require trained laboratory staff; the sample collection is noninvasive (unlike venipuncture); the analysis is fast; results are quickly available and easy to read; and the procedure is less costly. There are numerous noninvasive evidential breath testing (EBT) devices on the market. These devices are often used in emergency departments and law enforcement agencies because officers can carry the portable breath analyzers in their patrol cars. Along with field sobriety tests, breath results may be used as legal evidence in Driving While Intoxicated/Impaired (DWI) or Driving Under the Influence (DUI) cases. The Food and Drug Administration has also approved a saliva test for monitoring alcohol use.[12,18]

▮▮▮▮ COLLECTING BLOOD SPECIMENS FOR ALCOHOL LEVELS

Many states have provisions under which drivers suspected of being intoxicated must consent to the performance of certain laboratory assays to determine the level of blood alcohol. In some states, this statute applies only to the testing of urine and breath samples. Therefore, it is advisable to determine the medically acceptable manner for obtaining blood specimens from patients in each state. If blood alcohol specimens are collected by

---

Box 16–6   Alcohol and Drunk Driving

Alcohol-related motor vehicle crashes:

- kill someone every 30 minutes
- killed 17,448 individuals in 2001 in the U.S., representing 41 percent of all traffic-related deaths
- caused the arrest of approximately 1.5 million drivers in 2000 for driving under the influence of alcohol or narcotics
- cost more than $51 billion in 2000[18,19,20,21,22]

Alcohol intoxication is defined by the blood alcohol concentration (BAC), expressed as grams per deciliter. Since alcohol is unchanged as it goes through the bloodstream, when it gets to the lungs it is exhaled and can be measured on the breath. The legal limit now adopted by most states is 0.08 (0.08 grams of alcohol per 100 ml of blood, or 0.08 percent), even though the federal definition is a level of 0.1 percent. Each person's response to alcohol is different; generally, when the blood alcohol percentage reaches .02 to .03 percent one may feel "high"; when it reaches .05 to .10 percent one generally has reduced muscular coordination, a longer reaction time, and impaired judgment; when it reaches 0.4 percent the average person becomes unconscious; and reduced breathing and heart rate or even death may occur if the level is above 0.5 percent. A 160-pound man will have a BAC of about 0.04 percentage one hour after consuming two 12-ounce beers or two standard drinks on an empty stomach. Drunk driving becomes very hazardous due to impaired functions such as eye movement, glare resistance, visual perception, reaction time, steering tasks, and information processing.

There are several types of breath alcohol testing devices based on different principles; however, they all have a mouthpiece, a tube through which the subject blows air, and a sample chamber for analysis. The test can be performed after waiting at least 15 minutes after the last drink and at least 1 minute after smoking. Results are read from an electronic or manual meter.

venipuncture, all procedures are similar to routine collections except that the phlebotomist must use a nonalcoholic disinfectant to cleanse the site. If an alcohol wipe is used to cleanse the site it may interfere with test results. Correct identifications, precautions, and labeling procedures apply to these situations as well. The National Committee for Clinical Laboratory Standards (NCCLS) published *Blood Alcohol Testing in the Clinical Laboratory: Approved Guideline,* which provides technical and administrative guidance on laboratory procedures associated with blood alcohol testing, including specimen collection, analytic methods, quality assurance, and result reporting.[23]

NEONATAL DRUG TESTING

There are many health problems associated with neonatal drug exposure, including premature birth, low birth weight, impaired neurological functioning, and a higher risk of abuse and neglect.[6] Neonatal drug exposure is determined by using the maternal history, newborn clinical symptoms, and laboratory toxicology testing of the mother and infant. Cocaine is the drug most often identified in neonatal drug testing. Other drugs that are detected are opiates (including heroin, morphine, codeine, and other narcotics such as hydromorphone and hydrocodone), amphetamine and methamphetamines, and phencyclidine (PCP).

Urine is the specimen most often used for neonatal drug exposure. Collection is possible by using neonatal urine collection bags and collecting the urine during the first 24 hours after birth. If the infant's urine is positive, it generally means that the mother used drugs 24 to 72 hours prior to childbirth. Meconium, the first intestinal discharge of a neonate, is greenish and consists of epithelial cells, mucus, and bile. Meconium is also used for drug analysis; the specimen is easier to collect than urine. Since meconium accumulates in the fetal bowel at approximately 16 weeks of gestation, a positive result indicates drug exposure to the neonate months before the birth. Other specimens used are amniotic fluids, cord blood, and gastric fluid; however, they are less suitable due to poor recovery of drugs from these samples.[6]

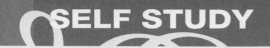

KEY TERMS

adulteration

chain-of-custody

Custody and Control Form (CCF)

Department of Health and Human Services (HHS)

erythropoietin (EPO)

forensic specimens

"gateway drugs"

illicit drugs

meconium

qualitative tests

quantitative tests

toxicology

trace evidence

STUDY QUESTIONS

The following questions may have more than one answer.

1. Substance abuse in the workplace accounts for which of the following?
   a. theft
   b. cancer
   c. assault and violence
   d. costly losses

2. Specimens that can be used in forensic analysis include:
   a. hair
   b. urine
   c. blood
   d. nails

3. "Gateway drugs" include:
   a. alcohol
   b. tobacco
   c. heroin
   d. cocaine

4. Forensic specimens are those involved in which of the following?
   a. routine testing for diabetes
   b. legal cases/criminal investigations
   c. urine screening for preemployment physicals
   d. Pap smears

5. What is the purpose of a chain-of-custody process?
   a. maintain control of the donor who gives the specimen
   b. account for a specimen from point of collection to final disposition
   c. specimen identification
   d. provide privacy to the donor

6. Urine specimen containers used in the federal workplace testing usually have which of the following?
   a. tamper-evident seals
   b. temperature strips
   c. aliquot identification
   d. confidentiality notices

7. Which of the following agencies/organizations are likely to have workplace drug testing programs?
   a. NFL
   b. college baseball teams
   c. airline security guards
   d. international chemical company

8. Workplace drug-testing programs are useful to employers for which of the following reasons:
   a. decrease the chance of hiring a drug user/abuser
   b. provides for a means to investigate accidents/incidents
   c. protects safety and well being of employees
   d. provides rehabilitation

9. Skin preparation for blood alcohol levels must be cleansed with which of the following?
   a. 70 percent ethyl alcohol
   b. iodine
   c. 70 percent isopropyl alcohol
   d. nonalcoholic disinfectants

10. Breath analysis for alcohol is used most often by which health care group:
    a. hospital laboratories
    b. postal workers
    c. fire fighters
    d. law enforcement officers

References

1. Office of Applied Studies, Substance Abuse and Mental Health Services Administration (SAMHSA): National Survey on Drug Abuse, 2001 State Estimates of Substance Use, www.samhsa.gov/oas/nhsda/2k1State/vol1/ch2.htm, accessed November 9, 2003.

2. Office of Applied Studies, Substance Abuse and Mental Health Services Administration (SAMHSA): National Survey of Substance Abuse Treatment Services, 2002, www.samhsa.gov/oas/2k3/YouthFacilities/YouthFacilities.cfm, accessed November 9, 2003.

3. National Institute on Drug Abuse (NIDA): Diagnosis and Treatment of Drug Abuse in Family Practice—Epidemiology, http://165.112.78.61/DiagnosisTreatment/Diagnosis3html, December 1997.

4. Office of Applied Studies, Substance Abuse and Mental Health Services Administration (SAMHSA): National Survey on Drug Use and Health, Drugged Driving, 2002 Update, www.samhsa.gov/oas/2k3/DrugDriving/DrugDriving.cfm, accessed November 9, 2003.

5. Substance Abuse and Mental Health Services Administration (SAMHSA): Workplace Substance Abuse, Related Violence and Security Issues, www.drugfreeworkplace.gov/WPResearch?WPViolence?WPSecurity.html, accessed November 9, 2003.

6. Soo, VA: Neonatal drug testing. *Adv Med Lab Professional,* July 3, 2000: 19–23.

7. Weedn, VW: Elementary, my dear Watson: Technological advances will fuel laboratory-based forensic science into the next millennium. *Adv Med Lab Personnel,* February 8, 1999; 8–11.

8. Weedn, VW, Rogers, GS, Henry, BE: DNA testing in the forensic laboratory. *Lab Med.,* 1998; 29(8): 484–489.

9. Collins, KA: The laboratory's role in detecting sexual assault. *Lab Med.,* 1998; 29(6): 361–365.

10. Substance Abuse and Mental Health Services Administration (SAMHSA): Urine Specimen Collection Handbook for the New Federal Drug Testing Custody and Control Form, US Department of Health and Human Services, www.drugfreeworkplace.gov/DrugTesting/SpecimenCollection/UrnSpcmnHndbk.html, accessed November 9, 2003. OMB No. 0930-0158; exp. date: June 30, 2003.

11. Massey, LD: Federal workplace drug testing, where urine specimen collection has a whole new meaning. *Adv Med Lab Professional,* September 25, 2000: 14–19.

12. Substance Abuse and Mental Health Services Administration (SAMHSA): Employer Tip Sheet, US Department of Health and Human Services, http://ncadi.samhsa.gov/, accessed on November 12, 2003.

13. Dufour, DR: Drugs-of-abuse testing adulteration. *Med Lab Observ,* April, 1999: 10.

14. National Collegiate Athletic Association (NCAA): NCAA Drug-Testing Program, www.ncaa.org/library/sports_sciences/drug_testing_program/2002-03/, accessed on November 9, 2003.

15. Briefings: Industry. *Lab Med.,* 2001; 32(2): 60.

16. Thomas, C, Olander, R: Keeping collegiate sports drug use in check. *Adv Med Lab Professional,* October 9, 2000: 30–32.

17. Fuller, DC, Orsulak, PJ: The broader view of drug testing. *Adv Lab Professional,* April 10, 2000: 8–12.

18. National Institute on Alcohol Abuse and Alcholism (NIAAA): Alcohol alert, No 31 PH 362, January 1996, www.niaaa.nih.gov/publications/aa31.htm, accessed November 10, 2003.

19. Intoximeters Incorporated: About Alcohol Testing, www.intox.com/about_alcohol_testing.asp, accessed November 10, 2003.

20. Medical Encyclopedia, U.S. National Library of Medicine: Breath Alcohol Test www.nlm.nih.gov/medlineplus/ency/imagepages/9134.htm, last updated October 8, 2003; accessed November 10, 2003.

21. Freudenrich, CC: How Breathalyzers Work, in How Stuff Works, http://science.howstuffworks.com/breathalyzer.htm/, accessed November 10, 2003.

22. Centers for Disease Control and Prevention (CDC), National Center for Injury Prevention and Control: Impaired Driving, www.cdc.gov/ncipc/factsheets/drving.htm, last reviewed November 6, 2003, accessed November 10, 2003.

23. National Committee for Clinical Laboratory Standards (NCCLS): Blood Alcohol Testing in the Clinical Laboratory: Approved Guideline, T-DM6-A. (940 West Valley Road, Ste. 1400, Wayne, PA 19087-1898, (610) 688-1100): NCCLS, 1997.

Home Care Collections

Mr. Albert A. Thomson, a 55-year-old white man, was released from Nicholson Community Hospital on March 25. He had been in the hospital for 14 days as a result of undergoing cardiac bypass surgery and experiencing some complications. On March 29, Ms. Terry Alright, a home health care phlebotomist from Nicholson Community Hospital, saw that her schedule included a visit to Mr. Thomson for blood collection for the following laboratory tests:

- Chemistry screen
- Protime
- CBC
- APTT
- Calcium, ionized

When she arrived at Mr. Thomson's home and began her preparations for blood collection, she noticed that Mr. Thomson had hematomas in both antecubital fossa areas of the left and right arms. Thus, she checked the right hand and found a vein that looked suitable for collecting blood with a safety winged infusion set with small blood collection vacuum tubes. She prepared the site for blood collection, and using a 23-gauge safety winged infusion needle, she inserted the needle into the vein and first collected blood in a red-speckled-topped vacuum tube, followed by a purple-topped tube, two light blue–topped tubes, and then a green-topped tube. As she collected each tube, she mixed the blood and additive in the blood collection tube. After completing the blood collection, she labeled the tubes, discarded the biohazardous blood collection items in her biohazardous disposal container, and left Mr. Thomson's home with the collected blood and her blood collection items.

She traveled next to Ms. Jennifer Smith's home to collect blood from Ms. Smith for a digoxin assay and a plasma potassium level determination. Ms. Smith, an 85-year-old African American woman, was homebound because of arthritis and a cardiac arrhythmia problem. Collecting blood from the median cubital vein in Ms. Smith's left arm, the phlebotomist used a regular evacuated tube system (needle attached to the barrel). Ms. Alright drew 2 mL of blood in a small red-speckled-topped blood collection tube and 3 mL of blood in a small purple-topped blood collection tube. She labeled the tubes, discarded the biohazard blood collection items, and left Ms. Smith's house to travel to the hospital laboratory and drop off the blood specimens.

Questions

1. For each of the following laboratory tests, what color should the top of the blood collection tube be?

PHLEBOTOMY CASE STUDIES

Laboratory Assay	Color of Blood Collection Tube Top
Calcium, ionized	_____
APTT	_____
CBC count	_____
Protime	_____
Chemistry screen	_____
Digoxin	_____
Plasma potassium	_____

2. Did the home health care phlebotomist use the proper order of draw for Mr. Thomson's laboratory tests? If not, what was the proper order of draw?
3. Did the phlebotomist use the proper order of draw to fill tubes for Ms. Smith's laboratory tests? If not, what was the proper order of draw?

Bedside Glucose Testing

A 59-year-old Hispanic woman having non-insulin diabetes mellitus tested her glucose level at home on March 14, 2003, and obtained a glucose reading of 320 mg/dL using a test strip. Because she was having symptoms of sweating, feeling bad, and feeling lightheaded, the woman went to her physician the next day. Her physician immediately hospitalized her for treatment of uncontrolled diabetes. During the hospitalization, the following glucose meter v. clinical laboratory comparisons were performed:

Date	Glucose Meter Results (mg/dl)	Laboratory Test Results (mg/dl)
3/15/03	151	198
3/16/03	192	238
3/17/03 (a.m.)	96	267
3/17/03 (p.m.)	120	246

From product performance specifications, hospital personnel determined that the comparisons for March 15 and March 16 were within the acceptable product performance variation range. The last two comparisons, however, fell outside the acceptable range. The patient indicated that she followed the preventive maintenance schedule described in the documentation packaged with the glucose meter. The calibration was checked weekly, and the last calibrator reading, which was performed on March 17, was in range. A control run on March 16 resulted in a reading of 129 mg/dL, with confidence limits of 90 to 120 mg/dL.

Questions

1. What is the problem in this case study?
2. What troubleshooting technique(s) should have been implemented to resolve this problem?

Newborn Nursery Collections

Two health care workers oversee blood collections in the newborn nursery on Saturday and Sunday of each week. On Sunday morning, the clinical laboratory scientist (CLS) overseeing the clinical chemistry section noticed that the bilirubin value for Baby McPherson was as follows:

Day	Time	Bilirubin Value (mg/dL)
Friday		15
Saturday	8:15 p.m.	12
Sunday	7:10 a.m.	2

Knowing that the ultraviolet light on newborn Baby McPherson could not make the bilirubin value decrease that dramatically from Saturday to Sunday, the CLS called in the health care worker who had collected the Sunday morning blood sample to ask him questions regarding the collection.

Questions

1. What type of microcollection container should have been used to collect the bilirubin sample?
2. Does taking the blood immediately to the laboratory for testing make any difference?
3. Describe two preanalytical variables that could cause the Sunday bilirubin value for Baby McPherson was so different from the values of the previous 2 days.

Collecting Blood from an Infant

The phlebotomist, Sherry Wiggins, had to collect blood from the infants in the critical care unit of the children's hospital. For Infant Jim Jenkins, the requested laboratory tests were hemoglobin, potassium, and thyroxine. The hospital protocol for this infant's age was to collect blood by skin puncture from the heel.

Questions

1. What blood collection equipment was required for this infant's blood collection?
2. What was the proper "order of draw" for this microcollection?

Blood Donor Complications

The father of a hospitalized patient went to the blood donor room to give blood. He was slightly overweight. A phlebotomist who had only worked there 2 weeks was assigned to collect his blood. The phlebotomist was able to palpate a vein but when she stuck the needle in, she had to manipulate it slightly and go deeper to withdraw blood. As the blood entered the tub, she noticed that it was bright red and appeared to "pulse" into the tubing; she was very relieved to get the blood flowing. As the supervisor walked by, he immediately noticed the circumstance and halted the procedure.

Questions

1. Why did the supervisor halt the procedure?
2. What might have happened to the father who was trying to donate blood if the procedure had not been stopped?
3. What actions need to be taken with the phlebotomist?

Answers for all case study questions can be found in Appendix 12.

Appendix 1

FINDING A JOB

Finding a job that is a good fit for both the applicant and the employer is a time-consuming, often challenging process. However, the time and effort spent researching and applying for a position can have a wonderful payoff in terms of job satisfaction, salary, benefits, how pleasant the environment is, and how gratified one is with the work. The key to finding the right job is to spend time searching, be prepared with documentation and with questions during the interview, and keep an open mind. Here are some essential factors to think about. This list can actually be used as a checklist for your application process.

Places to Seek Employment	Newspaper, professional journals, and Internet
	Health care organizations
	Friends & relatives
	School faculty & advisors
	Bulletin boards
	Employment agencies
Contacting an Employer	Check empoyer's website
	Call for an appointment
	Send a cover letter (see example below)
	Send a resume (see example below)
	Complete a job application (provided by employer)
Cover Letter	Be neat and use correct spelling
	State where you heard about the job
	State the specific job for which you are applying
	State why you are qualified for this position
	Give brief summary of your education, experience, and qualifications
	Refer to your resume
	Request an interview
	Give your name, address, and phone number
Resume	List name, address, phone number(s), and e-mail address
	Career plans (1–3 goal statements of where you want to be in a few years)
	Education (high school & beyond)
	Work experience (part-time or full-time, dates, duration of employment)
	Volunteer activities (community service, religious activities, etc.)

	Interests (sports, music, art, hobbies)
	Special skills and abilities (computer skills with particular software, telephone expertise, use of special equipment, etc.)
	Reference names and contact information (always ask permission to use someone as a reference before listing them)
Interview	Be well groomed & do not chew gum
	Dress neatly & professionally
	Be on time or a few minutes early
	Greet the interviewer with your name & a smile
	Shake hands firmly
	Stand until you are asked to sit
	Answer questions truthfully & sincerely
	Prepare a few questions about the job
	Avoid discussing personal problems
	Be enthusiastic & maintain eye contact
	Do not criticize former employers/teachers
	Thank the interviewer for his/her time and leave promptly
After the Interview	Send a thank-you letter to the interviewer

Jane Doe
8200 West Jersey Avenue
Lubbock, Texas 79452
511-799-9990
jdoe@nnn.com

January 20, 2004

Ms. A. D. Jones
Director, Laboratory Services
Muncy Hospital
P.O. Box 22333
San Antonio, Texas 78277

Dear Ms. Jones,

I am responding to an advertisement in the San Antonio Press on January 5, 2004, for an entry-level phlebotomy technician. I graduated from Lamar High School in 1999. Since then I have worked part-time and been a part-time student at the community college. I recently completed a phlebotomy training program, and my goal is to utilize my skills while pursuing additional studies in laboratory sciences.

I have enclosed my resume, which includes a list of skills and experience. I feel that I am well qualified for this position because of my work with adults and children coupled with my organizational skills. I hope to arrange an interview as soon as is convenient for you. Please feel free to contact me at 511-799-9990 to schedule an interview or for additional information. Thank you.

Sincerely,

Jane Doe

Sample Cover Letter for Job Inquiry

Jane Doe
8200 West Jersey Avenue
Lubbock, Texas 79452
511-799-9990
jdoe@nnn.com

Career Plans	To become an experienced phlebotomist while continuing my education in laboratory sciences
Experience	1999–present Community college phlebotomy student and part-time library assistant; responsibilities include clerical duties (filing, answering multiple telephone lines, word processing), greeting customers, and providing assistance in locating reference materials.
	1998–1999 Part-time caretaker for 3 children; responsibilities included carpooling, providing after-school snacks, assistance with homework, monitoring activities.
	1996–1998 Part-time employee at ABC Grocery; responsibilities included assisting customers in locating products, restocking groceries, checking out grocery items at cash register, assisting with inventory.
Education	1999 Graduated from Lamar High School
Skills/Strengths	Excellent communication skills in Spanish Computer skills include proficiency with both MAC and PC word processing, Internet research, Excel, and Power-Point
Interests	Reading, Camping, Art, Church Youth Group, Girl Scouts
References	Available on request

Sample Resume

THE BASICS OF VITAL SIGNS

Vital signs are indicators of the body's functioning, using measures of temperature, pulse, and respiration rate (TPR) and blood pressure. The body is considered to be in homeostasis when vital signs are within normal limits; if vital signs are not within normal limits, it is an indication that there is a clinical problem. Health care workers often have responsibilities that involve measurement of vital signs. Accuracy in the measurement and recording of results is critical to proper treatment decisions for each patient.

TEMPERATURE

Temperature is a measure of body heat, and is influenced by factors that cause the body to *retain heat,* such as exercise, ingestion of food, exposure to hot temperatures, illness, infection, excitement, and anxiety, or to *lose heat,* such as sleep, fasting, exposure to cold, certain illnesses, decreased muscle activity, depression, and mouth breathing.

There are several types of thermometers (instrument used to measure temperature) available, including the following:

Glass thermometer—a hollow glass tube with calibration lines marking the outside; it is filled with mercury. Mercury is heat sensitive and rises up the hollow tube when exposed to the heat of the patient. The patient's temperature is then read when the mercury stops rising after several minutes. Glass thermometers are specially designed to take temperatures orally or rectally. Glass thermometers designed for taking oral temperature should not be used to take rectal temperature, and vice versa.

Aural thermometer—used primarily for babies and children, a sensor is placed in the ear to measure temperature. Can also be used if patient is having trouble breathing such that oral thermometer is uncomfortable.

Chemically treated or plastic thermometer—temperature is measured by a color change on a strip of treated paper/plastic. The treated strip is placed on the skin and disposed of after one use.

Electronic/digital thermometers—widely used thermometer that has a probe that can be covered with disposable protective shields after each use. Temperature is read easily and very quickly from a digital screen. Manufacturer's instructions should be closely followed. (see Procedure A2–1.)

There are four sites used to take body temperature:

Oral (by mouth)—the safest, most common, convenient and comfortable site to take temperature. Normal oral temperature is 98.6°F or 37°C. (See Procedure A2–1.)

Rectal (by insertion 1.5 inches into the rectum)—the most accurate temperature is from this site. This site is used when use of the mouth is difficult, for example when patients have trouble breathing, are weak or confused, are being given oxygen, or have paralysis of the face caused by stroke or accident. Normal rectal temperature is 99.6°F or 38°C.

Aural (ear canal)—also safe and accurate site for patients who are less than 6 years old, or have the same conditions listed for rectal temperatures. Normal aural temperature is 98.6°F or 37° C. (See Procedure A2–2.)

Axillary(in the armpit)—the axillary temperature is the *least* accurate and should only be used when other sites are not easily accessed due to clinical conditions. Normal axillary temperature is 97.6°F or 36.4°C. (See Procedure A2–3.)

PULSE

Pulse is the number of times the heart beats in 1 minute. It is a measure of how well the blood is circulating through the body and is done by placing fingers over an artery and squeezing gently against the bone. The pulsating feeling is actually pressure of the blood against the wall of the artery as the heart contracts and relaxes. Pulse or pressure points are indicated in Figure A2–4. The pulse rate should be the same at all pulse points. The most common site to count the pulse rate is at the radial artery near the wrist.

Average pulse rates are as follows:

Age	Rate per minute
Before birth	140–150
At birth	90–160
First year of life	115–130
Childhood	80–115
Adult	60–80

BLOOD PRESSURE

Blood pressure is the force of blood pushing against the walls of blood vessels and is measured and reported using two numbers, one for the systolic pressure and one for the diastolic pressure. *Systolic* blood pressure (SBP) is exerted when the heart is contracting and is the greatest force on the wall of the arteries. *Diastolic* blood pressure (DBP) is the least force exerted on the walls of the arteries as the heart relaxes between contractions. There are many factors that increase blood pressure, such as loss of elasticity, exercise, eating, stimulant drugs, and anxiety; and factors that decrease blood pressure, such as hemorrhage, inactivity, fasting, suppressant drugs, and depression.

Normal blood pressure is measured by an instrument called a sphygmomanometer, or blood pressure (BP) cuff. Values on the instruments relate to "millimeters of mercury" (mm Hg) in a tube at certain points. There are 3 types of sphygomomanometers: mercury (now almost obsolete due to the hazardous nature of mercury), aneroid (cloth-covered bladder that fills with air as the bulb is squeezed and inflated), and electronic/digital type. When taking blood pressure, one must do two important things simultaneously—listen to the heartbeat and watch the guage—to take a reading at precise moments. (See Procedure A2–5.)

SBP, the highest value, is reported first and the DBP, the lowest value, is reported second. The average normal adult reading of 120/80, is read as "120 over 80." Normal systolic pressure ranges between 90 and 140 mm Hg; and normal diastolic pressure ranges between 60 and 90 mm Hg. If the blood pressure is above normal range, it is called hypertension or high blood pressure; conversely, if it is below normal range, it is called hypotension or low blood pressure.[1] Refer to Table A2–1.

1. Always follow Standard Precautions prior to, during, and after the procedure.

2. Assemble equipment by placing plastic covers near the electronic thermometer (remember that blue probes are for oral and red for rectal). Note there are several types of thermometers commercially available.

3. Identify the patient and explain the procedure.

4. Place the plastic thermometer cover over the probe.

5. Insert probe under the tongue gently. Position the thermometer to the side of the lips (Figures A2-1a & b ■).

6. Hold in place for 15 seconds or until sound is emitted to indicate that the body temperature is displayed.

7. Read temperature (Figure A2-1c ■).

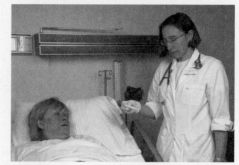

Figure A2–1c

8. Remove plastic cover and discard (Figure A2-1d ■).

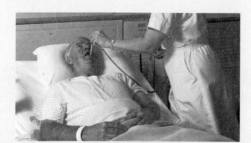

Figure A2–1a

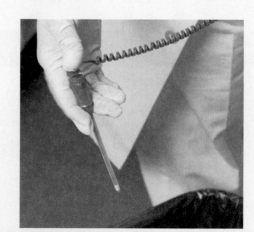

Figure A2–1d

9. Record temperature and, if elevated, report to appropriate personnel.

10. Position patient for comfort and thank him or her for cooperating.

11. Wash hands and return thermometer to storage place.

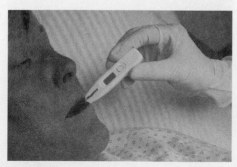

Figure A2–1b

Procedure A2-2 Taking Aural Temperature

1. The steps for taking aural temperature are essentially the same as for oral procedures.

2. The aural electronic thermometer is assembled using a disposable probe cover (Figure A2-2a ■).

3. Aural thermometer is inserted gently into the ear canal and held for 15 seconds or until a signal is emitted (Figure A2-2b ■). The temperature is then recorded and the plastic sheath removed and discarded.

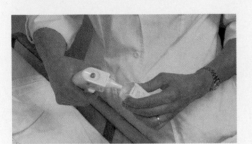

Figure A2–2a

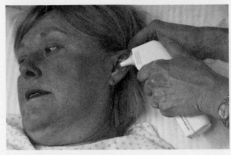

Figure A2–2b

Procedure A2-3 Taking Axillary Temperature

1. The steps for taking axillary temperature are similar to oral procedures, except the device may differ. Chemically treated strips can be used on the axillary site (Figure A2-3a ■).

2. Alternatively, digital or other models of thermometers can be used. Insert the

thermometer into the axilla (armpit) and keep it there for approximately 5 minutes (Figure A2-3b ■). Record the temperature and discard the plastic sheath.

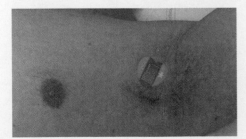

Figure A2–3a

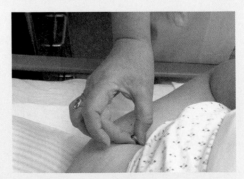

Figure A2–3b

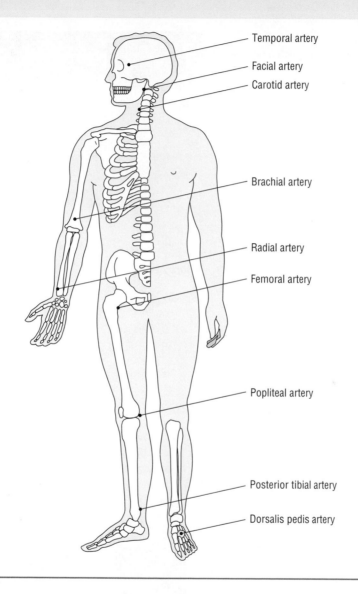

Figure A2–4. Pulse or Pressure Points

Temporal artery

Facial artery

Carotid artery

Brachial artery

Radial artery

Femoral artery

Popliteal artery

Posterior tibial artery

Dorsalis pedis artery

1. Wash hands.
2. Assemble equipment (watch with a second hand, pad, and pen).
3. Identify the patient and explain what you are going to do.
4. Place fingers on the patient's radial artery at the base of his/her thumb (or other pulse point) (Figure A2-5a ■). Do not use your own thumb to measure pulse.

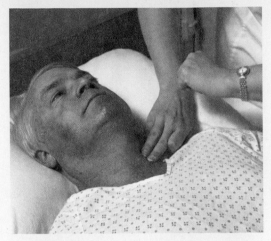

Figure A2–5b

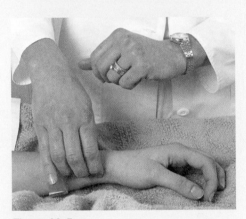

Figure A2–5a

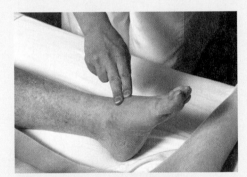

Figure A2–5c

5. Alternative sites include the carotid antery (neck), the dorsalis pedis or posterior tibial arteries (foot). (See Figures A2–5b-d ■.)
6. Count the number of pulsations that occur within one minute.
7. Record pulse rate immediately.
8. Wash hands and thank the patient for cooperating.
9. Record pulse rate on other necessary records.
10. Report any unusual observations or abnormal rates immediately.

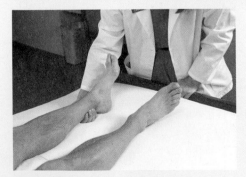

Figure A2–5d

1. Wash hands.
2. Blood pressure should be taken with a properly calibrated and validated instrument. Persons should be seated quietly for at least 5 minutes in a chair (rather than an exam table), with feet on the floor and arm supported at heart level.
3. Assemble equipment (alcohol wipes, sphygmomanometer, stethoscope, pad, pen). An appropriate size cuff (cuff bladder encircling at least 80% of the arm) should be used. (Figure A2–6a ■.)
4. Identify patient and explain what you are going to do. Plan to take at least 2 measurements.
5. Support the patient's arm on a firm surface.
6. Apply cuff correctly according to manufacturer instructions around the upper arm and over the brachial artery. Note there are various types available. Aneroid sphygmomanometers come in many sizes and are inflated with air as the bulb is squeezed and deflated as the valve is released. Mercury devices are older and are slowly being replaced (Figure A2-6b ■).
7. Clean earpieces on the stethoscope and place in ears.
8. Place the stethoscope over the artery distal to the cuff, then inflate the cuff until the

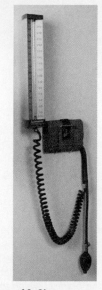

Figure A2–6b

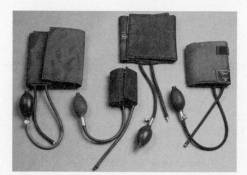

Figure A2–6a

(continued)

TABLE A2–1. Classification of Blood Pressure for Adults[2]

BP CLASSIFICATION	SBP (mm HG)	DBP (mm HG)
Normal	<120	and <80
Prehypertension	120–139	or 80–90
Stage 1 Hypertension	140–159	or 90–99
Stage 2 Hypertension	>160	or >100

pressure reads 170 mm. At this point, the brachial artery collapses, the flow of blood stops and the sound of the pulse disappears. (Figure A2-6c ■).

cuff and the other hand on the stethoscope diaphragm over the brachial artery. Keep eyes on the readings from the instrument (Figure A2-6d ■).

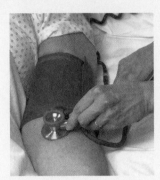

Figure A2–6c

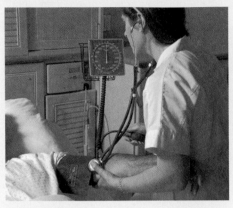

Figure A2–6d

9. Open the valve slowly to let the air out of the cuff. At first, blood enters only at peak systolic pressure and the stethoscope picks up the sound of blood pulsing through the artery. As air is removed from the cuff the sounds change because the artery is remaining more open. When the cuff pressure decreases to less than diastolic pressure, blood flow becomes continuous, and the sound of the pulse becomes muffled or disappears completely. *The SBP reading is the point at which the first of two or more sounds is heard, that is, the sound when the pulse appears corresponds to the peak systolic pressure (the first number reported). When the pulse fades, the pressure reading has reached diastolic level (DBP is the second number reported).* Keep one hand on the bulb to inflate/deflate the

10. Record readings on pad and repeat if possible.

11. Wash hands and thank the patient for his or her cooperation.

12. Wash earpieces on stethoscope, and put equipment away.

13. Record blood pressure on other necessary documents.

14. Report any abnormal results to the appropriate personnel.

Note: Blood pressure changes frequently and is an important vital sign. Health care workers must be accurate in their measurements and recording of results, and report any abnormalities immediately.

RESPIRATION RATE

Respiration rate is the measure of how many times one breathes in and out (inspiration and expiration, respectively) within one minute. It is usually taken at the same time or just after the pulse rate. Often a health care worker can count the pulse rate and the respiration rate while the temperature is being taken. The observation of the rise and fall of the patient's chest constitutes one respiration. The respirations can be counted for 1 minute. Factors that cause the respiration rate to increase are exercise, anxiety, respiratory diseases, medications, pain, and heart disease, conversely, factors that cause the rate to decrease are relaxation, depression, head injury, or medications. Normal adult rate is 14 to 18 respirations per minute. Any abnormalities such as difficulty breathing, irregular breathing, breathing that has stopped, or bubbling/rattling sounds during breathing should be reported.[2]

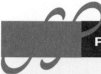

Procedure A2-6	Measuring Respiration Rate

1. While a patient's temperature is being taken, count the number of respirations in 1 minute (rise and fall of chest = 1 respiration).

2. Record the measurement and proceed with taking other vital signs.

REPORTING VITAL SIGNS

Temperature, pulse, and respiration (TPR) are most often reported in the same order. Blood pressure is the fourth vital sign and is usually reported in a designated spot on the patient's medical record/chart near the other vital signs. A common notation for TPR would be 98.6/73/15, meaning oral temperature of 98.6, a pulse rate of 73, and respiration rate of 15. Rectal temperatures are indicated by a R (in a circle), axillary temperatures by an AX next to the reading, and sometimes aural temperatures are indicated by a T next to the reading, e.g., 99.6R or 97.6AX or 98.6T.

Accurate reading and reporting of vital signs is an important function that all members of the health care team rely on. Abnormal results should be immediately reported.

References

1. Badasch, SA, and Chesebro, DS: Introduction to Health Occupations, *Today's Health Care Worker,* 5th ed. Upper Saddle River, NJ: Prentice Hall Health, 2000.
2. National Heart, Lung, and Blood Institute (NHLBI): The 7th Report of the Joint National Committee on Prevention, Detection, Evaluation, and Treatment of High Blood Pressure, NIH Publication No. 03-5233. Bethesda, MD: National Institutes of Health (NIH), May 2003. www.nhlbi.nih.gov.

Appendix 3

CDC GUIDELINE FOR HAND HYGIENE IN HEALTH-CARE SETTINGS

PART A: RECOMMENDATIONS TO IMPROVE HAND-HYGIENE PRACTICES

The following recommendations excerpted from the complete CDC report promote improved hand hygiene and hand antisepsis to reduce transmission of pathogens to patients and health care workers (HCWs). The complete guideline and report is available for free at www.cdc.gov.

CATEGORIES

These recommendations are designed to improve hand-hygiene practices of HCWs and to reduce transmission of pathogenic microorganisms to patients and personnel in health-care settings. This guideline and its recommendations are not intended for use in food processing or food-service establishments, and are not meant to replace guidance provided by FDA's Model Food Code.

As in previous CDC/HICPAC guidelines, each recommendation is categorized on the basis of existing scientific data, theoretical rationale, applicability, and economic impact. The CDC/HICPAC system for categorizing recommendations is as follows:

Category IA. Strongly recommended for implementation and strongly supported by well-designed experimental, clinical, or epidemiologic studies.

Category IB. Strongly recommended for implementation and supported by certain experimental, clinical, or epidemiologic studies and a strong theoretical rationale.

Category IC. Required for implementation, as mandated by federal or state regulation or standard.

Category II. Suggested for implementation and supported by suggestive clinical or epidemiologic studies or a theoretical rationale.

No recommendation. Unresolved issue. Practices for which insufficient evidence or no consensus regarding efficacy exist.

RECOMMENDATIONS

1. Indications for handwashing and hand antisepsis
   a. When hands are visibly dirty or contaminated with proteinaceous material or are visibly soiled with blood or other body fluids, wash hands with either a non-antimicrobial soap and water or an antimicrobial soap and water (IA).
   b. If hands are not visibly soiled, use an alcohol-based hand rub for routinely decontaminating hands in all other clinical situations described in items 1c–j (IA). Alternatively, wash hands with an antimicrobial soap and water in all clinical situations described in items 1c–j (IB).

c. Decontaminate hands before having direct contact with patients (IB)

d. Decontaminate hands before donning sterile gloves when inserting a central intravascular catheter (IB).

e. Decontaminate hands before inserting indwelling urinary catheters, peripheral vascular catheters, or other invasive devices that do not require a surgical procedure (IB).

f. Decontaminate hands after contact with a patient's intact skin (e.g., when taking a pulse or blood pressure, and lifting a patient) (IB).

g. Decontaminate hands after contact with body fluids or excretions, mucous membranes, nonintact skin, and wound dressings if hands are not visibly soiled (IA).

h. Decontaminate hands if moving from a contaminated-body site to a clean-body site during patient care (II).

i. Decontaminate hands after contact with inanimate objects (including medical equipment) in the immediate vicinity of the patient (II).

j. Decontaminate hands after removing gloves (IB).

k. Before eating and after using a restroom, wash hands with a non-antimicrobial soap and water or with an antimicrobial soap and water (IB).

l. Antimicrobial-impregnated wipes (i.e., towelettes) may be considered as an alternative to washing hands with non-antimicrobial soap and water. Because they are not as effective as alcohol-based hand rubs or washing hands with an antimicrobial soap and water for reducing bacterial counts on the hands of HCWs, they are not a substitute for using an alcohol-based hand rub or antimicrobial soap (IB).

m. Wash hands with non-antimicrobial soap and water or with antimicrobial soap and water if exposure to *Bacillus anthracis* is suspected or proven. The physical action of washing and rinsing hands under such circumstances is recommended because alcohols, chlorhexidine, iodophors, and other antiseptic agents have poor activity against spores (II).

n. No recommendation can be made regarding the routine use of nonalcohol-based hand rubs for hand hygiene in health-care settings. Unresolved issue.

2. Hand-hygiene technique

a. When decontaminating hands with an alcohol-based hand rub, apply product to palm of one hand and rub hands together, covering all surfaces of hands and fingers, until hands are dry (IB). Follow the manufacturer's recommendations regarding the volume of product to use.

b. When washing hands with soap and water, wet hands first with water, apply an amount of product recommended by the manufacturer to hands, and rub hands together vigorously for at least 15 seconds, covering all surfaces of the hands and fingers. Rinse hands with water and dry thoroughly with a disposable towel. Use towel to turn off the faucet (IB). Avoid using hot water, because repeated exposure to hot water may increase the risk of dermatitis (IB).

c. Liquid, bar, leaflet or powdered forms of plain soap are acceptable when washing hands with a non-antimicrobial soap and water. When bar soap is used, soap racks that facilitate drainage and small bars of soap should be used (II).

d. Multiple-use cloth towels of the hanging or roll type are not recommended for use in health-care settings (II).

3. Surgical hand antisepsis
   a. Remove rings, watches, and bracelets before beginning the surgical hand scrub (II).
   b. Remove debris from underneath fingernails using a nail cleaner under running water (II).
   c. Surgical hand antisepsis using either an antimicrobial soap or an alcohol-based hand rub with persistent activity is recommended before donning sterile gloves when performing surgical procedures (IB).
   d. When performing surgical hand antisepsis using an antimicrobial soap, scrub hands and forearms for the length of time recommended by the manufacturer, usually 2–6 minutes. Long scrub times (e.g., 10 minutes) are not necessary (IB).
   e. When using an alcohol-based surgical hand-scrub product with persistent activity, follow the manufacturer's instructions. Before applying the alcohol solution, prewash hands and forearms with a non-antimicrobial soap and dry hands and forearms completely. After application of the alcohol-based product as recommended, allow hands and forearms to dry thoroughly before donning sterile gloves (IB).
4. Selection of hand-hygiene agents
   a. Provide personnel with efficacious hand-hygiene products that have low irritancy potential, particularly when these products are used multiple times per shift (IB). This recommendation applies to products used for hand antisepsis before and after patient care in clinical areas and to products used for surgical hand antisepsis by surgical personnel.
   b. To maximize acceptance of hand-hygiene products by HCWs, solicit input from these employees regarding the feel, fragrance, and skin tolerance of any products under consideration. The cost of hand-hygiene products should not be the primary factor influencing product selection (IB).
   c. When selecting non-antimicrobial soaps, antimicrobial soaps, or alcohol-based hand rubs, solicit information from manufacturers regarding any known interactions between products used to clean hands, skin care products, and the types of gloves used in the institution (II).
   d. Before making purchasing decisions, evaluate the dispenser systems of various product manufacturers or distributors to ensure that dispensers function adequately and deliver an appropriate volume of product (II).
   e. Do not add soap to a partially empty soap dispenser. This practice of "topping off" dispensers can lead to bacterial contamination of soap (IA).
5. Skin care
   a. Provide HCWs with hand lotions or creams to minimize the occurrence of irritant contact dermatitis associated with hand antisepsis or handwashing (IA).
   b. Solicit information from manufacturers regarding any effects that hand lotions, creams, or alcohol-based hand antiseptics may have on the persistent effects of antimicrobial soaps being used in the institution (IB).
6. Other aspects of hand hygiene

a. Do not wear artificial fingernails or extenders when having direct contact with patients at high risk (e.g., those in intensive-care units or operating rooms) (IA).
b. Keep natural nails tips less than 1/4-inch long (II).
c. Wear gloves when contact with blood or other potentially infectious materials, mucous membranes, and nonintact skin could occur (IC).
d. Remove gloves after caring for a patient. Do not wear the same pair of gloves for the care of more than one patient, and do not wash gloves between uses with different patients (IB).
e. Change gloves during patient care if moving from a contaminated body site to a clean body site (II).
f. No recommendation can be made regarding wearing rings in health-care settings. Unresolved issue.

7. Health-care worker educational and motivational programs
    a. As part of an overall program to improve hand-hygiene practices of HCWs, educate personnel regarding the types of patient-care activities that can result in hand contamination and the advantages and disadvantages of various methods used to clean their hands (II).
    b. Monitor HCWs' adherence with recommended hand-hygiene practices and provide personnel with information regarding their performance (IA).
    c. Encourage patients and their families to remind HCWs to decontaminate their hands (II).

8. Administrative measures
    a. Make improved hand-hygiene adherence an institutional priority and provide appropriate administrative support and financial resources (IB).
    b. Implement a multidisciplinary program designed to improve adherence of health personnel to recommended hand-hygiene practices (IB).
    c. As part of a multidisciplinary program to improve hand-hygiene adherence, provide HCWs with a readily accessible alcohol-based hand-rub product (IA).
    d. To improve hand-hygiene adherence among personnel who work in areas in which high workloads and high intensity of patient care are anticipated, make an alcohol-based hand rub available at the entrance to the patient's room or at the bedside, in other convenient locations, and in individual pocket-sized containers to be carried by HCWs (IA).
    e. Store supplies of alcohol-based hand rubs in cabinets or areas approved for flammable materials (IC).

Reference

CDC: Guideline for Hand Hygiene in Health Care Settings, Morbidity and Mortality Weekly Report, October 25, 2002; 51(RR-16). Complete report available at www.cdc.gov.

Part B: Antimicrobial Spectrum and Characteristics of Hand-Hygiene Antiseptic Agents

GROUP	GRAM-POSITIVE BACTERIA	GRAM-NEGATIVE BACTERIA	MYCOBACTERIA	FUNGI	VIRUSES	SPEED OF ACTION	COMMENTS
Alcohols	+++	+++	+++	+++	+++	Fast	Optimum concentration 60%–95%; no persistent activity
Chlorhexidine (2% and 4% aqueous)	+++	++	+	+	+++	Intermediate	Persistent activity; rare allergic reactions
Iodine compounds	+++	+++	+++	++	+++	Intermediate	Causes skin burns; usually too irritating for hand hygiene
Iodophors	+++	+++	+	++	++	Intermediate	Less irritating than iodine; acceptance varies
Phenol derivatives	+++	+	+	+	+	Intermediate	Activity neutralized by nonionic surfactants
Triclosan	+++	++	+	−	+++	Intermediate	Acceptability on hands varies
Quaternary ammonium compounds	+	++	−	−	+	Slow	Used only in combination with alcohols; ecologic concerns

Note: +++ = excellent; ++ = good, but does not include the entire bacterial spectrum; + = fair; — = no activity or not sufficient.

*Hexachlorophene is not included because it is no longer an accepted ingredient of hand disinfectants.

LABORATORY ASSAYS AND THE REQUIRED TYPES OF ANTICOAGULANTS

TEST NAME	SPECIMEN TUBE (CLOSURE TYPE/COLOR)	WHOLE BLOOD, MINIMUM VOLUME FOR ADULTS (ml)
A_{1c} hemoglobin (see Glycosylated hemoglobin)		
ABG (See Blood gases)		
ABO group and Rh typing	Whole blood (pink)	6 (adult); 1 (child)
Acetazolamide	Serum (speckled) or plasma (purple or green)	3
Acetaminophen (Tylenol)	Serum (speckled)	1
Acetone (ketones)	Serum (speckled)	2
Acetylcholine receptor-binding antibodies	Serum (speckled)	3
Acid hemolysis (PNH)	Plasma (light blue)	3
Acid phosphatase, total	Serum (speckled) or plasma (green)	1
Acidified serum test (see Hamm's test)		
ACTH (adrenocorticotropic) hormone	Plasma (purple) Critical frozen	3
Activated partial thromboplastin time (see Partial thromboplastin time)		
Activated Protein C Resistance (APCR)	Plasma (blue) Freeze immediately	2
Adenovirus antibody	Serum (speckled)	3
Adrenal cortical antibody	Serum (speckled)	3
Adrenalin (see Catecholamines)		
Albumin	Serum (speckled)	2
Alcohol (ethanol)	Whole blood (gray)	3
Aldolase	Serum (speckled)	2
Aldosterone	Serum (speckled) or plasma (green)	1
	*Collect at 8 am. Patient should be on normal diet 2 weeks prior to test.	
	*Patient should be recumbent for at least 30 minutes prior to blood collection	

TEST NAME	SPECIMEN TUBE (CLOSURE TYPE/COLOR)	WHOLE BLOOD, MINIMUM VOLUME FOR ADULTS (ml)
Alkaline phosphatase (Alk p'tase)	Serum (speckled)	2
Alkaline phosphatase isoenzymes	Serum (speckled)	2
Alpha$_1$-antitrypsin (AAT)	Serum (speckled)	1
Alpha-fetoprotein (AFP)	Serum (speckled)	3
AFP tumor marker	Whole blood (speckled)	3
Alpha$_2$-macroglobulin	Serum (speckled)	1
Aluminum	Serum (royal blue)	3
Amebiasis	Serum (speckled)	3
Amikacin	Serum (speckled)	1
Amino acids	Whole blood (green)	3
Amiodarone	Serum (red)	2
Amitriptyline	Serum (red)	3
Ammonia	Plasma (green) on ice, deliver immediately	3
Ampicillin	Serum (red)	5
Amylase	Serum (speckled)	2
Amylase Isoenzymes	Serum (speckled)	2
Androstenedione	Serum (speckled)	3
Angiotensin-converting enzyme (ACE)	Serum (speckled) or plasma (purple)	1
Antibody to hepatitis A virus (anti-HAV)	Serum (speckled)	5
Antibody to hepatitis B core antigen (Anti-HBc)	Serum (speckled)	5
Antibody to hepatitis BE antigen	Serum (speckled)	3.5
Antibody to hepatitis B surface antigen (Anti-HBs)	Serum (speckled)	4
Antibody identification	Whole blood (pink)	6
Antibody screen and blood grouping	Whole blood (pink)	6 (adult) 3 (child)
Antibody titer	Whole blood (red, pink, or purple)	5
Anti-cardiolipin antibodies	Whole blood (speckled)	3
Antidiuretic hormone (ADH, vasopressin)	Plasma (purple) Critical frozen	3
Anti–DNase B	Serum (speckled)	3
Anti-ds-DNA	Whole blood (speckled)	3
Anti-microsomal antibody (thyroid peroxidase antibody) TPO	Whole blood (speckled)	4
Anti-mitochondrial antibody (AMA)	Whole blood (speckled)	4
Anti-neutrophil cytoplasmic antibody (CANCA)	Whole blood (speckled)	4

TEST NAME	SPECIMEN TUBE (CLOSURE TYPE/COLOR)	WHOLE BLOOD, MINIMUM VOLUME FOR ADULTS (ml)
Antinuclear antibodies (ANA)	Whole blood (speckled)	5
Anti–smooth muscle antibody (ASMA)	Serum (speckled)	3
Anti-thyroid antibodies (ATA)	Whole blood (speckled)	2
Antithrombin III (AT III)	Plasma (light blue)	5
Anti-thyroglobulin	Whole blood (speckled)	3
Apolipoprotein A–1	Serum (speckled) Fasting required	2
APTT	Plasma (light blue)	1.8
Arboviruses (St. Louis encephalitis)	Serum (speckled)	3
Arsenic (As)	Whole blood (royal blue)	7
Ascorbic acid (see Vitamin C)		
ASO (anti-streptolysin O) titer	Whole blood (speckled)	3
Aspirin (see Salicylate)		
Autologous blood	Whole blood (red)	5
Bactrim (see Sulfonamides)		
Barbiturates	Serum (speckled)	2
B-cell antigen	Whole blood (red)	3
Benzodiazepines	Serum (speckled)	2
Beta$_2$-microglobulin	Serum (speckled)	1
Bile acids total	Serum (speckled)	0.5
Bilirubin, total and direct	Serum (speckled) Protect blood from light	2
Blastomycosis, complement fixation (fungal serology)	Serum (speckled)	4
Bleeding time	Patient	Test performed on patient's arm
Blood cell count, CBC survey (WBC, RBC, Hgb, Hct, MCV, MCH, MCHC)	Whole blood (purple)	3
Blood cell count, differential	Blood smear	Blood smear
Blood cell count, eosinophil	Whole blood (purple)	3
Blood cell count, erythrocyte (RBC)	Whole blood (purple)	3
Blood cell count, leukocyte (WBC)	Whole blood (purple)	3
Blood cell count, platelets	Whole blood (purple)	3
Blood cell count, reticulocyte	Whole blood (purple)	3
Blood gases, arterial (ABG) (pH, pCO$_2$, pO$_2$, HCO$_3^-$, base excess [BE])	Arterial blood (heparinized syringe)	0.6
Blood packed red blood cells	Whole blood (red)	5

TEST NAME	SPECIMEN TUBE (CLOSURE TYPE/COLOR)	WHOLE BLOOD, MINIMUM VOLUME FOR ADULTS (ml)
Bordetella pertussis antibody (whooping cough)	Serum (red)	3
Borrelia burgdorferi antibody (Lyme disease)	Serum (red)	3
Bromide	Serum (speckled)	2
Brucella	Serum (speckled)	4.5
BUN (blood urea nitrogen)	Whole blood (speckled)	1
CA 125 (cancer antigen 125)	Serum (speckled)	1
Cadmium (Cd)	Whole blood (royal blue)	7
Calcitonin	Plasma (purple) or serum (speckled)	1
Calcium	Serum (speckled)	5
Calcium, ionized	Whole blood (green) DELIVER IMMEDIATELY	
Candida serology, qualitative	Serum (speckled)	3
Carbamazepine (see Tegretol)		
Carbon dioxide (CO_2)	Serum (speckled)	1
Carcinoembryonic antigen (CEA)	Serum (speckled)	3
Cardiac troponins (cTnl, cTnT)	Serum (speckled)	3
Cardiolipin antibodies (anti-cardiolipin antibody IgG and IgM)	Serum (speckled)	3
Carotene	Serum (speckled)	3
Catecholamines (Adrenalin; Epinephrine)	Plasma (green) (Patient must be calm or supine for 30 min before collection *Ice needed for transportation	4
CD4-CD8 (T-cell subsets)	Whole blood (purple)	5
Ceruloplasmin	Serum (speckled)	3
Chemistry screen (T. protein, Alb, Ca, Glu, BUN, Creat, T.bil, Alk p'tase, AST ALT, potassium, creatinine, chloride, sodium, CO_2)	Serum (speckled)	3
Chickenpox titer	Whole blood (speckled)	3
Chlamydia antibody	Serum (speckled)	1
Chloramphenicol	Serum (speckled)	4
Chloride	Whole blood (speckled)	1
Cholesterol (total)	Serum (speckled) (FASTING)	1
Cholinesterase	Plasma (green or purple)	5
Chromium (Cr)	Serum (royal blue) *Avoid glass containers	2
Chromosome analysis	Sterile whole blood (green) (Na heparin)	5

TEST NAME	SPECIMEN TUBE (CLOSURE TYPE/COLOR)	WHOLE BLOOD, MINIMUM VOLUME FOR ADULTS (ml)
Circulating anticoagulants	Plasma (light blue)	3
Clonazepam	Serum (red) or plasma (purple)	2
CMV, IFA serology	Serum (speckled)	3
Coccidioides immitis (San Joaquin fever)	Serum (speckled)	3
Cold agglutinins	Whole blood (speckled) *Place in warm water and deliver immediately	3
Colloid osmotic pressure (COP)	Whole blood (green)	3
Complement, total	Serum (speckled)	5
Complement—C3	Serum (speckled)	5
Complement—C4	Serum (speckled)	5
Comprehensive allergy profile	Serum (speckled)	5
Coombs' test, direct (direct antiglobulin test) (DAT)	Whole blood (purple or pink)	5
Copper (Cu)	Serum (speckled)	3.5
Cortisol	Plasma (green)	1
Coxsackievirus (Bornholm disease)	Serum (speckled)	3
Coxiella burnetii (Q fever)	Serum (speckled)	3
C-peptide	Serum (speckled)	3
Creatine kinase (CK)	Serum (speckled)	1
CK isoenzymes (CK-MB)	Serum (speckled)	3
C-reactive protein	Serum (speckled)	2
Creatinine	Serum (speckled)	1
Cross-match	Whole blood (pink)	6
Cryofibrinogen	Whole blood (speckled) and whole blood (purple) Immediately after collecting, place in warm water	10
Cryoglobulin	Serum (speckled) *Immediately place in warm water and transport to lab	10
Cyclic AMP, plasma	Plasma (purple)	1
Cryptococcal antigen	Serum (red)	3
Cyclosporine	Whole blood (purple)	5
Cystic fibrosis DNA Test	Whole blood (purple)	5
Cytomegalovirus (CMV), IFA serology	Serum (speckled)	3
D-dimer (D-D$_{1M}$)	Whole blood (blue)	3.5
Dengue virus antibody (breakbone fever)	Serum (speckled)	3

TEST NAME	SPECIMEN TUBE (CLOSURE TYPE/COLOR)	WHOLE BLOOD, MINIMUM VOLUME FOR ADULTS (ml)
Deoxycorticosteroids	Serum (speckled) or plasma (green)	3
Depakene (see Valproic acid)		
Desipramine	Serum (red) or plasma (green or purple) Test not appropriate after imipramide administration	2
DHEA (Dehydroepiandrosterone)	Serum (speckled) *Morning sample preferred	10
Diazepam (see Valium)		
Digoxin (Lanoxin)	Serum (speckled)	2
Dilantin (phenytoin)	Serum (speckled)	1
Dilute Russell viper venom (DRVV)	Whole blood (light blue) Deliver immediately. Indicate if the patient is on any type of anticoagulant	5
Direct antiglobulin test (DAT)	Whole blood (purple or pink)	5 (adult) 3 (child)
DNA single strand IgG antibody	Serum (speckled)	1
Donath-Landsteiner antibody	Whole blood (special collection)	6
Dopamine (catecholamines fractionated)	Plasma (green)	4
Drug screen	Serum (red)	6
EBV (Epstein Barr virus) by PCR	Serum (red) Keep Sterile	3
EBV-NA	Serum (speckled)	3
EBV-VCA, IgM	Serum (speckled)	3
EBV-VCA, IgG	Serum (speckled)	3
Electrolytes (Na, K, Cl, HCO_3)	Plasma (green) or whole blood (green)	2
Electrophoresis (hemoglobin)	Whole blood (purple)	2
Electrophoresis (SPE)	Serum (speckled)	3
Entamoeba histolytica	Serum (speckled)	3
Eosinóphil count	Whole blood (purple)	2
Epinephrine (see Catecholamines)		
Erythropoietin	Serum (speckled)	2
ESR (sedimentation rate, sed rate)	Whole blood (purple)	5
Estradiol (E_2)	Serum (speckled)	3
Estrone	Serum (speckled) or plasma (green)	1
Estrogen, fractions	Serum (speckled)	2
Ethanol (alcohol)	Whole blood (gray)	2
Ethosuximide (Zarontin)	Whole blood (speckled)	1

TEST NAME	SPECIMEN TUBE (CLOSURE TYPE/COLOR)	WHOLE BLOOD, MINIMUM VOLUME FOR ADULTS (ml)
Ethylene glycol	Serum (speckled)	2
Euglobulin lysis	Plasma (blue) Deliver immediately	4.5
Factor assays	Plasma (blue) Test not valid if patient on hepanin	4.5
Fasting blood glucose (FBG)	Plasma (gray) or whole blood (green)	1
Fatty acids, free	Serum (speckled) Critical Frozen	1
Ferritin	Serum (speckled)	2
Fetal hemoglobin	Whole blood (purple)	1
Fibrin Split products (FSP)	Plasma (blue)	2
Fibrinogen	Plasma (blue)	3.5
Fibrinogen antigen	Blood (blue)	4.5
Fitzgerald factor	Blood (blue) Patient must not be on heparin	4.5
Flecainide	Serum (red)	1.5
Fletcher factor (prekallinkrein)	Blood (blue)	4.5
Fluoride	Serum (red)	6
Fluxetinet norfluoxetine	Serum (red) or plasma (lavender or green)	3
Folate, serum	Serum (speckled)	3
Folate, whole blood (RBC and serum)	Whole blood (purple)	3
Follicle-stimulating hormone (FSH)	Serum (speckled) or plasma (green)	3
Food allergy profile	Serum (speckled)	5
Fragile X DNA mutation	Whole blood (purple)	10
Free erythrocyte porphryn (FEP)	Whole blood (purple) (royal blue EDTA)	1
Free, T$_4$ (see Thyroxine, free)		
Free thyroxine index (see Thyroid studies)		
Fungal serology	Serum (speckled)	1
Gamma-glutamyl transferase (GGT) (GT)	Serum (speckled)	1
Gastrin	Serum (speckled)	7
Gentamicin	Serum (speckled)	1
Giardia lambia antibody	Serum (speckled)	3
Glucagon	Whole blood (purple)	3
Glucose (FBS and tolerance)	Whole blood (green)	1

TEST NAME	SPECIMEN TUBE (CLOSURE TYPE/COLOR)	WHOLE BLOOD, MINIMUM VOLUME FOR ADULTS (ml)
Glucose-6-phosphate dehydrogenase (G6PD), quantitative	Whole blood (green)	2
Glucose, 2-hour postprandial	Whole blood (green)	1
Glycosylated hemoglobin	Whole blood (purple)	1
Gonadotropin HCG-beta (immuno test)	Serum (speckled)	5
Growth hormone (HGH)	Serum (speckled) or plasma (purple)	1.5
Hamm's test (PNH) confirmation	Whole blood (lavender and blue)	5
Haptoglobin	Blood (speckled)	5
HDL (high-density lipoprotein) cholesterol	Serum (speckled)	3
Heinz body preparation	Whole blood (purple or green)	3
Helicobacter pylori antibody (H. pylori)	Blood (speckled)	4
Helper T	Whole blood (purple)	2
Hematocrit	Whole blood (purple)	5
Hematology profile (Hct, Hgb, WBC, RBC, MCV, MCH, MCHC)	Whole blood (purple)	5
Hemoglobin	Whole blood (purple)	5
Hemoglobin S solubility	Whole blood (purple)	5
Hemoglobin, Free	Plasma (green)	2
Hemoglobin electrophoresis	Whole blood (purple)	2
Heparin	Plasma (blue)	3
Hepatitis A Ab IgM (Anti-HAV-IgM)	Serum (speckled)	5
Hepatitis B core antibody (HB$_c$Ab) (Anti-HB$_c$)	Serum (speckled)	3
Hepatitis B surface Ab (Anti-HB$_s$)	Serum (speckled)	4
Hepatitis B surface antigen (HB$_s$Ag)	Serum (speckled)	3
Hepatitis Be antibody	Serum (speckled)	3.5
Hepatitis Be antigen	Serum (speckled)	2
Hepatitis C Ab (Anti-HCV)	Serum (speckled)	5
HCV PCR quantitative	Blood (speckled)	5
Hepatitis delta antibody	Serum (speckled) or plasma (purple)	1
Hepatitis G virus, PCR	Plasma (purple)	10
Herpes simplex, virus serology	Blood (speckled)	5
Heterophile antibody (see Monospot)		

TEST NAME	SPECIMEN TUBE (CLOSURE TYPE/COLOR)	WHOLE BLOOD, MINIMUM VOLUME FOR ADULTS (ml)
Histamine	Whole blood (purple or green)	1
Histoplasmosis (antibody)	Serum (speckled)	1
HI titer (St. Louis encephalitis)	Serum (speckled)	1
HIV-1/HIV-2 antibody screen	Blood (speckled)	5
HIV-1, PCR	Whole blood (purple)	5
HLA B27	Whole blood (green) Critical maintain room temperature	5
Homocysteine	Serum (speckled)	1
Human chorionic gonadotrophin (HCG)	Serum (speckled)	6
Human growth hormone (HGH) (see Growth hormone)		
Human T-cell lymphotropic virus type I antibody	Blood (speckled)	5
17 Hydroxyprogesterone	Serum (speckled)	3
Ibuprofen	Serum (red) or plasma (gray)	2
IgA	Serum (speckled)	5
IgD	Serum (speckled)	1
IgFI (Insulin like growth factor 1) Somatomedin C	Serum (speckled) or plasma (purple)	0.5
IgG	Blood (speckled)	5
IgM	Serum (speckled)	5
Imipramine (Tofranil)	Serum (red) or plasma (purple or green)	3
Immune complex panel (RAJI Cell, C1Q binding)	Serum (speckled)	3
ImmunoFixation (IFE)	Blood (speckled)	5
Infectious mononucleosis (Monospot)	Blood (speckled)	4
Influenza A & B virus antibody	Serum (speckled)	1
Inhalant profile	Serum (speckled)	3
Insulin	Serum (speckled)	1
Intrinsic factor blocking antibody	Serum (speckled)	1
Iron profile (iron, TIBC, and saturation)	Blood (speckled) Avoid Hemolysis	1
Ketones	Blood (speckled)	2
Kleihauer-Betke stain (fetal hemoglobin stain	Blood (purple)	1
Lactate dehydrogenase (LD) and LD isoenzymes (LD-1)	Serum (speckled)	2
Lactic acid (on ice)	Blood (gray) Avoid hemolysis	1

TEST NAME	SPECIMEN TUBE (CLOSURE TYPE/COLOR)	WHOLE BLOOD, MINIMUM VOLUME FOR ADULTS (ml)
Lanoxin (see Digoxin)		
LDL (low-density lipoprotein) cholesterol	Serum (speckled)	1
Lead, blood	Blood (royal blue) or (purple)	7
Legionnaires' serology	Serum (speckled)	1
Leishmania antibody	Serum (speckled)	3
Leptospira antibody	Serum (speckled)	3
Leucine aminopeptidase (LAP)	Plasma (purple) or serum (speckled)	1
Leukocyte alkaline phosphatase (LAB) stain	Blood (green)	5
LGV-psittacosis titer (See Chlamydia antibody)		
LH (see Luteinizing hormone)		
Lidocaine	Blood (speckled)	5
Lipase	Blood (speckled)	3
Lipid profile	Blood (speckled)	3
Lithium	Serum (speckled)	1
Low-density lipoprotein (LDL) cholesterol	Serum (speckled)	3
Lupus anticoagulant	Blood (blue) *Deliver immediately; indicate if patient on anticoagulant therapy	5
Luteinizing hormone (LH)	Blood (speckled)	3
Lyme antibody	Serum (speckled)	1
Magnesium, serum	Blood (speckled)	3
Malaria Prep	Blood (purple)	Blood smear
Manganese (Mn)	Whole blood (royal blue) or serum	2
Methanol	Serum (red) *Use acid-washed syringes	7
Methemoglobin	Whole blood (heparinized syringe) Deliver immediately	2
Methotrexate	Blood (speckled)	10
Mexiletine	Serum (red)	1.5
Molecular diagnostic lab tests	Whole blood (purple) *Immediately transport in ice slurry	3 × 10 mL
Monocyte antigens	Whole blood (purple)	2
Mumps Antibody	Blood (speckled)	3
Mycoplasma pneumoniae antibody	Serum (speckled)	1

TEST NAME	SPECIMEN TUBE (CLOSURE TYPE/COLOR)	WHOLE BLOOD, MINIMUM VOLUME FOR ADULTS (ml)
Myocardial antibody IgG	Serum (speckled)	1
Myoglobin	Blood (speckled)	2
Neisseria gonorrhoeae	Serum (red)	1
NAPA (see Procainamide)		
5′ -Nucleotidase	Serum (speckled)	1
Nutritional panel	Blood (speckled)	2
Osmolality, serum	Blood (speckled)	3
Osteocalcin antibody	Serum (speckled)	0.5
PAP (Prostatic acid phosphatase)	Blood (speckled)	3
Parathyroid hormone (PTH)	Blood (purple)	5
Partial thromboplastin time (PTT) (APTT)	Blood (blue) Indicate if patient on anticoagulant	5
Pentobarbital	Serum (red)	3
Peroxidase (leukocyte peroxidase) stain	Blood (purple)	3
pH, blood (see Blood gases)		
Phenobarbital	Serum (red)	3
Phenylalanine	Whole blood *Filter paper with low background fluorescence	Droplets used to saturate filter paper (<0.5)
Phenytoin (Dilantin)	Blood (speckled)	1
Phenytoin (free)	Blood (red)	5
Phosphorus	Blood (speckled)	1
Plasminogen	Plasma (blue)	1
Platelet antibody screen	Whole blood (red)	6
Platelet count	Whole blood (purple)	2
Pneumococcal antibody	Serum (speckled)	1.5
Porphyrins, plasma fractionation	Plasma (green)	3
Potassium (k)	Whole blood (green) or blood (speckled)	1
Prealbumin	Blood (speckled)	3
Pro-BNP (N-terminal pro-brain natriuretic peptide)	Serum (speckled)	3
Procainamide, N-acetylprocainamide (NAPA)	Blood (speckled)	2
Progesterone	Serum (speckled)	2
Proinsulin	Serum (speckled)	1
Prolactin	Blood (speckled)	2
Pronestyl (procainamide)	Blood (speckled)	2
Prostatic acid phosphatase (PAP) (see PAP)		
Prostatic specific antigen (PSA)	Blood (speckled)	1
Protein, total	Blood (speckled)	1

TEST NAME	SPECIMEN TUBE (CLOSURE TYPE/COLOR)	WHOLE BLOOD, MINIMUM VOLUME FOR ADULTS (ml)
Protein C total	Plasma (blue)	2
Protein electrophoresis (see electrophoresis)		
Prothrombin consumption time	Serum (speckled)	3
Protime (International Technidyne Corporation) (prothrombin time, PT)	Plasma (blue)	2
PSA (see prostatic specific antigen)		
PTH (see Parathyroid hormone)		
Pyruvate	Whole blood (gray) *Transport immediately in ice water	5
Q fever antibodies	Serum (speckled)	1
Quinidine	Blood (speckled)	1
Rabies virus antibody	Serum (speckled)	3
RAST allergens	Serum (speckled)	0.25/allergen
Renin activity	Plasma (purple) *Transport immediately in ice water	1
Reptilase time	Whole blood (blue)	3.5
Reticulocyte count (RBC)	Whole blood (purple)	5
Rheumatoid factor assay	Serum (speckled)	2
Rocky mountain spotted fever, IgG, IgM	Serum (speckled)	1
RPR	Blood (speckled)	5
Rubella antibody	Blood (speckled)	4
Rubeola antibody	Blood (speckled)	4.5
Salicylate (aspirin)	Whole blood (speckled)	2
Salmonella antibody	Serum (speckled)	5
Sedimentation rate (ESR) (erythrocyte sedimentation rate)	Whole blood (purple)	5
Selenium (Se)	Plasma, whole blood, serum (royal blue with heparin or EDTA or no anticoagulant) AVOID GLASS	2
Serotonin blood (5-hydroxytryptamine)	Serum (speckled)	1
SGOT (AST)	Serum (speckled)	1
SGPT (ALT)	Serum (speckled)	1
Sickling screen	Whole blood (purple)	5
Sjögren's antibody	Serum (red)	7
Sodium, blood	Blood (green)	1
SPE (serum protein electrophoresis)	Serum (speckled)	3

TEST NAME	SPECIMEN TUBE (CLOSURE TYPE/COLOR)	WHOLE BLOOD, MINIMUM VOLUME FOR ADULTS (ml)
Sucrose hemolysis test (sugar water test)	Whole blood (blue)	5
Sulfonamides	Serum or plasma (red, purple, or green)	2
Suppressor	Whole blood (purple)	3
Syphilis (RPR)	Serum (speckled)	5
T-Cell subsets T_4/T_3 (CD_4/CD_8)	Blood (purple)	5
T_3 uptake	Serum (speckled)	2
Tegretol (carbamazepine)	Serum (speckled)	2
Teichoic acid antibody	Serum (speckled)	5
Testosterone	Blood (speckled)	6
Theophylline (aminophylline)	Serum (speckled)	1
Thiamine	Whole blood (green)	3
Thiocyanate	Serum (speckled) or plasma (purple)	1
Thrombin time	Plasma (blue)	3
Thyroglobulin	Serum (speckled)	5
Thyroid antibodies	Serum (speckled)	3
Thyroid studies (T_3, T_4, TSH)	Serum (speckled)	3
Thyroiditis, antithyroglobulin, and antimicrosomal fraction	Serum (speckled)	5
Thyroxine (T_4)	Serum (speckled)	2
Thyroxine (T_4), free	Serum (speckled)	3
Tobramycin	Serum (speckled)	1
Tofranil (see Imipramine)		
TORCH titers	Serum (speckled)	5
Total T_3 (triiodothyronine)	Serum (speckled)	2
Toxoplasmosis antibody	Serum (speckled)	5
Transaminase (ALT, SGPT)	Serum (speckled)	1
Transaminase (AST, SGOT)	Serum (speckled)	1
Transferrin	Serum (speckled)	5
Trichinella antibody	Serum (speckled)	0.5
Tricyclic antidepressants (amitriptyline, nortriptyline)	Serum (speckled)	3
Triglycerides (fasting)	Serum (speckled)	1
Troponin I (cTnI)	Serum (speckled)	3
Troponin T (cTnT)	Serum (speckled)	3
TSH (thyroid-stimulating hormone, or thyrotropin)	Serum (speckled)	2
Tylenol (see Acetominophen)		
Urea nitrogen (BUN)	Serum (speckled)	1
Uric acid	Serum (speckled)	1
Valium (diazepam)	Serum (red)	2

TEST NAME	SPECIMEN TUBE (CLOSURE TYPE/COLOR)	WHOLE BLOOD, MINIMUM VOLUME FOR ADULTS (ml)
Valproic acid (Depakene)	Serum (speckled)	5
Vancomycin	Serum (speckled)	1
Varicella-zoster immune status	Serum (speckled)	2
Varicella-zoster IgG antibody	Serum (speckled)	5
Vitamin A	Serum (speckled) *Protect blood from light	1
Vitamin B_6	Whole blood (purple)	1
Vitamin B_{12} (Cyanocobalamin)	Serum (speckled)	2
Vitamin B_{12} binding capacity	Serum (speckled)	1
Vitamin C (ascorbic acid)	Whole blood (green)	2
Vitamin D (25-OH)	Serum (speckled) Protect from light	1
Vitamin E level	Serum (speckled)	1
von Willebrand's factor assay (Ristocetin cofactor)	Whole blood (blue) *Deliver immediately	5
Zinc	Serum (Royal blue) Avoid glass	1

Update for this edition courtesy of Memorial Hermann Hospital Laboratory.

GUIDE FOR MAXIMUM AMOUNTS OF BLOOD TO BE DRAWN FROM PATIENTS YOUNGER THAN 14 YEARS

PATIENT'S WEIGHT		MAXIMIM AMOUNT TO BE DRAWN AT ANY ONE TIME (ml)	MAXIMUM AMOUNT OF BLOOD (CUMULATIVE) TO BE DRAWN DURING A GIVEN HOSPITAL STAY (1 MONTH OR LESS) (ml)
Pounds	*Kilograms*		
6–8	2.7–3.6	2.5	23
8–10	3.6–4.5	3.5	30
10–15	4.5–6.8	5	40
16–20	7.3–9.1	10	60
21–25	9.5–11.4	10	70
26–30	11.8–13.6	10	80
31–35	14.1–15.9	10	100
36–40	16.4–18.2	10	130
41–45	18.6–20.5	20	140
46–50	20.9–22.7	20	160
51–55	23.2–25.0	20	180
56–60	25.5–27.3	20	200
61–65	27.7–29.5	25	220
66–70	30.0–31.8	30	240
71–75	32.3–34.1	30	250
76–80	34.5–36.4	30	270
81–85	36.8–38.6	30	290
86–90	39.1–40.9	30	310
91–95	41.4–43.2	30	330
96–100	43.6–45.5	30	350

Courtesy of Memorial Hermann Hospital Laboratory, with permission.

Appendix 6

OCCUPATIONAL SAFETY & HEALTH ADMINISTRATION (OSHA) U.S. DEPARTMENT OF LABOR LABELING REQUIREMENTS

ITEM	NO LABEL NEEDED IF UNIVERSAL PRECAUTIONS ARE USED AND SPECIFIC USE OF CONTAINER OR ITEM IS KNOWN TO ALL EMPLOYEES	BIOHAZARD LABEL		RED CONTAINER
Regulated waste container (e.g., contaminated sharps container)		X	or	X
Reusable contaminated sharps container (e.g., surgical instruments soaking in a tray)		X	or	X
Refrigerator/freezer holding blood or other potentially infectious material		X		
Containers used for storage, transport, or shipping of blood		X	or	X
Blood/blood products for clinical use	**No labels required**			
Individual specimen containers of blood or other potentially infectious materials remaining in facility	X	X	or	X
Contaminated equipment needing service (e.g., dialysis equipment; suction apparatus)		X Plus a label specifying where the contamination exists		

ITEM	NO LABEL NEEDED IF UNIVERSAL PRECAUTIONS ARE USED AND SPECIFIC USE OF CONTAINER OR ITEM IS KNOWN TO ALL EMPLOYEES		BIOHAZARD LABEL		RED CONTAINER
Specimens and regulated waste shipped from the primary facility to another facility for service or disposal			X	or	X
Contaminated laundry	X*	or	X	or	X
Contaminated laundry sent to another facility that does not use Universal Precautions			X	or	X

*Alternative labeling or color coding is sufficient if it permits all employees to recognize the containers as requiring compliance with Universal Precautions.

From OSHA website: http://www.osha.gov/SLTC/nursinghome_ecat/laundry/label.html. Accessed June, 2003.

Appendix 7

WHOLE BLOOD OR APHERESIS PROCEDURE

Gulf Coast Regional Blood Center
1400 La Concha
Houston, TX 77054

Uncontrolled
Reference Copy

DC SOP 301.06V7
Implementation Date: 5/7/02
Page 1 of 18

301.06V7 Phlebotomy

PURPOSE

1.0 To provide instructions for the following:

1.1 Preparation for phlebotomy; confirmation of donor's identity, final pre-phlebotomy check of the donor record, inspection of collection bags and vacutubes, BUI verification;

1.2 Selection and preparation of venipuncture site;

1.3 Preparation of collection bag(s);

1.4 Proper performance and documentation of the venipuncture procedure;

1.5 Discontinuing a phlebotomy, including removal of the needle from the donor's arm; filling test sample tubes; rechecking the labels on the donor record, primary and satellite bags, and sample tubes; and documenting the end of the phlebotomy;

1.6 Post-phlebotomy cleaning of the donor's arm, and providing proper information for post-donation instructions.

1.7 Performing and documenting a second phlebotomy when the first venipuncture on a particular donor is unsuccessful;

1.8 Recognizing, handling and documenting whole blood and apheresis collections that do not meet the standards established for acceptable collections.

SCOPE

1.0 This procedure will be performed by trained phlebotomists or apheresis operators for each donor who undergoes a whole blood or apheresis donation procedure.

MATERIALS

- Donor Form
- Black or blue pen
- Purple top sample vacutubes

- Black indelible marker
- Gloves
- Lab coat
- Face mask (optional)
- Rubber bands
- Tape
- Donor Scale calibrated to collect the appropriate volume of blood (450 mL or 500 mL)
- SampLink Access Device
- Test tube rack

- Plastic bags
- Blood Pack Unit containing the LabSite Sampling Site (**LSSS**) and DonorCare Needle Guard
- Hematron
- Hemostats
- Bio-Sharps container
- Quarantined Component tag
- Designated blood cooler
- Blood pressure cuff
- Red top sample vacutubes
- Crimper
- Grommetts
- Hand sealer

Gulf Coast Regional Blood Center
1400 La Concha
Houston, TX 77054

Uncontrolled
Reference Copy

DC SOP 301.06V7
Implementation Date: 5/7/02
Page 2 of 18

PROCEDURE

PREPARATION FOR PHLEBOTOMY (WHOLE BLOOD AND APHERESIS PROCEDURES)

1.0   Greet the donor as he/she enters the phlebotomy area and show him/her to a donor chair or bed.

2.0   Ask the donor, "What is your name?" or "Please state your full name", or a similar statement that helps to establish positive identity of the donor.

     2.1   Verify that the name is the same as the one on the **Donor Form**.

     2.2   If you cannot understand the donor's pronunciation, ask him/her to spell the name.

     2.3   If the donor has to leave the room between the completion of the screening process and phlebotomy, upon the donor's return, verify the donor's identity as described above.

3.0   Review the following parts of the **Donor Form** for completeness, accuracy, and legibility:

- Donor demographics (including the recorded weight of the donor).
- **Donor Disqualification Directory** or computer check,
- Medical history interview,
- Physical examination,
- Blood unit identification number.
- Ensure that the donor has signed the informed consent statement and that the interviewer has signed and placed his/her employee ID# in the appropriate area of the **Donor Form**.
  Note: Verify signature on the informed consent statement matches the name in the demographic section of the donor form if legible.

     3.1   If any section is incomplete, <u>confidentially</u> ask the donor for or obtain the missing information, where applicable and generate a **Quality Improvement Report,** (hereafter referred to as a **"QIR").**
  SEE: Quality Assurance SOP "Reporting An Incident".

         a.   If vital signs are missing, incomplete, and/or illegible, take/retake as applicable the donor's vital signs and generate a **QIR**.
  NOTE: Ensure all documentation is in accordance with Q.A. Department Document Preparation and Review Standards.

     3.2   If any reason for deferral is identified that was not identified by the screener, document this in the deferral section of the **Donor Form** and defer the donor according to the appropriate SOP.
  NOTE: If the discrepancy is discovered during or after the collection procedure, quarantine the unit as appropriate.

4.0   Once the review is done, place the **Donor Form** near the donor for the duration of the phlebotomy procedure.

5.0   Inspect the blood bags and vacutubes for expiration date, defects, cracks or contamination.

6.0   Verify that all bar coded and eye-readable labels on the **Donor Form**, any applicable procedure record, blood/component bags and vacutubes are identical and have been appropriately placed.
  NOTE: It is the responsibility of the phlebotomist to ensure that this information is identical.

- ***When performing collection using the Donor ID system, all necessary steps for registering a donor with the use of a palm pilot should be applied here.***

Gulf Coast Regional Blood Center
1400 La Concha
Houston, TX 77054

Uncontrolled
Reference Copy

DC SOP 301.06V7
Implementation Date: 5/7/02
Page 3 of 18

SELECTION OF VENIPUNCTURE SITE (WHOLE BLOOD AND APHERESIS)

7.0   Apply a tourniquet or pressure cuff snugly around the donor's arm. Have the donor squeeze a hand grip intermittently. Select a vein for venipuncture.
NOTE: Avoid areas that are scarred or that have pits or dimples associated with prior phlebotomies since these areas are difficult to clean and bacteria is harder to remove.

7.1   Ask the donor if he / she is allergic to iodine.

a.   If the donor is not allergic to iodine, use the Routine Scrub (PVP Iodine Solutions) procedure.
b.   If the donor is allergic to iodine, refer to the Non-routine scrub procedure.

7.2   You may mark the location of the vein with the stick end of an iodine scrub, so that the vein can be easily located.

7.3   If a vein is located, loosen the tourniquet or blood pressure cuff and proceed to clean the intended venipuncture site with the appropriate solutions as defined in this SOP.

7.4   If you are not able to find an adequate vein, ask another phlebotomist and/or consult the Supervisor for assistance. If no veins can be found, defer the donor and document the deferral. Record in the Comments section of the **Donor Form**, "suitable vein not located" or a similar statement.

PREPARATION OF VENIPUNCTURE SITE (WHOLE BLOOD AND APHERESIS)

NOTE: Proper preparation of the venipuncture site helps to assure that the phlebotomy procedure will be as aseptic as possible. The scrub process helps remove possible contaminates such as dead skin cells and bacteria, leaving an aseptic area.

Routine Scrub

PVP Iodine Solutions

8.0   Using the 0.75% PVP-iodine scrub solution, scrub the intended phlebotomy site and an area approximately 3 inches in diameter around the site, continuously and randomly for at least 30 seconds.

9.0   Using the 1-% PVP-iodine solution swab, start at the intended venipuncture site and move the swab in an outward spiral. Cover the entire 3" diameter area that was initially scrubbed. DO NOT reswab any area that has already been swabbed. You may cover the venipuncture area with sterile gauze if the venipuncture is not going to be performed immediately.
NOTE: When applying the gauze, precautions should be taken to avoid contamination of the intended venipuncture site, and avoid applying pressure during application and/or removal of gauze.

9.1   Allow the iodine solution to stand for at least 30 seconds; this allows time for the iodine to properly decontaminate the venipuncture site.

9.2   DO NOT touch or repalpate the area after it has been cleaned. Do not wipe the iodine off the scrubbed area. If the area is touched or otherwise compromised, repeat the entire arm prep procedure.

NON-ROUTINE SCRUB (SOAP/ALCOHOL SOLUTIONS)

10.0   Using the tincture of green soap swab, scrub the intended phlebotomy site and an area approximately 3" in diameter around the site continuously and randomly for at least 2 minutes.

Gulf Coast Regional Blood Center
1400 La Concha
Houston, TX 77054

Uncontrolled
Reference Copy

DC SOP 301.06V7
Implementation Date: 5/7/02
Page 4 of 18

11.0   Using the acetone alcohol swab, start at the intended venipuncture site and move the swab in an outward spiral. Cover the entire 3" diameter area that was initially scrubbed. DO NOT reswab any area that has already been swabbed. Cover the venipuncture area with sterile gauze.
        NOTE: When applying the gauze, precautions should be taken to avoid contamination of the intended venipuncture site, and avoid applying pressure during application and/or removal of gauze.

   11.1   Allow the alcohol to stand for one minute or until dry; this allows time for the alcohol to properly decontaminate the venipuncture site.

   11.2   DO NOT touch or repalpate the area after it has been cleaned. If the area is touched or otherwise compromised, repeat the entire arm prep procedure.

PREPARATION OF THE BAG (WHOLE BLOOD)

NOTE: May be performed prior to performing scrub.

12.0   Write "ASA" on the upper right side of the primary bag base label if it is indicated in the medical history section of the **Donor Form** that the donor has taken aspirin or Piroxicam or medications containing either of these drugs in the past 2 days. Do not write over the bar code on the base label.

13.0   Write the blood type, if known, in the appropriate area of the primary bag base label. Do not write over the bar code on the base label.

14.0   Record the lot number of the blood bag pack in the appropriate area of the **Donor Form**.
        NOTE: It is not necessary to perform steps 12.0, 13.0 and 14.0 when using the Donor ID system.

15.0   After properly labeling the bag, place the bag on a platform scale, shaker, or weight monitor depending on the donor's weight and the donation location.

   15.1   **Platform Scales** - If the donor weighs between 110 pounds and 121 pounds, place the primary bag on the platform scale.

   15.2   **Shakers** - If the donor weighs 122 pounds or more, place the primary bag flat on the shaker platform.

        a. Thread the two (2) standing metal leg supports attached to the platform through the side loop of the bag closest to the donor bed and thread the metal leg support located at the end of the metal platform through the slit at the bottom of the bag.

        b. Hang the satellite bags on the leg support located at the back of the shaker platform.

        c. Secure the labeled vacutubes through the side loops of a satellite bag.

   15.3   **Weight Monitors -** If the donor weighs 122 pounds or over, hang the bag on the weight monitor from the slit at the bottom of the bag; this will allow the blood to travel from the tubing up into the bag through the anticoagulant.

        a. Thread the tubing as soon as possible through the cut-off groove on the Fenwal weight monitor (trip scale) or adjustable knob weight monitor and pull the tubing back and forth through the groove to ensure that it is not pinched.

        b. Hang the satellite bags from the peg on the end of the weight monitor.

        c. Secure the labeled vacutubes through the side loops of a satellite bag.

PREPARATION FOR APHERESIS COLLECTION

16.0   See the appropriate SOP for proper installation of the kits / sets for each apheresis procedure.

Gulf Coast Regional Blood Center
1400 La Concha
Houston, TX 77054

Uncontrolled
Reference Copy

DC SOP 301.06V7
Implementation Date: 5/7/02
Page 5 of 18

VENIPUNCTURE (WHOLE BLOOD)

17.0   Place a loop in the blood tubing below the LSSS.

18.0   Apply a hemostat to the blood tubing between the LSSS and the donor needle.
         NOTE: The Donor Care needle guard device should be positioned between the hemostat and the needle, closer to the needle.

   18.1   Apply adequate pressure with the tourniquet or the blood pressure cuff. Have the donor squeeze the handgrip.

19.0   Remove the cap from the needle, retract the skin firmly below the scrubbed area, and insert the needle through the skin and into the vein in one smooth motion.
         NOTE: During the collection process, the donor should be in a reclined position. If the donor is unable to be placed in a reclining position, contact the Medical Director for instructions.

20.0   While holding the needle hub, switch hands and continue to hold/stabilize the needle hub.

21.0   Release the hemostat, instruct the donor to unclench his/her fist, and watch for blood flow into the tubing.

22.0   If the initial venipuncture does not produce blood flow or an adequate blood flow, check for crimps in tubing, adjust the needle or ask for assistance.
         Do not probe in the donor's arm.

23.0   When stripping the unit to observe blood flow, strip the tubing away from the donor in a downward motion. **Never strip toward the donor.**

24.0   If the adjustment is unsuccessful, discontinue the phlebotomy.
         See: Repeat Phlebotomy - Double Stick Procedure in the Special Procedures SOP.

25.0   Engage the needle guard by sliding the device up the tubing and over one half to two thirds of the needle hub.

26.0   Secure the needle guard and tubing to the donor's arm by taping over the raised arrow.

27.0   Re-cover the venipuncture site with the gauze.

28.0   Ask the donor to open and close his/her hand slowly and continuously throughout the collection.

   28.1   Loosen / readjust the tourniquet, if necessary, for the donor's comfort.

DOCUMENTATION OF VENIPUNCTURE

NOTE: Not necessary when using Donor ID System

29.0   Document whole blood venipuncture procedure appropriately according to the *Donor Form Documentation* SOP.

   29.1   Document apheresis venipuncture procedure appropriately according to the *Apheresis Documentation* SOP.

30.0   Document the time, in military time, that the whole blood collection procedure began on the upper right side of the primary bag base label. Do not write over the bar code on the base label.

   30.1   If satellite bags are attached to the primary bag, also write the time, in military time, the collection began on the upper right side of the appropriate satellite bag.
            NOTE: On "double" bags, the time will be placed on the satellite bag with the paper label. On "triple" or "quad" bags, the time will be placed on the satellite bag with the preservation solution.

31.0   Perform the following functions as appropriate for the type of collection device being used:

Gulf Coast Regional Blood Center
1400 La Concha
Houston, TX 77054

Uncontrolled
Reference Copy

DC SOP 301.06V7
Implementation Date: 5/7/02
Page 6 of 18

31.1   If using an electric bag shaker, turn the shaker on.

31.2   <u>If using a Weight Monitor (trip scale), platform scale or adjustable knob weight monitor</u>, mix the blood and anticoagulant immediately after blood flow begins by gently inverting the bag several times. **Agitate the bag several times during the collection procedure.**

32.0   Refer to chart below for the approximate unit range (after hematroning). The weight of the primary bag should not differ significantly from the target unit range listed.
NOTE: For autologous donors who weigh less than 110 pounds, SEE: Special Procedures SOP.

Donor Weight	Target Unit Range At End Of Collection
110 - 121 lbs.	574 gms. - 606 gms.
122 lbs. – over	574 gms. - 667 gms

33.0   To identify the target weight for each apheresis procedure, see the specific apheresis procedure SOP.

34.0   Monitor the flow of blood.
NOTE: The frequent gentle inversion / agitation of the bag to mix the blood and anticoagulant, during a whole blood phlebotomy procedure, is essential to prevent clots and to provide quality blood components.

34.1   If it appears the blood flow has slowed or stopped, use strippers to check the flow. DO NOT USE HEMOSTATS.
NOTE: Excessive stripping of tubing can cause the vein to collapse and can hemolyze cells.

34.2   If palpation of the vein after the insertion of the needle is necessary, it is recommended that the procedure be done only with a GLOVED finger above the site of insertion.

34.3   Adjust the needle, if necessary, to restore blood flow.
NOTE: Turning the needle slightly will often be adequate.

35.0   If an adequate blood flow cannot be restored, discontinue phlebotomy as described in this SOP and refer to procedure for repeat phlebotomy.
NOTE: Always observe donors for adverse reactions during and after their phlebotomies.

Gulf Coast Regional Blood Center
1400 La Concha
Houston, TX 77054

Uncontrolled
Reference Copy

DC SOP 301.06V7
Implementation Date: 5/7/02
Page 7 of 18

DISCONTINUATION OF PHLEBOTOMY AND COLLECTION OF SAMPLE TUBES

NOTE: This process is performed following collection of appropriate amount of blood in the primary bag. WEAR GLOVES ON BOTH HANDS.

36.0 Clamp the donor tubing with a hemostat below the SampLink sampling site.

37.0 Instruct the donor to stop squeezing the handgrip.

38.0 If using grommets and crimper or heat sealer, apply two grommets or two heat seals, on the tubing below the SampLink sampling site.

39.0 If using grommets, close the grommets with the crimper.

40.0 Alternatively, discontinue the phlebotomy by tightening the loop in the tubing to form a tight knot approximately one inch below the SampLink sampling site.
NOTE: The tightening of the loop in the tubing will prevent air contamination of the blood and ensures that samples are being collected from the donors vein yielding blood samples undiluted with anticoagulant.

41.0 Verify knot is tied, grommets are closed or that heat seals are intact.

42.0 Remove the hemostat below the SampLink sampling site.

43.0 Remove the SampLink Access Device from the sterile package, using aseptic technique.
NOTE: The SampLink Access Device must not be removed from the package until ready for immediate use.

44.0 Mount the SampLink Access Device on the SampLink sampling site.

45.0 Align the "⌐" shaped slots of the SampLink Access Device with the tubing on both sides of the SampLink sampling site.

46.0 Rotate the SampLink Access Device clockwise until it stops.

47.0 Remove the vacutubes from the satellite bags.
Note: If the donor is complaining about the tourniquet being too tight before vacutubes are collected, you may loosen the tourniquet, but do not remove it until sample collection is complete.

48.0 Insert a purple vacutube, stopper first, so that the needle pierces the concave center of the vacutube.

49.0 Once the tube is full, pull the sample tube to remove it from the needle protector device.

50.0 Insert the red vacutube.

51.0 Remove the tube, and insert the next two purple vacutubes until all four vacutubes have been collected.

52.0 Gently invert each purple-top vacutube several times after filling.

53.0 Release the tourniquet or the blood pressure cuff on the donor's arm after all vacutubes have been collected.

54.0 Whenever blood cannot be collected in the vacutube(s),:

- Send the labeled vacutube(s) back with the unit as normal.
- Document in the Comment Section of the **Donor Form** what has occurred with the vacutube(s).

55.0 If any tube does not fill:

- Get another tube of the same type and fill it.
- Apply a bar coded identification number sticker to the tube.

Gulf Coast Regional Blood Center
1400 La Concha
Houston, TX 77054

Uncontrolled
Reference Copy

DC SOP 301.06V7
Implementation Date: 5/7/02
Page 8 of 18

> ***NOTE: Fill no more than 5, 7 mL vacuum tubes per SampLink Access Device, preventing blood leakage into the SampLink Access Device. Never reuse a SampLink Access Device.***

56.0 If an extra sticker is not available:

- Remove the label from the tube that did not fill; and apply it to the new tube.
- Have the supervisor or another person witness as you apply the barcode to the additional tube(s).
- Clear adhesive tape may be used to secure the number.
- Release tourniquet or blood pressure cuff after last tube is filled.

57.0 See procedure **Obtaining a Sample if SampLink Collection Fails**, if unable to obtain any vacuum tubes from the donor.

58.0 Dispose of the unfilled tubes in a biohazard sharps container.

59.0 Apply a hemostat to the blood tubing below the DonorCare Needle Guard and above the SampLink sampling site.

60.0 Lift gauze and view angle of needle placement.

61.0 Hold the DonorCare Needle Guard with thumb and forefinger at the raised arrow end.

62.0 Hold donor tubing below hemostat with thumb and two to three fingers.

    62.1 Ask the donor to apply pressure to the venipuncture site immediately after hearing the clicking sound of the needle guard (if the donor is able to do so).

63.0 Pull swiftly (following same angle as needle placement) until needle is removed from the donor's arm and you hear the needle click and lock in the needle guard.
NOTE: When pulling donor tubing to remove needle and needle guard, make sure to pull at the same angle as the donor needle is placed in the arm/vein. Pulling at a different angle or direction may cause donor discomfort and/or hematoma.

64.0 Remove the tape and needle guard from the donor's arm.

    64.1 If the donor is able, have the donor raise his/her arm straight up and hold pressure over the venipuncture site with his/her other hand for approximately two minutes. If the donor is not able to apply pressure, have the donor bend his/her arm for approximately two minutes. If venipunctures were performed in both arms, the donor may bend both arms for approximately two minutes.

65.0 Securely loop the red and purple top tubes to the primary blood bag.

66.0 Insert the needle guard with attached needle into the Samplink access device.

67.0 If there is a blood spill or needle injury, follow guidelines in the Blood Center Safety Manual for reporting a blood spill or needle injury.

RECHECK LABELING

68.0 At the donor's bed, check the bar coded unit identification numbers on the **Donor Form**, primary and satellite bags, and test sample tubes. Verify that all numbers are identical and present in each required location.

    68.1 If an omission is noted, notify the supervisor/designee. Have him/her witness as you apply a bar code to the appropriate area and generate a QIR.

    68.2 If a discrepancy that cannot be corrected at the bedside is noted, initiate an investigation to determine the cause. Attach a **Quarantined Component Tag** to the unit(s) that may be implicated in the discrepancy and generate a QIR.

Gulf Coast Regional Blood Center
1400 La Concha
Houston, TX 77054

Uncontrolled
Reference Copy

DC SOP 301.06V7
Implementation Date: 5/7/02
Page 9 of 18

DOCUMENTATION OF DISCONTINUANCE OF PHLEBOTOMY

NOTE: Not necessary when using Donor ID System

69.0 Document the discontinuation of the phlebotomy procedure appropriately according to the *Donor Form Documentation* SOP and/or *Apheresis Procedure Documentation* SOP.

69.1 When applicable, appropriately complete and attach a **Quarantined Component Tag**.
NOTE: If a Double Stick is performed, indicate this on the Donor Form and write "DS" in the center right side of the base label of the primary bag from the first venipuncture.

69.2 Take the unit, test sample tubes, and **Donor Form** to the hematroning area.

69.3 Perform hematroning procedure appropriately. SEE "Unit Storage Preparation and Disposition" SOP.

70.0 One employee should not perform all the procedures involved in the collection of a unit of whole blood (screen, collect and hematron). However, in circumstances when it is necessary for one employee to perform all of these procedures, another employee must be available to review the **Donor Form**, the unit of blood, and the test samples for potential discrepancies or errors.

POST-PHLEBOTOMY CARE

71.0 Check the venipuncture site after at least two minutes of applied pressure to ensure the bleeding has stopped and that there are no visible signs of a hematoma. In the event of an arterial stick or a hematoma.
SEE: Donor Collections Donor/Visitor Incidents: Recognition, Treatment, and Documentation procedures.

71.1 Re-apply pressure to the site, if bleeding has not stopped.

71.2 Clean the donor's arm around the venipuncture site with alcohol, once bleeding has stopped.
NOTE: DO NOT use iodine removal pads to clean donors arm.

72.0 Apply a clean pressure bandage to the venipuncture site.

72.1 Once the donor has rested and exhibits no sign(s) of an adverse reaction, they may be released from the phlebotomy area.

- Assist the donor to a sitting position.
- **Do not leave a donor unattended!**
a. Prior to releasing the donor, explain the post donation instructions.
b. If the donor feels ready and exhibits no symptoms of a donor reaction, assist the donor off the bed supporting the arm in which the venipuncture was performed. Release and direct the donor to the refreshment area and recommend that he/she consume refreshments. If possible, escort the donor to the area.
c. If the donor does not feel well or exhibits symptoms of a donor reaction, have the donor remain on the bed until symptoms subside. Follow instructions provided in "Recognition and Treatment of Adverse Reactions" procedures, as necessary.
d. Thank the donor for his/her donation.

NON-ROUTINE COLLECTION PROCEDURES

Dry Sticks (Plateletpheresis Procedures only) – A procedure in which no blood was collected in the disposable or sample pouch, and the final product volume is less than 1 mL.

Gulf Coast Regional Blood Center
1400 La Concha
Houston, TX 77054

Uncontrolled
Reference Copy

DC SOP 301.06V7
Implementation Date: 5/7/02
Page 10 of 18

NOTE: If this donation type is used, a Double Stick should not be performed.

73.0   Dry Stick plateletpheresis procedures should be performed in the following manner:

73.1   Write "Dry Stick" or "Dry" in the ABO area of both of the platelet storage containers and labeled sample tubes below the BUI number.

73.2   Place the storage container and labeled vacutubes in an appropriately labeled plastic bag, then in the aerated basket.

73.3   Draw a single line through the donation type on the front page of the **Donor Form**, and document "Dry" or "Dry Stick" adjacent to the original product type. Initial and date the documentation.

73.4   Document the reason for the dry stick in the Comment Section of the **Donor Form** along with your initials and date.

73.5   Change the donation type in SafeTrace to "Dry Stick" to properly reconcile the change in the phlebotomy area and Donor Form.

DOUBLE STICK-- IF FIRST COLLECTION PROCEDURE IS UNSUCCESSFUL:

74.0   If a second venipuncture will be performed, do not collect samples from the first unit. However, after needle removal apply the needle protection device over the needle and follow procedure for discontinuance of phlebotomy as described in this SOP.

74.1   Prior to the performance of a second venipuncture, weigh the unit and tubing from the initial venipuncture. If the total weight is **166 gms.** or less, a second venipuncture may be performed with the donor's consent.

74.2   Ask the donor if he/she is willing to have a second venipuncture; do not pressure the donor.

a.   If the donor is not willing to have a second venipuncture performed, the first venipuncture will be considered a QNS. Refer to instructions described in this SOP for documentation and labeling of a QNS.

74.3   If the donor is willing, examine the arm opposite the one in which the first venipuncture was performed to determine arm suitability. The second venipuncture MUST be done in the opposite arm; unless otherwise authorized by the Medical Director.

WHOLE BLOOD DOUBLE STICK

75.0   Transfer the first whole blood bag to the hematron area.

a.   Package the first venipuncture bag for transport to the laboratory by folding the primary blood bag over the satellite bags; and wrapping the in-line tubing snugly around the primary bag.

b.   Place the blood bag pack and labeled vacutubes in an appropriately labeled plastic bag, then in the aerated basket.

c.   If the donor leaves the phlebotomy area between the first and second venipuncture, upon the donor's return, verify the donor's identity as described in this SOP.

d.   Complete the appropriate information on the Donor Form.
       NOTE: Not necessary when using Donor ID System

e.   Write "DS" in the center right side of the base label of the primary bag from the first venipuncture.

f.   Place an "X' over the original bar code number and the "Phlebotomy 1" area on the Donor Form with black or blue indelible ink, and initial and date. Write "Double stick performed" or a similar statement, in the Comments Section of the **Donor Form**. Initial and date the documentation.

Gulf Coast Regional Blood Center
1400 La Concha
Houston, TX 77054

Uncontrolled
Reference Copy

DC SOP 301.06V7
Implementation Date: 5/7/02
Page 11 of 18

g. Mark "QNS" as the "Completion Code" in the "Phlebotomy 1 area" for the initial phlebotomy procedure

h. Follow the procedures for preparation of the second blood bag as described in Review and Labeling SOP. **DO NOT** peel off the bar coded label set from the back of the first blood bag.

- Obtain a new bag. Obtain a new bar coded label set and apply the new bar coded stickers to the base labels of the new bags and *Donor Form*.

- Obtain a new set of vacutubes and apply the new bar coded stickers as described in Review and Labeling Procedures.

i. Record the lot number of the new bag in the appropriate area of the *Donor Form*. *NOTE: Not necessary when using Donor ID System*

j. Follow the appropriate procedures for vein selection, arm preparation, and venipuncture.

k. Once the second venipuncture has been performed, mark and/or record as applicable the following phlebotomy information in the appropriate sections of the *Donor Form*.

- Left and right arm

- Collection device number

- Start time of phlebotomy

- Your initials and employee ID number, which identifies you as the second phlebotomist.

NOTE: 1) The DC time of the first stick need not be recorded when a double stick is performed.

- *Step H not necessary when using Donor ID System*

2) If the second attempt also resulted in a "QNS", do not attempt a third venipuncture. Routinely the donor must be placed on a 56-day rest for any subsequent whole blood donations.

l. If the repeat phlebotomy-double stick is unsuccessful, discontinue the phlebotomy as described in this SOP. *NOTE: In the "SafeTrace" system, if a "QNS" occurs, and a double stick has been performed, the first venipuncture attempt will be indicated as "No Yield" in the "Donor Count Summary" screen.*

APHERESIS DOUBLE STICK

NOTE: 1) Whenever an apheresis venipuncture is performed on a donor and an Apheresis Kit and/or venipuncture site is changed, or a donor is moved to another instrument, it is considered a "Double Stick".

2) IF ANY BLOOD VOLUME HAS BEEN COLLECTED IN THE SAMPLE POUCH OR THE IN-LINE TUBING, A SECOND VENIPUNCTURE MAY NOT BE PERFORMED.

76.0 If a second apheresis blood venipuncture is attempted or the disposable set is changed (or if the donor is moved to a different apparatus).

a. Seal and remove the storage container from the initial kit.

b. Write "DS" in the upper right hand corner of the storage container.

c. Place an "X' over the original bar code number which is attached to the storage container with black or blue indelible ink, and initial and date.

d. Apply the BUI number set to the back of the storage container.

e. Place the storage container and labeled vacutubes in an appropriately labeled plastic bag, then in the aerated basket.

f. Remove the old Apheresis Kit from the instrument and discard appropriately.

Gulf Coast Regional Blood Center
1400 La Concha
Houston, TX 77054

Uncontrolled
Reference Copy

DC SOP 301.06V7
Implementation Date: 5/7/02
Page 12 of 18

g. If the donor leaves the phlebotomy area between the first and second venipuncture, upon the donor's return, verify the donor's identity as described in this SOP.

h. Retrieve a new Apheresis Kit and install onto instrument or move the donor to another apheresis instrument as outlined in the appropriate SOP.
   - Follow the instructions listed in the appropriate SOP for moving a donor from one apheresis instrument to another instrument.
   - If the technician moving the donor from the initial instrument is not trained for the instrument the donor is being moved to, a technician which is trained for the second instrument must assist in the move, write the explanation in the comment section, and initial and date the explanation.

i. Retrieve a new Blood Unit Identification label set.
   - Place an "X" over the original bar code number and the "Phlebotomy 1" area of the **Donor Form**. Initial and date the documentation.
   - Place the new bar code number in the appropriate area of the **Donor Form**.
   - On the specific apheresis device procedural records. place an "X" over the original bar code number, initial and date.
   - Place the new bar code number in the appropriate area of the apheresis procedural record.
   - For plateletpheresis, on the **Evaluation of Apheresis Platelet Products Form**, place an "X" over the original bar code number, initial and date.
   - Place the new BUI barcode sticker on the **Evaluation of Apheresis Platelet Products Form** and complete all required information on this form.
   - Return the **Evaluation of Apheresis Platelet Products Form**, and any specific apheresis procedure record, along with the product samples, to the laboratory.

j. Apply the new bar code stickers to the apheresis product bags.

k. Obtain a new set of vacutubes and apply the new bar coded stickers as described in the appropriate SOP.

l. If the procedure was a two-arm procedure and the second venipuncture fails, the donor may be moved to a single arm plasma procedure only, using the first venipuncture.
   NOTE: It is unnecessary to document the DC time of the second venipuncture from the initial two-arm procedure when the donor is being moved to a single arm plasma procedure. However, the DC time from the single arm plasma procedure must be documented appropriately in the PHLEBOTOMY section of the Donor Form.
   - This procedure is considered a "Double Stick" and should be handled and documented in the same manner as outlined in the steps listed above.
   - The transfer must be documented in the Comments Section on the back of the **Donor Form** (EXAMPLE: "Donor started on two arm procedure, second venipuncture failed, moved to single arm plasma using first venipuncture") or a similar statement, then initial and date.
   - Draw one line through the previously recorded information, and record the new information in all appropriate areas on the **Donor Form** and the appropriate apheresis procedural record. Initial and date all changes.

m. Follow the procedures for vein selection, arm prep, and venipuncture. Once the second venipuncture has been performed, record the following phlebotomy information in the appropriate sections of the "PHLEBOTOMY 2" section: left or right arm, scale number, time phlebotomy begun, and employee ID number of the second phlebotomist.

IF A WHOLE BLOOD OR APHERESIS REPEAT PHLEBOTOMY/DOUBLE STICK WILL NOT BE PERFORMED:

Gulf Coast Regional Blood Center
1400 La Concha
Houston, TX 77054

Uncontrolled
Reference Copy

DC SOP 301.06V7
Implementation Date: 5/7/02
Page 13 of 18

77.0 If a second venipuncture will not be performed:
NOTE: In the "SafeTrace" system, if a "QNS" occurs (a double stick has not been performed), the venipuncture attempt will be indicated as "No Yield" in the "Donor Count Summary" screen.

    77.1 Mark "QNS":on:

        a. Appropriate section of the **Donor Form.**

        b. WHOLE BLOOD -on the **Quarantined Component Tag** and attach tag to the primary bag.

        c. APHERESIS - on the **Quarantined Component Tag** (which is attached to the apheresis product bag) and the appropriate apheresis procedural record and Cumulative Data Sheet.

        d. Sample tubes.

    77.2 Record on the **Donor Form** the time (military time) the needle was removed from the donor's vein.

        a. Record your initials and employee ID number appropriately on the **Donor Form**.

    77.3 Record your employee initials, ID number, and date appropriately on the **Quarantined Component Tag**.

    77.4 Transfer the donor record, and collection bag/kit as applicable to the hematron area following appropriate documentation and review.
NOTE: In apheresis procedures, place the needle into a nearby sharps container

WHOLE BLOOD COLLECTIONS THAT DO NOT MEET STANDARDS

General Information

78.0 How to determine if unit is QNS:

    a. The unit is **acceptable** if it weighs:

      - Approximately 574 gms. to 606 gms. for donors weighing 110-121lbs.
      - Approximately 574 gms. to 667 gms. for donors weighing 122 lbs. and over prior to discontinuance of phlebotomy.

    b. The unit is **not acceptable** if:

      - A unit in which the **WHOLE BLOOD** primary bag and its contents weigh **less than** 574 **gms.** (after hematroning has been performed; without the weight of the test tubes) will be considered **QNS**.

    c. **For apheresis procedures** - If the weight is less than required, record the weight of the unit in the appropriate area of the appropriate apheresis procedural record, if applicable.

      - For **PLATELET COMPONENTS**, units weighing **0-99 gms.** will be considered **QNS**; units weighing **100-500 gms.** will be considered a **Complete Unit**.
      - For **PLASMA** components, units weighing: **0-179 gms.** will be considered **QNS**; units weighing **180-600 gms.** will be considered a **Complete Unit**.
      - For **SPLIT PLATELET PRODUCTS,** the product weight limit is **100-500 gms**.

79.0 How to determine if unit is An Over Draw (OD).

    a. An overdraw is a unit in which the **WHOLE BLOOD** primary bag and its contents (after hematroning has been performed; without the weight of the test tubes) weigh more than:

Gulf Coast Regional Blood Center
1400 La Concha
Houston, TX 77054

Uncontrolled
Reference Copy

DC SOP 301.06V7
Implementation Date: 5/7/02
Page 14 of 18

- **606 gms.** for donors weighing 110-121 lbs. In this case, try to record the exact donor weight in the comments section of the donor record and in the appropriate area of the *Quarantined Component Tag*.
- **667 gms**. for donors weighing 122 lbs. and over.

80.0 Attach a *Quarantined Component Tag* to the primary bag of all whole blood units that do not meet standards.
NOTE: This excludes Double Sticks – "DS".

80.1 Obtain and complete a *Quarantined Component Tag.*

80.2 Appropriately mark, record or affix the following on or to the tag:

a. Unit #.

b. Reason the unit was quarantined.
- If a unit is quarantined due to an overdraw, document the donor's weight in the appropriate area of the *Quarantined Component Tag.*
- If a unit is quarantined because information obtained indicated the donor was not acceptable, also mark as applicable "Medical Information" and/or "Vital Signs".

c. Comments (if applicable).

d. Initials and/or ID number of person who completes the *Quarantined Component Tag.*

e. Date unit tagged.

f. If the unit is leaking, wrap the *Quarantine Component Tag* around the outside of the appropriately labeled plastic bag and secure with a rubber band.

g. If the blood bag has a defective canula (blood from the primary bag is leaking into a satellite bag), tape the tubing and attach a note and send the unit to the laboratory. Document in Comments Section of the *Donor Form* - "Defective Canula". Initial and date the documentation.

QUANTITY NOT SUFFICIENT (QNS)

NOTE: See "Unit Storage and Preparation" SOP

81.0 If a unit is suspected to be usable for transfusion.

81.1 Hematron the unit as you would for a routine collection.

81.2 Appropriately complete and attach a *Quarantined Component Tag* to the unit.

81.3 Place the bag in an aerated basket.

81.4 Place the tubes in tube rack and cooler for final transport to laboratory.

OVERDRAW (OD)

82.0 If a unit is suspected to be an "OD" (bag apparently filled beyond capacity), hematron the unit as you would for a routine whole blood collection.

82.1 Mark 'OD" in the appropriate area of the *Donor Form*.

82.2 Place the sample tubes in the rack. Place the rack, with tubes, into a refrigerator / refrigerated blood cooler; this is recommended within one hour of collection.
CAUTION: extended time at room temperature will destroy the virus and could give a false negative reading.

82.3 Appropriately complete and attach a *Quarantined Component Tag* to the primary bag of the unit.

Gulf Coast Regional Blood Center
1400 La Concha
Houston, TX 77054

Uncontrolled
Reference Copy

DC SOP 301.06V7
Implementation Date: 5/7/02
Page 15 of 18

82.4 Appropriately complete and attach a *Quarantined Component Tag* to the primary bag of the unit.

82.5 Place the bag in an aerated basket until final transport.

DIFFICULT STICKS (DIFF)

83.0 Phlebotomies in which the needle had to be readjusted or repositioned several times or the in-line tubing was constantly checked, by stripping, for an adequate blood flow (regardless of the actual bleed time) are considered difficult sticks. RBCs and plasma for manufacturing use can be prepared from these units. However, platelets, cryoprecipitate, and fresh frozen plasma cannot.

83.1 Mark "DIFF" on the *Quarantined Component Tag* and attach the tag to the primary bag of the unit.

83.2 Hematron the unit as you would a routine whole blood collection.

83.3 Place the sample tubes in the rack. Place the rack, with tubes, into a refrigerator / refrigerated blood cooler; this is recommended within one hour of collection. **CAUTION: extended time at room temperature will destroy the virus and could give a false negative reading.**
SEE: Appendix 1.0 for appropriate temperature parameters.

83.4 Place the bag in an aerated basket until ready for transport to the laboratory.

SLOW DRAW

84.0 Phlebotomies which take longer than 15 minutes, without frequent needle adjustments or excessive stripping are considered slow draw.

84.1 Document "Slow Draw" or similar statement in the comment section of the Donor Form. Initial and date the documentation.

84.2 Mark "Other" on the *Quarantined Component Tag* and attach the tag to the primary bag of the unit.

84.3 Hematron the unit as you would a routine whole blood collection.

84.4 Place the sample tubes in the rack. Place the rack, with tubes, into a refrigerator / refrigerated blood cooler; this is recommended within one hour of collection. **CAUTION: extended time at room temperature will destroy the virus and could give a false negative reading.**
SEE: Appendix 1.0 for appropriate temperature parameters.

84.5 Place the bag in an aerated basket until ready for transport to the laboratory.

QUARANTINED COMPONENTS (Q)

85.0 Quarantined Components ("Q") - a component of blood which may not be used because of one of the following occurrences:

- Unit was contaminated with air.
- Blood bag is leaking after venipuncture has been performed.
- Donor was drawn inappropriately - information from medical history indicated that donor should not have been eligible to donate.
- Unknown information (medication, medical condition, immunizations, etc..) approved by the supervisor on site.
- Donor volunteered information during or after phlebotomy that disqualifies donor from donation eligibility.

85.1 Hematron the unit as you would for a routine whole blood collection. Write "Q" on the sample tubes.

Gulf Coast Regional Blood Center
1400 La Concha
Houston, TX 77054

Uncontrolled
Reference Copy

DC SOP 301.06V7
Implementation Date: 5/7/02
Page 16 of 18

85.2 Document the appropriate reason for the "Q" on the **Donor Form,** and the apheresis procedural record, if applicable. Initial and date the documentation.

85.3 Place the sample tubes in the rack. Place the rack, with tubes, into a refrigerator / refrigerated blood cooler; this is recommended within one hour of collection. **CAUTION: extended time at room temperature will destroy the virus and could give a false negative reading**.

85.4 Appropriately complete and attach a **Quarantined Component Tag** to the primary bag of the unit.

85.5 Place the bag in an aerated basket until later transport back to the laboratory for disposal.

    a. Do not place any separated blood segments from the unit in the labeled vacutubes. It is important that the blood segments remain attached to the unit. Whenever no blood is collected in the vacutubes, send the labeled vacutubes back with the unit as normal. Note in the Comment Section of the **Donor Form** what has occurred with the vacutubes. Initial and date the documentation.

NOTES

None

REFERENCES

1.0 Vengelen-Tyler, ed. Technical Manual. Bethesda, MD: American Association of Blood Banks.

2.0 Code of Federal Regulations. Current edition. Washington, DC: U.S. Government Printing Office.

3.0 American Association of Blood Banks Association Bulletin #96-6, regarding Bacterial Contamination of Blood Components, August 7, 1996.

4.0 AABB Monthly Newsletter

5.0 Baxter Fenwal Insert Needle/Tube Sampling Protector.

6.0 Documentation Preparation and Review - SOP#217.00

7.0 Reporting An Incident With The Quality Improvement Report Procedure - SOP #267.00

8.0 Donor Form Documentation - SOP #301.02

9.0 Donor Deferment - SOP #301.05

10.0 Unit Storage Preparation and Disposition - SOP#301.07

11.0 Donor/Visitor Incident Recognition Treatment and Documentation - SOP #301.08

12.0 Special Procedures - SOP #301.09

13.0 Review and Labeling - SOP #301.10

14.0 Obtaining a Sample if SampLink Collection Fails - SOP #301.12

15.0 Apheresis Documentation - SOP #414.00

16.0 Redi Product Suggested Procedure for Venipuncture Site Preparation (Operand Topical Povidone Iodine Gel)

17.0 The Blood Center Safety Manual

Gulf Coast Regional Blood Center
1400 La Concha
Houston, TX 77054

Uncontrolled
Reference Copy

DC SOP 301.06V7
Implementation Date: 5/7/02
Page 17 of 18

RECORDS, REPORTS OR JOB AIDS

1.0   Donor Record (GC 300)-(GC302)

2.0   Evaluation of Apheresis Platelet Products Form - (GC 358)

APPENDICES

None

DOCUMENT INFORMATION

Document Owner: DC

Document ID #: 301.06

Version #: 7

CURRENT DATA

Author: RCHAPA

Validation Date: 3/12/02

Approval Date: 4/10/02

Training Date: 5/2/02

Implementation Date: 5/7/02

Authorized Copy Identification: AUDI, METHODIST HOSPITAL; 1 COPY EACH

BCET – 5 COPIES, DCF/M – 43 COPIES

Procedure Records/Report/Job Aid ID #s: GC 300,GC302,GC 358. Blood Center Safety Manual

Referenced Procedures ID #s: Documentation Preparation and Review - SOP#217.00
Reporting An Incident With The Quality Improvement Report - SOP #267.00
Donor Form Documentation - SOP #301.02
Donor Deferment - SOP #301.05
Unit Storage Preparation and Disposition - SOP#301.07
Donor/Visitor Incident Recognition Treatment and Documentation - SOP #301.08
Special Procedures - SOP #301.09
Review and Labeling - SOP #301.10
Obtaining a Sample if SampLink Collection Fails - SOP #301.12
Apheresis Documentation - SOP #414.00

REGULATORY STANDARDS

GCRBC: QA Quality Plan

AABB: Current

FDA: 606.100(B), 606.160, 640.3, 640.63, 640.21

Other (specify):
RETIRED DOCUMENTS

Document ID #s 301.06V6
REVISION HISTORY

Date Original SOP Implemented: 12/02/98

Date Revision Implemented/V4 – 3/6/00; Delete instructions to tag rare donor units, instructions to use
Change Description: new gel arm scrub,
Date Revision Implemented/V5 – 8/17/00- Date Revision Implemented/V6 – Scope procedure steps –
Change Description: 1.0, 3.1a, 7.4, 24.1, 33.0, 34.0 –
Date Revision Implemented/V7 SampLink procedure, venipunture section changed, Step 3.0 added note,
Change Description: STEPS 17.0 THROUGH 28.1, and STEPS 36.0 THROUGH 69.0, Changed unit weight
range tables, STEP 32.0 TABLE, 78.0 a & b, removed step 38.0 and re-numbered, 79.0A
THROUGH 79.1A, Deleted "scissors" from Materials section, changed note to step 56.0
number of sample tubes from 6 to 5, added step 58.0, removed steps 66.0 and 67.0

Date Revision Implemented/
Change Description **Step 3.0** - Added a note to this step that requires that the signature on the informed consent statement be verified and matches the name in the demographic section of the donor form, if legible. (If the signature is not legible you should ask the donor if that's their signature.)

Step 32.0 - Table was revised to include a new minimum weight of a blood bag to 574 grams.

Step 38.0 - Removed the step that required that the whole blood unit and satellite bags be removed from the scales and placed at the foot of the donor bed to draw samples. (Re-numbered remaining steps.)

Step 47.0 - Revised step to require that tourniquet remain on the donors arm during sample collection.

Steps 48.0 - 51.0 - Changed the order in which tubes should be drawn. You should now collect a **purple** top tube first, then a **red** top and complete the sample procedure by drawing the last **two purple top tubes**.

Step 62.1 - added "if donor is able to do so" in parenthesis.

Step 78.0 a and b - changed the minimum weight to 574 grams.

Appendix 8

UNITS OF MEASUREMENT AND SYMBOLS

The JCAHO has published 2004 National Patient Safety Goals that call for compliance with a "minimum list of dangerous abbreviations, acronyms and symbols." In addition, the Institute for Safe Medication Practices (ISMP) has published a "List of Error-Prone Abbreviations, Symbols, and Dose Designations" with additional abbreviations. The aim is to eliminate misinterpretations of written information. Selected recommendations from both have been incorporated into this appendix as they may apply to phlebotomy practices, however this list is not exhaustive. For more comprehensive information, consult their websites, www.jcaho.org and www.ismp.org, respectively.

a	alpha
Å	angstrom
amp	ampere (unit of electric current)
and	formerly written as symbol "&", should now be a written word
at	formerly written as symbol "@", should now be a written word
c	centi- (10^{-2})
°C	degrees centigrade or Celsius (unit of temperature)
cubic centimeter	(same as ml) formerly written as "cc", it should not be abbreviated
cd	candela (unit of luminous intensity)
cm	centimeter
cu mm	cubic millimeter
d	deci- (10^{-1})
discharge	formerly written as "D/C", it should not be abbreviated
discontinue	formerly written as "D/C", it should not be abbreviated
dl	deciliter (1/10 of a liter)
°F	degrees Fahrenheit (unit of temperature)
g or gm	gram (1/1000 of a kilogram, unit of mass)
G%	grams in 100 mL
h	hecto- (10^{2})
hpf	high-power field on microscope
international unit	formerly written as "IU", it should not be abbreviated
k	kilo- (10^{3})
°K	degrees Kelvin (thermodynamic temperature)
kg	kilogram (1000 g, or 2.2 lb)
l	liter (1000 ml, unit of volume)
less (greater) than	formerly written as symbols, "< or >", or should now be written words
lpf	low-power field on microscope
mcg	microgram (1/1000 mg)

m	meter (unit of length)
m	milli- (10^{-3})
mCi	millicurie
mEq or meq	milliequivalent
mg	milligram (1/1000 g)
mg%	milligrams in 100 ml (same as dl)
min	minutes
mL	milliliter (1/1000 L, same as a cubic centimeter)
mm	millimeter (1/10 cm)
mm^3	cubic millimeter
mm Hg	millimeters of mercury
mmole	millimole
mol, M	mole (unit of substance)
mOsm	milliosmol
µm	micrometer (formerly called a micron), (1/1000 of mm)
N	normality
n	nano- (10^{-9})
ng	nanogram (1/1000 mg)
p	pico- (10^{-12})
pg	picogram (1/1000 ng)
QNS	quantity not sufficient
sec or s	second (unit of time)
sp g	specific gravity
TPN	total parenteral nutrition
TPR	temperature, pulse, respirations
Unit	formerly written as "U", it should not be abbreviated
WNL	within normal limits
WNR	within normal range
wt	weight
w/v	weight/volume

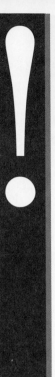

Clinical Alert: Trailing Zeros, Decimal Points, Periods, Spacing, and Latin Abbreviations

Be particularly mindful when you are hand writing data or reading handwritten information. The following symbols are often misread and can lead to errors in patient care. If you read symbols that are unclear, you should ask for clarification prior to proceeding with any type of phlebotomy procedure.

Trailing zeros: do not use a zero alone *after* a decimal point because the reader may not notice the decimal point. (For example: 3.0 ml might be mistaken for 30 ml; instead write 3 ml)

Decimal point: always use a zero before a decimal point when the measurement is less than a whole unit so the reader notices the decimal point. (For example: .5 ml might be mistaken for 5 ml; instead write 0.5 ml)

Periods: do not use a terminal period after a symbol for a unit of measurement because it may be interpreted as another symbol. (For example: 7 ml. might be mistaken for 7 ml1, which is meaningless; instead write 7 ml)

Spacing: use adequate space between numbers and letter symbols so that they will not run together. (For example: 8ml might be mistaken as 8001 if the "m" is mistaken for zeros; instead write 8 ml)

Latin abbreviations: use exact meaning of words rather than Latin abbreviations. (For example: instead of the terms "q.i.d., q.o.d., t.i.d.", refer to "once daily, every other day, three times per day," respectively and they should be written as such.)

Appendix 9

FORMULAS, CALCULATIONS, AND METRIC CONVERSION

Area   square meter (sq m or m^2)

Blood volume   Total blood volume = weight (kg) × average blood volume per kg (defined by age)

Clearance   liter/second (l/s)

Concentration and conversions

  Mass   kilogram/liter (kg/l)

  Substrate   mole/liter (mol/l)

% w/v to M or vice versa:

$$M = \frac{\% \text{ w/v} \times 10}{\text{molecular wt (mol wt)}}$$

% w/v to N or vice versa:

$$N = \frac{\% \text{ w/v} \times 10}{\text{eq wt}}$$

mg/dl to mEq/l or vice versa:

$$\text{mEq/l} = \frac{\text{mg/dl} \times 10}{\text{eq wt}}$$

M to N:

$$N = M \times \text{valence}$$

N to M:

$$M = \frac{N}{\text{valence}}$$

Density   kilogram/liter (kg/l)

Dilutions   Final concentration = Original concentration × dilution 1 × dilution 2, etc.

Hematology math   Mean corpuscular volume (MCV) = average volume of red blood cells (RBCs); expressed in cubic microns (μm^3) or femtoliters (fL)

$$\text{MCV} = \frac{\text{Hct} \times 10}{\text{RBC count (in millions)}}$$

Hct = hematocrit value

Mean corpuscular hemoglobin (MCH) = Average weight of hemoglobin in RBC; expressed in picograms (pg)

$$MCH = \frac{\text{hgb (g)} \times 10}{\text{RBC count (in millions)}}$$

$$\text{hgb} = \text{hemoglobin value}$$

Mean corpuscular hemoglobin concentration = Hemoglobin concentration of average RBC

$$MCHC = \frac{\text{hgb (g)}}{\text{Hct}} \times 100\%$$

RBC distribution width (RDW) = numerical expression of variation of RBC size, dispersion of RBC volumes about the mean

$$RDW = \frac{\text{SD (standard deviation) of RBC size}}{\text{MCV}}$$

Metric Conversions
  Length or Distance

1 inch (in) = 2.54 centimeters (cm)
1 foot (ft) = 30.48 centimeters (cm)
39.37 inches (in.) = 1 meter (m) (Note: 1 meter is slightly more than 3 feet.)
1 mile (mi) = 1.61 kilometers (km)

  Mass or Weight

1 ounce (oz) = 28.35 grams (g)
1 pound (lb) = 453.6 grams (g)
2.205 pounds (lb) = 1 kilogram (kg)

  Volume (Cubic centimeter, cc, is interchangeable with milliliter, ml, e.g., 1 cc = 1 mL)

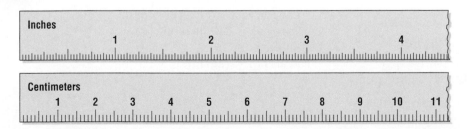

Figure A9–1. Comparison of Standard and Metric Units of Length

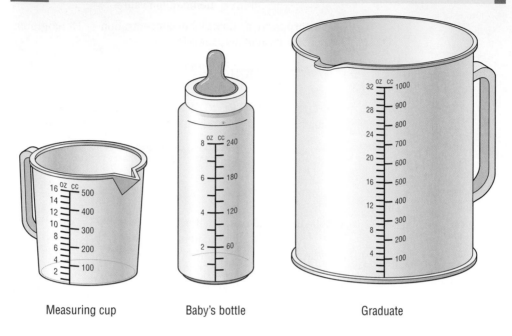

Measuring cup   Baby's bottle   Graduate

- They are all calibrated.
- They are made of metal, glass, or plastic.
- They are used for measuring liquids in cubic centimeters (cc).
- They are used for measuring liquids in ounces (oz).
- The measuring cup is used to measure liquids in the home.
- The baby's bottle is used to measure liquids in the home.
- The calibrated graduate is used to measure fluid in the health care institution.

1 fluid ounce (fl oz) = 29.57 milliliters (ml) (Note: 1 ounce is about 30 ml = 30 cc.)

1.057 quarts (qt) = 1 liter (liter or l)

1 gallon (gal) = 3.78 liters (liter or l)

Military Time	See Appendix 10
Pressure	Pascal (Pa) $= (kg/m)s^2$

Quality control math:

Variance (s^2)

$$s^2 = \frac{(x - \bar{x})^2}{n - 1}$$

Standard deviation (s)

$$s = \sqrt{s^2}$$

% Coefficient of variation

$$\% \text{ CV} = \frac{s}{\bar{x}} \times 100$$

Relative centrifugal force (rcf)

Measures force of centrifugation acting on blood components and allowing them to separate. Can be used to calibrate centrifuges.

$$\text{rcf} = 1.118 \times 10^{-5} \times 4 \times n^2$$

$$r = \text{rotating radius (centimeters)}$$

$$n = \text{speed of rotation (revolutions per minute)}$$

Specific gravity (sp g):

$$\text{sp } g = \frac{\text{wt of solid or liquid}}{\text{wt of equal volume of } H_2O \text{ at } 4°C}$$

Temperature:

Celsius or Centigrade

$$°C = K - 273.15; °C = °F - 32 \times 0.555$$

Kelvin

$$°K = °C + 273.15 \text{ or } \frac{5}{9}(°F) + 255.35$$

Fahrenheit

$$°F = (°C \times 1.8) + 32$$

Box A9–1	Fahrenheit and Celsius Selected Comparisons

FAHRENHEIT (DEGREES)	CELSIUS/CENTIGRADE (DEGREES)
32	0
95	35
96	35.5
96.8	36
98.6	37
99.6	37.5
100.4	38
102.2	39
104	40

Volume

deciliter (dl) $= \frac{1}{10}$ of a liter
10 dl $= 1\,l$
centiliter (cl) $= \frac{1}{100}$ of a liter
100 cl $= 10\text{ dl} = 1\,l$
milliliter (ml) $= \frac{1}{1000}$ of a liter
1000 ml $= 100\text{ cl} = 10\text{ dl} = 1\,l$

Appendix 10

MILITARY TIME
(24-HOUR CLOCK)

Military time uses a 24-hour time clock and eliminates the need for the "A.M." or "P.M." designations that are used in "civilian," or Greenwich time (12-hour time clock). The 24-hour clock is particularly useful in health care settings so that confusion is eliminated when documenting time for treatment procedures, specimen collections, tests, drug administration, surgical procedures, etc. It is important that all health care workers understand and use it correctly.

Military time is expressed by four numerals; the first pair is "hours" (00 to 24) and the second set is "minutes" (00 to 59). Each day begins at midnight, 0000, and ends at 2359.

The first 12 hours are equivalent in Greenwich and military time; that is, 3:00 A.M. is equivalent to 0300 in military time, but conversion of afternoon and evening times from a 12-hour clock to military time requires adding 12 to each hour (2:00 P.M. is 1400 in military time).

Examples:
- 1:00 A.M. = 0100
- 5:00 A.M. = 0500
- 10:00 A.M. = 1000
- 11:00 A.M. = 1100
- 12:00 noon = 1200
- 1:00 P.M. = 1300
- 4:00 P.M. = 1600
- 9:00 P.M. = 2100
- 10:00 P.M. = 2200
- 12:00/midnight = 2400/0000

Military time is usually stated in terms of hundreds (e.g., 1500 is stated as "fifteen hundred hours"; 0300 is stated as "zero three hundred").

Reference

Badasch, SA, and Chesebro, DS: Introduction to Health Occupations, *Today's Health Care Worker,* 5th ed. Upper Saddle River, NJ: Prentice Hall Health, 2000.

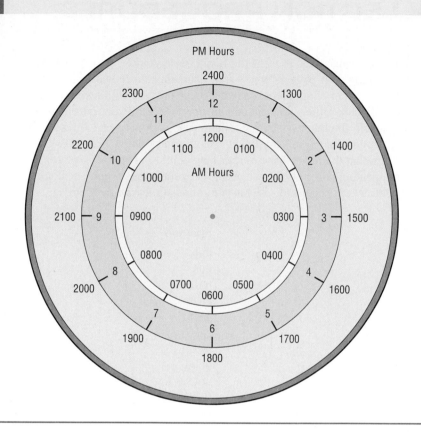

BASIC SPANISH FOR SPECIMEN COLLECTION PROCEDURES

The following translations present the health care worker with a very basic means of communicating with patients who speak Spanish. Before speaking with patients, the health care worker should practice using these phrases with someone who knows the correct pronunciation. Otherwise, the patient may become even more confused. Remember that in Spanish, the letter *h* is always silent. Also, if a word ends in *a* it is usually feminine gender; if it ends in "o" it is masculine. Another alternative is to have the key phrases printed on cards that the health care worker may point to or use as a reference when he or she is communicating with the patient. Also, use your hands when speaking; pantomime, point, or use facial expressions to assist in communicating your message.

English	Spanish
one	uno
two	dos
three	tres
four	cuatro
five	cinco
six	seis
seven	siete
eight	ocho
nine	nueve
ten	diez
twenty	veinte
thirty	treinta
forty	cuarenta
fifty	cincuenta
sixty	sesenta
seventy	setenta
eighty	ochenta
ninety	noventa
one hundred	ciento/cien
Hello.	Hola.
Good day.	Buenos dias/Buendia.
Good morning.	Buenos dias.
Good afternoon.	Buenas tardes.
Good evening.	Buenas noches.
Mother	Madre/mama
Father	Padre/papa

Sister	Hermana
Brother	Hermano
Son	Hijo
Daughter	Hija
Husband	Esposo/marido
Wife	Esposa/marida
Infant/baby	Niño/niña
Grandfather	Abuelo
Grandmother	Abuela
Friend	Amigo/Amiga
Mister	Señor
Mrs.	Señora
Miss	Señorita
Doctor	Doctor/medico
Technician	Técnico
Nurse	Enfermera
alcohol	alcohol
fasting	enayunas
gloves	guantes
needle	aguja
sterile	estéril
syringe	jeringa
tourniquet	torniquete
pathology	patología
procedure	procedimiento
hematology	hematología
complete blood count (CBC)	biometría hemática complete
blood bank	banco de sangre
coagulated	coagulado
reports	reportes
specimen	muestra
tubes	tubos
My name is . . .	Me llamo . . . /Mi nombres . . .
I work in the laboratory.	Trabajo en el laboratorio.
I speak . . .	Hablo . . .
We are going to analyze	Vamos analizar
. . . your blood.	. . . su sangre.
. . . your urine.	. . . su orina.
. . . your sputum.	. . . su esputo.
Do you understand?	¿Entiende usted (ud.)?
I do not understand.	No entiendo.
Please (pls.)	Por favor (p.f.)
Thank you.	Gracias.

You are welcome.	De nada.
Speak slower, pls.	Hable mas despacio, p.f.
Repeat, pls.	Haga me el favor de repetir, p.f.
Can you hear me?	¿Puede oírme?
Can you speak?	¿Puede hablar?
Relax.	Relajese.
What is your name?	¿Como se llama?
What is your address?	¿Que es su domicillo?
What is your birth date?	¿En que fecha nacio?
How old are you?	¿Cuantos años tiene ud.?
Have you been here before?	¿Ha estado ud. aquí antes?
Who is your doctor?	¿Quien es su doctor?
Your doctor wrote the order.	El doctor/la doctora escribio la orden.
Here is the bathroom.	Aquí esta el baño.
Here is the call light.	Aquí esta la luz de emergencia.
You may not eat/drink anything except water.	No debe de comer/beber nada solamente agua.
You may not smoke.	No puede fumar.
Have you had breakfast?	¿Ya tomo el desayuno?
We need a blood/urine/stool sample.	Necesitamos una muestra de su sangre/orina/del excremento.
Please stay in bed.	Por favor, quédese en la cama.
Please do not eat after midnight.	Por favor, no coma después de medianoche.
Please	Haga me el favor de
. . . make a fist.	. . . cerrar el puño.
. . . bend your arm.	. . . doblar el brazo.
. . . roll up your sleeve.	. . . levantarse la manga.
. . . open your hand.	. . . abrir la mano.
. . . sit down here.	. . . sientese aquí.
. . . change your position.	. . . cambiarse de posición.
. . . turn over.	. . . voltearse.
. . . change to the left.	. . . cambiarse a la izquierda.
. . . change to the right.	. . . cambiarse a la derecha.
I am going to lift your sleeve.	Voy levantar la manga.
I need to	Necesito
. . . take a blood sample.	. . . sacar una muestra de sangre.
. . . stick/prick your finger.	. . . picarle su dedo.
. . . two tubes of blood.	. . . dos tubos de sangre.
Open your hand.	Abra la mano.
It will hurt a little.	Le va a doler un poquito.
Please do not move.	No se mueva, por favor.
This is done quickly.	Esto se hace rapido.

The needle will stay in your arm while I am collecting the blood sample.

La aguja se quedara en su brazo/durante el tiempo necessario para obtener la muestra.

I am finished. Thank you.

Ya termine. Gracias.

Press this gauze on your arm/finger until I can make sure that the bleeding has stopped.

Comprese esta banda en su brazo/su dedo hasta que pare la sangre.

I am going to put a bandage on you.

Voy a ponerle una cinta adhesiva/un curita/un bandaid.

Are you lightheaded?

¿Esta usted mareado/mareada?

Do you feel as if you are going to faint?

¿Se siente como si se va a desmayar?

Do you feel all right?

¿Se siente bien?

You must lie down.

Necesita acostarse.

Collect the midstream portion of the urine in the container or bottle.

Coleccione la porción del medio de la orina en el vaso.

Void a little, then put urine in this cup.

Orine un poco, luego ponga la orina en esta taza.

Source: Joyce, EV, Villanueva, ME: *Say It in Spanish, A Guide for Health Care Professionals,* 2nd ed. Philadelphia: W.B. Saunders Co, 2000.

Appendix 12

ANSWERS TO SELF-STUDY QUESTIONS AND CASE STUDY QUESTIONS

SELF-STUDY ANSWERS FOR CHAPTERS 1–4

CHAPTER 1

1. a, c,	6. c, d	11. a, b, c, d
2. a, b, d	7. a, b	12. a, b, c, d
3. a, b, c	8. a, b, c, d	13. a, b, c, d
4. a, b, c	9. a, b, c, d	
5. d	10. a, b, d	

CHAPTER 2

1. b	4. d	7. b
2. e	5. c	
3. a	6. d	

CHAPTER 3

1. a, b, c	5. a, b	9. d
2. c	6. a, b, d	10. b, c
3. b	7. b	11. b
4. a, c, d, e	8. c	12. a

CHAPTER 4

1. a, b, c	5. c, d, e	9. d
2. a	6. a, b, c, d	10. a, b, c, d
3. a, c	7. a, b	
4. a	8. b	

CASE STUDY ANSWERS

CAREER PATHWAYS: SMOOTH OR STORMY

1. Derek can seek advice from within his current organization and begin to network outside his organization. Because he is well-liked by his coworkers and supervisors, he would likely be able to approach them for ideas about job opportunities and reference letters in support of his next job application. Derek could also re-evaluate his competence in various job responsitbilities and begin to "brush-up" on areas where his skills may be weaker due to lack of experience. He might consider taking continuing education courses through professional organizations, begin reading more about current events in laboratory technology, updating his computer skills, and/or written and verbal communication skills.

2. Derek should begin his job search by compiling a resume, a cover letter to accompany job inquiries, and a list of possible employers. He should begin searching for the right fit for his educational background and experience.
3. There are many professional organizations that can help by providing job opportunities either in their publications or on their websites; they can provide continuing education opportunities in class or online; and they may provide networking opportunities by getting involved in committees focused on one's interests.

CHANGING RESPONSIBILITY IN PHLEBOTOMY PRACTICE

1. Ms Hansen should engage in stress reducing activities outside of work because obviously the major change that will occur seems to affect her profoundly. She has many character and professional traits to be proud of that will smooth out the change once she becomes accustomed to the idea and the new staff she will work with. She should also realize that the stakeholders she provides services to will essentially remain the same.
2. She already has very positive personality traits and work habits that should contribute to the team concept in a productive manner. She should remember the following skills needed for effective teams:
   - Understand the mission of the organization.
   - Know basic skills for group process and team dynamics (e.g., active listening, setting norms, etc.).
   - Understand relevance and commitment to team goals.
   - Be reliable and dependable in work assignments.
   - Be able to communicate ideas and feelings
   - Actively participate in decision making.
   - Learn how to be flexible in decision making.
   - Constructively manage conflicts.
   - Contribute to the cohesion of the team.
   - Contribute to problem solving strategies.
   - Support and encourage other team members.
3. She has numerous positive attributes that will help her in her new role. These are efficiency in blood collection, her willingness to provide assistance, her attention to details, and her ability to communicate effectively with patients. These types of traits and work habits are universally beneficial no matter what type of health care setting she is in.

COLLECTION FROM THE DORSAL SIDE OF THE HAND

1. Dorsal (proximal) refers to the back of the hand in this case. The anterior hand or wrist should NOT be used for venipuncture.
2. Supine means lying on the back, face upward.
3. An orthopedic floor is for patients with bone and joint disorders.

COMMUNICATION AND CULTURAL SENSITIVITY: KEYS TO SUCCESS

1. The fact that Elizabeth does not speak Spanish or that Mrs. Rodriguez does not speak English well is a major barrier to effective communication between them. This barrier needs to be addressed before a successful and comfortable scenario can be achieved. In addition, having so many family members present, including the child, may also be somewhat of a distraction.

2. Mrs. Rodriguez obviously wants or needs a support group of her family members to be with her during this encounter. She may be fearful or nervous about the procedure, or she may believe that her family can help her understand what is going to happen. She may believe that if any major medical decisions need to be made, her family members can help with the decisions.

3. As mentioned in Chapter 1, communication strategies may involve the following:
   - Seek the assistance of a translator
   - Utilize written instructions in Spanish for reinforcing the messages
   - Show empathy through body language and facial expressions
   - Show respect for privacy
   - Build trust by trying to explain carefully using a model, symbols, or body language
   - Establish rapport with the patient and her family members
   - Listen actively to the patient and her family members
   - Provide as much feedback as possible

4. In this case, one or more of the family members may be able to help with the translation of various parts of the conversation. Even the child may be able to assist with some basic translations and information. They may hold her hand or comfort her as the procedure is taking place. If possible, let them participate in helping her to relax.

5. Elizabeth may want to familiarize herself with medical terms in Spanish. She could use the translations in the Appendix to practice basic requests for venipuncture and urinalysis. She could take a medical terminology course in Spanish. She could find out more about Hispanic cultures and the diversity among Hispanic cultures through their music, literature, and popular media.

COMMUNICATION AND CONSENT

1. The phlebotomist should check with the floor nurse to determine whether Ms. Garcia speaks English and/or whether she has a hearing disability. If the patient speaks only Spanish, an interpreter or a written description of the phlebotomy procedure should be available in Spanish to assist in this situation. If the patient has a hearing disability, efforts should be made to write down instructions for the patient.

2. If a patient has a hearing disability, writing tools should be kept at the bedside of the patient. If a large segment of the patient population speaks another language, the hospital should provide interpreters who know the basic use of that language. Also, instruction sheets on phlebotomy steps should be made available in other languages for patients who do not speak English.

3. The patient has not consented to the venipuncture, nor did she appear to understand the verbal communication. The efforts mentioned in the above answers will facilitate seeking consent and minimize the risk of legal or financial loss to the hospital. Above all, these efforts will provide a cooperative, professional interaction for the patient and health care worker.

AN ETHICAL DILEMMA

1. and 2. Marty took the correct action by informing the nurse in charge. However, in this case, it is important to share the incident with another supervisor because of possible legal ramifications later. More importantly, it is impossible to tell from the scenario how long the identification was incorrect and there could have been other procedures, treatments, or care plans that were performed with the patients incorrectly identified. Thus, someone else may be able to trace all possible errors associated with the mix-up and remedy the situation before any harsh outcomes for either of the patients has occurred. Marty should make sure the corrections have been made and then continue with her careful evaluation of the patient and venipuncture procedure.

3. There are several ethical issues associated with this case. The first involves the relationship between the two employees. It appears that Ms. Daley was using her friendship with Marty to cover up her own mistake and not report it. These actions were unethical. Secondly, Marty had to make a decision about whether or not to report Ms. Daley's mistake to another supervisor or third party, thereby directly violating Ms. Daley's request. The ethical and professional decision would be for Marty to report it to another supervisor and document the incident, even though she would jeopardize her friendship.

   There are many legal, ethical, and most importantly, clinical consequences that can be extremely damaging to both of the patients, both employees, and the health care organization itself. The clinical consequences of misidentifying a patient can result in severe injury, including death. Legal consequences might include malpractice, negligence, and large financial penalties to all parties involved. Ethical consequences involve violations of institutional policy, negative feelings toward both employees and their families, and negative afterthoughts for many years.

SELF-STUDY ANSWERS FOR CHAPTERS 5–8

CHAPTER 5

1. c, d	4. d, e, f	7. a, b
2. c, b, d	5. b	8. b, c, d
3. b	6. c	

CHAPTER 6

1. c, d	4. a, c, d	7. c
2. a, b, d	5. a, b, c, d	8. b
3. a, b, c, d	6. b, d	9. b

CHAPTER 7

1. a, b, c, d	5. a, b, c, d	9. a
2. a, b, c, d	6. b	10. c
3. a, c, d	7. a, b, d	
4. a, b, c	8. a, b, c	

CHAPTER 8

1. a, b, c	5. c	9. a, b, c
2. d	6. b	10. c
3. a	7. a	
4. b	8. a	

CASE STUDY ANSWERS

RUNNING LATE ON THE DAY SHIFT

1. There were several fundamental problems in this case. First, John made the mistake of rushing his work because he was behind schedule. Secondly, John was not fully prepared, i.e., he should have had all the supplies he needed at the bedside in case something went wrong.

2. He might have called for back-up when he began to notice that he was falling behind schedule. His co-workers might have finished early and could have helped him. Or his supervisor might have notified someone else to help out.

A SUPERVISOR'S FOLLY

1. Since Helen "has never had any problems," she appears to feel immune to hazards that she is creating for both herself and patients. By using outdated (and reckless) practices, she is creating a significant legal risk for herself and her hospital. She may not be fully knowledgeable of updated Infection Control practices, Needlestick Prevention strategies, or Safety regulations. If this is the case, Helen needs to take some responsibility in her own education and her employer needs to provide her with training opportunities in these topic areas. If she has had the training, and continues to ignore current standards of practice, she could be subject to disciplinary actions for insubordination, for jeopardizing the safety of patients and herself. Adherence to infection control, needlestick prevention, and safety policies is a compliance and competency issue. She may be competent in the current practices but not complying thus opening herself to claims of "negligence."

2. Coworkers and subordinates have an ethical and professional duty to uphold professional standards of practice and institutional policies/procedures related to safety and infection control. Co-workers should continue to encourage Helen to change her practices, and even consider documenting the times that it has been mentioned to her. However, the "bottom line" is that non-compliant individuals should be reported to appropriate individuals (safety officer, infection control supervisor, or laboratory manager) and specific incidents documented so that further action is possible to protect all parties involved. While this may not be a popular action among coworkers, it is "the right thing to do."

3. Helen needs to review Infection Control and Universal Precaution practices related to hand washing and gloving to reinforce "breaking the chain of infections." She also needs to become more knowledgeable about needlestick hazards, infection rates from needlesticks and implement related safety practices, i.e., using safety needles and devices for venipuncture rather than syringe/needles. Ultimately, if she feels she cannot change her practices, she needs to change her career or retire.

STOCKING SUPPLIES IN PHLEBOTOMY PRACTICE

1. Barcode technology has many benefits and applications in the clinical laboratory. The technology has been proved to be fast and accurate. Bar codes are particularly valuable in large-volume laboratories. As mentioned in Chapter 6, bar codes can be used for the following:
   - Patients' names
   - Patients' identification numbers
   - DOB
   - Test codes
   - Specimen accession or log numbers
   - Expiration dates for inventory of supplies and equipment
   - Product codes for needles, syringes, specimen collection tubes, etc.
   - Billing codes to facilitate accounting
   - Sample identification numbers on laboratory analyzers

   The only drawbacks are the costs associated with starting up (equipment, software, scanners, printers, new labels) and the training time needed to teach all personnel how to operate the system.
2. Barcodes can help reduce preanalytical errors by saving transcription time and avoiding multiple entries of the same information, thereby reducing clerical errors substantially. It is faster to scan a bar code than to write down a patient's name and identification number. It is easier to scan a product bar code as it is delivered than to write down all the details of a receiving order for specimen collection supplies. Above all, identification of patients and specimens becomes more accurate and timely as each specimen works its way through the analytical phases of laboratory testing.

TRAUMATIC TRANSPORT

1. Hemolysis can be caused by a variety of physiological and artificially-induced factors:
   a. RBC diseases such as sickle cell
   b. Exposure to drugs or toxins
   c. Excessive shaking or mixing of the specimen
   d. Excessive vibration during transportation
   e. Transfusion reactions
   f. Artificial heart valves
   g. Infections
2. The first factor of concern is that the phlebotomist failed to label the specimen correctly. Since there were no initials indicated, it would require that various staff members be involved in trying to track down the individual who remembers collecting

the specimen. Once this person is identified, she or he must be questioned and counseled about the specimen and about the labeling omission. The laboratory supervisor who investigates this situation will also need to check on several "preanalytical" factors that may have caused the hemolysis. Factors would include inquiring about excessive mixing/shaking, conditions in the pneumatic tube system that may have caused excessive vibrations or jolts to the specimen, and the patient's clinical condition. Based on all the information gathered, a decision will be made about whether or not a "recollect" should be ordered.

ACCIDENTAL INJURY

1. Even though Sally was tired, she had a job to do. Her fatigue might have contributed to her inability to draw blood from Mr. Johnson on the first try, however, there is no way to substantiate that. She probably did the procedure correctly except she should have discarded the first needle and holder immediately after she used it. At that time she would have noticed that the biohazard container was full, and she could have notified the appropriate person for a replacement. She should not have stuffed the other needles into the full biohazard container!! However, she took the appropriate action by notifying her supervisor immediately of her injury.
2. Sally would have to review the exposure control plan, OSHA standards, universal precautions, and safety procedures for disposing of contaminated waste.
3. Aside from a thorough review of the procedures mentioned in Question 2, Sally would benefit from going to classes on the importance of being rested and healthy for work. In addition, it appears she needs additional practice on patients who are difficult to draw. She may benefit from observing other experienced phlebotomists while they perform difficult draws.

TRANSPORTING SPECIMENS FROM HOMEBOUND PATIENTS TO THE LABORATORY

1. Larry seemed so pleased that he successfully communicated with Mr. Gonzales that he forgot to be meticulous about checking the specimen integrity. He should have carefully placed each specimen in a leakproof plastic container in an upright position in the carrying container with absorbant material. He should have securely locked the container, and placed it in a safer place in his car, perhaps the floor.
2. Larry should be careful not to touch the contaminated area. He should report the spill immediately and find out the appropriate procedures for spill cleanups and decontamination procedures.

SELF-STUDY ANSWERS FOR CHAPTERS 9–11
CHAPTER 9

1. b, c	5. b, c, d	9. a, c, d, b
2. a, b, c, d	6. b, d	10. a, b
3. b	7. d	
4. a, c, d	8. b	

CHAPTER 10

1. a, b, c	5. c	9. a, b, c, d
2. b, d	6. b, c, d	10. c
3. c, d	7. b	
4. a, b, c, d	8. b	

CHAPTER 11

1. a, b, c, d	5. c	9. a
2. b, d	6. b	10. a, b
3. a, b, c, d	7. b	
4. c	8. a	

CASE STUDY ANSWERS

AMBULATORY HEALTH CARE COLLECTIONS

1. Under normal blood collection procedures with an evacuated tube system, the health care provider did use the proper order of draw for Mrs. Ragsdale's laboratory tests. The light blue-topped tube containing citrate should be collected prior to the red-speckled tube (gel separator tube). However, when using a winged-infusion blood collection set, the tubing in the assembly contains air and will underfill the first evacuated tube, leading to an erroneous protime result.

2. The health care provider used the proper collection procedure. A 21- or 23-gauge needle is better, however, than a 25-gauge needle because the small diameter of the 25-gauge needle may lead to hemolysis of the collected blood and erroneous laboratory tests' results.

3. The proper blood collection procedure was used for obtaining blood from Mr. Sadler. Often, hemophiliacs have sclerosed veins due to so many blood collections and transfusions. Thus, a butterfly needle assembly used on the hand or lower arm is appropriate. A "complete" assembly set, however, should be used rather than pieces from different manufacturers.

   Mismatched medical equipment has led to 50 percent of mucocutaneous blood-borne pathogen exposures of health care workers to HIV-positive and/or HCV infected patients.

VENIPUNCTURE SITE SELECTION

1. The preferred site would be the dorsal side of the left wrist, below the IV site. The preferred phlebotomy method would be to use a winged infusion set in combination with evacuated tubes that could handle a short draw in case of difficulty.

2. The right arm of Mrs. McDonald should never be used for venipuncture because of her partial mastectomy. This type of surgical procedure often results in removal of lymph nodes resulting in edematous areas. Since she is a diabetic, foot veins should be eliminated because of an increased likelihood of infectious complications. Since the left arm had an IV located below the anticubital area, this location could not be used

for venipuncture due to contamination with IV fluid. The area below the IV site is acceptable for tourniquet application and venipuncture. The winged infusion system is most effective for the smaller veins of the wrist. It is also less painful for the patient.

3. It would be helpful to the clinical laboratory and other members of the health care team to document that the blood sample was drawn from below the IV site since the patient was diabetic, had a mastectomy on the right side, and had an IV located in the left arm.

4. Site selection can be facilitated by the following: proper positioning, use of a pillow or towel under the wrist, rotation of the patient's arm, palpation, warming the site, and dangling the arm for a short while to increase blood flow to the area.

FINDING THE RIGHT SITE

1. The phlebotomist should clarify on which side the mastectomy was performed and draw from a vein in the other arm.

2. and 3. Often when a mastectomy is performed, lymph nodes are also removed from the area adjacent to the malignant site. Once they have been removed they never grow back. Since lymph nodes function to move lymph fluid throughout the body, the absence of lymph nodes causes fluid build-up in that region of the body. While the swelling probably is not significant after 5 years, even a minor fluid build-up might have a dilution effect on the specimen if it is collected from that side of the body.

TRICKY COMPLICATIONS WITH AN IV

1. Blood was likely collected above the IV site where chemotherapy drugs were being infused and probably diluted the specimen, thus causing a falsely low value of sodium.

2. There are several alternatives and Betty should have discussed these with her supervisor since she was not sure of the consequences. She might have considered using veins of the dorsal side of the hand below the IV infusion, or a finger puncture if microcollection supplies were available.

3. There are other options that could also have be considered in cases like this, especially after consultation with the physician, laboratory supervisor, and/or nursing staff:
   a. The specimen may have been used as drawn if a notation about the site had been indicated at the time, e.g., "specimen collected above IV infusion site"
   b. It is possible that the IV infusion could have been stopped prior to blood collection so that dilution would not be a factor, then the phlebotomist could use the preferred anticubital area.

SELF-STUDY ANSWERS FOR CHAPTERS 12–16

CHAPTER 12

1. a, b	5. a, d	9. a, b, c
2. b, d	6. d	10. b
3. a, b, d	7. b	11. a, b, c
4. c	8. a, b	12. d

CHAPTER 13

1. c	5. d	9. a
2. c	6. c	10. b
3. d	7. a	
4. a	8. b	

CHAPTER 14

1. c	5. d	9. a
2. d	6. b	10. c
3. b	7. b	
4. c	8. a	

CHAPTER 15

1. b	5. c	9. b
2. b	6. b	10. b
3. c	7. b	
4. c	8. c	

CHAPTER 16

1. a, c, d	5. b	9. b, d
2. a, b, c, d	6. a, b	10. d
3. a, b	7. a, b, c, d	
4. b	8. a, b, c, d	

CASE STUDY ANSWERS
HOME CARE COLLECTIONS

1. **Laboratory Assay** — **Color of Blood Collection Tube Top**

Laboratory Assay	Color of Blood Collection Tube Top
Calcium, ionized	green
APTT	light blue
CBC count	purple
Protime	light blue
Chemistry screen	red or red-speckled
Digoxin	red or red-speckled
Plasma potassium	green

2. The order of draw was incorrect for blood vacuum tube collections. The correct order should have been red, light blue, green, and purple. The correct order prevents contamination of nonadditive tubes by additive tubes, and minimizes cross-contamination between the different anticoagulants.

3. The order of draw should have been the same as for vacuum tubes; therefore, the order of draw for this specimen was correct. Care should have been taken to mix the purple-topped tube immediately after filling it.

BEDSIDE GLUCOSE TESTING

1. The problem in this bedside glucose testing case is that the patient's meter was reading outside the control confidence limits. Thus, the glucose results are out of control and not considered accurate or reliable.
2. The phlebotomist, the nurse, and other health care providers involved in the bedside glucose testing for this patient should troubleshoot for:
   a. Correct timing of the analytic procedure.
   b. Reagents and controls stored at correct temperature and within appropriate expiration dates.
   c. Instrument blotting or wiping technique performed according to manufacturer's directions.

   In this case, the control solution had expired March 2, 2002.

NEWBORN NURSERY COLLECTIONS

1. Blood collected from a baby for a bilirubin determination should be collected in an amber microcollection tube or a tube covered with foil so that the microcollection tube is not exposed to light. Light breaks down bilirubin.
2. Because bilirubin breaks down in the presence of light, the longer a blood specimen is exposed to light, the more bilirubin is broken down. Thus, the bilirubin value will be falsely decreased.
3. Probably, the phlebotomist who collected Baby McPherson's blood on Sunday morning collected the blood in a clear microcollection tube and allowed it to remain in direct light for an extended period prior to delivering it to the clinical laboratory.

COLLECTING BLOOD FROM AN INFANT

1. For this microcollection, Ms. Wiggins needed to have the following equipment:
   a. Sterile automatic disposable pediatric safety lancet devices
   b. 70% isopropyl alcohol swabs in sterile packages
   c. Sterile cotton balls or gauze sponges
   d. Plastic microcollection containers
   e. Puncture-resistant sharps container
   f. Disposable sterile gloves (nonlatex if infant is allergic)
   g. Compress (towel or washcloth) to warm heel if necessary
   h. Marking pen
   i. Laboratory request slips or labels

   For the procedure, after Ms. Wiggins washes her hands outside of the nursery and then dons the gown, gloves, and mask, she picks up her blood collection tray with two clean paper towels and enters the nursery area. The tray is then placed on a diaper on the small metal cart next to the infant. Then, the infant must be identified properly. The phlebotomist then collects the blood after ensuring that the infant's heel is adequately warm for the collection.

2. For infant Jim Jenkins, the microcollection tube with EDTA was used first to collect blood for the hemoglobin procedure, then the microcollection tube with lithium heparin was used next to collect blood for the potassium test, and finally a microcollection tube without additives was used to collect blood for the thyroxine test.

BLOOD DONOR COMPLICATIONS

1. The phlebotomist punctured a deep artery. This was evident by the bright redness of the blood and the pulsating action as it was withdrawn.
2. If the supervisor had not halted the procedure, the puncture may have bled excessively either subcutaneously (hematoma) or on the surface of the skin, especially since a larger bore sized needle is used for blood donations. Bleeding from an artery is more difficult to stop than bleeding from a vein. Excessive blood loss might also have caused other complications such as syncope, and hazards associated with the phlebotomist being exposed to blood. In addition, deeper manipulation of the needle may have resulted in nerve damage.
3. The phlebotomist probably needs further training and education about blood donor collections and the hazards associated with her technique. She should be supervised more closely until she demonstrates competence in a variety of situations.

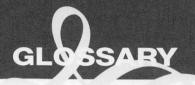

GLOSSARY

ABO blood group system a method by which red blood cell antigens are classified (e.g., individual's blood cells with type A antigens have type A blood; those with B antigens have type B blood, etc.).

acid-citrate-dextrose (ACD) an additive commonly used in specimen collection for blood donations to prevent clotting. It ensures that the RBCs maintain their oxygen-carrying capacity.

acidosis a pathologic condition existing when the blood pH decreases to less than 7.35.

active listening a set of skills that enables one to become a more effective listener. The skills include concentrating on the speaker, getting ready to listen by clearing one's mind of distracting thoughts, use of silent pauses when appropriate, providing reassuring feedback, verifying the conversation that took place, keeping personal judgments to oneself, paying attention to body language of the person speaking, and maintaining eye contact.

acute care health care delivered in a hospital setting that is associated with a hospital stay of usually less than 30 days.

additives substances (gels, clothing activators, or anticoagulants) that are added in small amounts to specimen collection tubes to alter the specimen so as to make it appropriate for laboratory analysis or handling.

administrative law a type of law that is initiated by the executive branch of government. Federal agencies write regulations that enforce laws created through the legislative body.

adrenals glands that produce hormones as a result of emotional changes like fright or anger. Hormone production causes an increase in blood pressure, widened pupils, and heart stimulation.

adulteration means of tampering with a specimen, usually urine, to make the specimen test negatively for drugs. Water is the most common substance added to the specimen or ingested to dilute the urine so that drug concentrations are below the detection limit.

age-specific care considerations providing services that are age-appropriate and considerate (e.g., special considerations are needed for differ-ent ages of children (toddler versus teen) and also for geriatric patients). Factors typically relate to age-related fears/concerns, communication styles, procedures for comforting the patient, and safety.

alcohol colorless liquid that can be used as an antiseptic.

alkalosis a pathologic condition that results when the blood pH increases to more than 7.45. In serious cases, it can lead to coma.

Allen test a procedure used prior to drawing specimens (for ABGs) from the radial artery. It assures that the ulnar and radial arteries are providing collateral circulation to the hand area. Basically, it entails compressing the arteries to the hand and emptying the hand of arterial blood, then releasing the compression to see if the circulation is immediately restored. A negative test would indicate that collateral circulation is not sufficient and an alternative artery (brachial or femoral) should be used for ABG collections.

aliquot a portion of a blood sample that has been removed/separated from the primary specimen tube.

alveolar sacs grapelike structures in the lungs that allow for diffusion between air and blood.

ambulatory care health care services that are delivered in an out-patient, or nonhospital, setting. It implies that the patients are able to ambulate, or walk, to the clinic to receive their services.

American Hospital Association (AHA) nonprofit group or alliance of member hospitals and health care organizations that promote the interests of hospitals. Annual state and national conferences are held each year to discuss important legislation, financial considerations, regulations, and accreditation issues that affect hospitals. AHA is an advocacy group for health care organizations, particularly hospitals.

American Nurses Association (ANA) professional organization for nurses.

American Society for Clinical Laboratory Scientists (ASCLS) professional organization for laboratory personnel that provides continuing education, conference activities, and certification examinations for specified groups.

American Society of Clinical Pathologists (ASCP) professional organization that certifies many types of laboratory personnel based on their passing a certification examination. ASCP offers clinical and research conferences, many types of continuing education activities, and ongoing certification programs.

amniotic fluid fluid from the amniotic sac (i.e., the membranes that hold a developing embryo and fetus).

amphetamines a type of drugs in tablet or capsule form that are "stimulants."

anabolism a body function whereby cells use energy to make complex compounds from simpler ones. It allows the synthesis of body fluids (e.g., sweat, tears, saliva, etc.).

analytic phase refers to the phase in laboratory testing whereby the specimen is actually assessed or evaluated, and results are confirmed and reported.

anatomic pathology major area of laboratory services whereby autopsies are performed and cytology procedures and surgical biopsy tissues are analyzed.

anatomy study of the structural components of the body.

anemia medical condition where by there is a reduction in hemoglobin thus lowering the O_2 carrying capacity of blood cells.

anterior surface region of the body characterized by the front (or ventral) area and including the thoracic, abdominal, and pelvic cavities.

anticoagulant substance introduced into the blood or a blood specimen to keep it from clotting.

antimicrobial chemical or therapeutic agent that destroys microorganisms such as bacteria, viruses, fungi, etc.

antiseptic hand rub applying/rubbing a waterless antiseptic product onto all surfaces of the hands to reduce the number of microorganisms present; the hands are rubbed until the product has dried.

antiseptic hand wash washing hands with soap and water or other detergents containing an antiseptic agent.

antiseptics chemicals (e.g., 70 percent isopropyl alcohol, iodine, chlorohexidine, chlorine, hexachlorophene, chlorooxylenol, quarternary ammonium compounds, and triclosan) used to clean human skin by inhibiting the growth of microorganisms.

aorta the largest artery in the body.

arterial blood gases (ABGs) analytical test that measures oxygen and carbon dioxide in the blood. Provides useful information about respiratory status and the acid–base balance of patients with pulmonary disorders.

arteries highly oxygenated blood vessels that carry blood away from the heart.

arterioles smaller branches of arteries.

assault a legal term referring to the unjustifiable attempt to touch another person or the threat to do so in circumstances that cause the other person to believe that it will be carried out, or to cause fear. An assault may be permissible if proper consent has been given (e.g., consent to obtain a blood specimen).

assessments a quality improvement measurement term referring to both the analytic (quantitative) and nonanalytic (qualitative) components of health care. In the clinical laboratory, assessments are used to ensure test sensitivity, specificity, precision and accuracy, and/or effective communication styles, timeliness, etc.

atria two of the four chambers of the heart.

autologous transfusion a patient donates his or her own blood or blood components for use later; this is the safest type of transfusion (i.e., using one's own blood). It prevents transfusion-transmitted infectious diseases and eliminates the formation of antibodies from other donors.

automated skin-puncture device a single-use apparatus that pierces the skin with a lancet that automatically retracts into a protective casing.

bacteremia presence of bacteria in the blood; an infection of the blood.

bar codes series of light and dark bands of varying widths that relate to alphanumeric symbols.

They can correspond to the patient's name and/or identification numbers.

basal state for phlebotomy procedures, this refers to the patient's condition in the early morning, approximately 12 hours after the last ingestion of food. In hospitals, most laboratory tests are analyzed on basal state specimens.

basilic vein vessel of the forearm that is acceptable for venipuncture.

battery a complex legal term referring to the intentional touching of another person without consent, and/or beating or carrying out threatened physical harm. "Battery" always includes an assault, and is therefore commonly used with the term in "assault and battery."

bevel slanted surface at the end point of a needle.

bioethics moral issues, dilemmas, or problems that are the result of modern medical practices, health care services, clinical research, and/or technology (often bioethical issues involve "life-and-death" situations). *Bio* refers to "life" and *ethics* refers to a branch of philosophy dealing with the distinction between right and wrong.

bleeding-time test test useful for assessing platelet plug formation in the capillaries. It is generally done along with other coagulation tests and often used as a preoperative (presurgical) screening test. Basically it utilizes an automated, sterile incision-making instrument to puncture the skin, and then the blood-clotting process is timed. Phlebotomists must be specially trained to perform this procedure accurately.

blood circulating fluid and cells in the cardiovascular system.

bloodborne pathogens (BBPs) pathogenic microorganisms, including hepatitis B virus and human immunodeficiency virus, that are present in human blood and can cause disease in humans.

blood cultures tests that aid in identifying the specific bacterial organism causing infections in the blood. In the case of a patient that is experiencing fever spikes, it is recommended that the blood culture specimens be collected before and after the fever spike, when bacteria are most likely present in the peripheral circulation. Care must be taken by the phlebotomist not to contaminate the specimen, so special preparation of the collection site is required.

blood-drawing chair chair specifically designed to hold a patient comfortably and safely in a proper position during and after a blood collection procedure. The design typically includes a moveable armrest on both sides of the chair.

blood gas analysis refer to *arterial blood gases.*

blood pressure assessment of the functioning of the cardiovascular system using an instrument called a sphygmomanometer or blood pressure cuff. It is measured as systolic pressure, when the heart receives blood, and diastolic pressure, when the heart's ventricles relax.

blood urea nitrogen (BUN) analytic testing procedure to determine the amount of urea in the blood.

blood vessels key component of the circulatory system, these vessels transport blood throughout the body.

blood volume the total amount of blood in an individual's body. This is particularly important in pediatric phlebotomies because withdrawing blood can cause a significant decrease in the total blood volume of a small infant, thus resulting in anemia. Blood volume is based on weight and can be calculated for any size person.

body planes imaginary dividing lines of the body that serve as reference points for describing distance from or proximity to the body. Body planes include the sagittal, frontal, transverse, and medial planes.

brachial artery an artery located in the cubital fossa of the arm and used as an alternative site for ABG collections. Phlebotomists must be specially trained to perform collections from this site.

breach of duty a legal term referring to an infraction, violation, or failure to perform.

buffy coat in blood specimens that contain anticoagulants, the WBCs and platelets form a thin white layer above the RBCs called the *buffy coat.*

butterfly system also called a winged infusion system or scalp needle set, the system can be used for difficult venipunctures due to small or fragile veins. The needle is typically smaller, and has a thin tubing with a Luer adapter at the end so that it can be used on a syringe or an evacuated tube system during venipuncture. Newer models have needle safety devices such as retractable needles and/or needle coverings/sheaths.

calcaneus heel bone.

cannula a tube that can be inserted into a cavity or blood vessel and used as a channel for transporting fluids. The term is most commonly used in dialysis for patients with kidney disease. The cannula is used to gain access to venous blood for dialysis or for blood collections. Specialized training and experience are required to draw blood from a cannula.

capillaries microscopic blood vessels that carry blood and link arterioles to venules.

capillary action a term used when referring to microcollection procedures that indicates the free flowing movement of blood into the capillary tube without the use of suction.

capillary blood a specimen from a skin puncture that contains a blend of blood from venules, arterioles, and tissue fluid.

capillary blood gas analysis using microcollection methods on infants (usually the heel site) to collect specimens for blood gas analyses; these analytical tests measure oxygen and carbon dioxide in the blood. Provides useful information about respiratory status and the acid–base balance of patients with pulmonary disorders.

capillary tubes disposable narrow-bore pipettes that are used for pediatric blood collections and/or microhematocrit measures. The tubes may be coated with anticoagulant such as heparin, and for safety reasons are usually made of plastic.

cardiac (striated involuntary) muscles muscles that make up the wall of the heart.

cardiopulmonary resuscitation (CPR) the method used to revive the heart and/or breathing of a patient whose heart or respiration has stopped. It is advisable for health care workers to be appropriately trained in the use of CPR.

cardiovascular system body system that provides for rapid transport of water, nutrients, electrolytes, hormones, enzymes, antibodies, cells, and gases to all cells of the body.

cartilage substance similar to bone except that cells are surrounded by a gelatinous material that allows for flexibility.

catabolism chemical reactions in the body that break down complex substances into simpler ones while simultaneously releasing energy. The process provides energy for all body functions.

cause-and-effect diagrams (Ishikawa) a quality improvement tool that uses diagrams to identify interactions between equipment, methods, people, supplies, and reagents.

Celsius scale temperature scale named after Anders Celsius, a swedish astronomer; see centigrade

Centers for Disease Control and Prevention (CDC) federal agency responsible for monitoring morbidity (disease) and mortality (death) throughout the country.

centigrade thermometer based on a 100 degree range from 0 as the freezing point to 100 as the boiling point for water.

central intravenous line a commonly used VAD. Refer to *vascular access devices.*

centrifugation phase period of time when a blood specimen is inside the centrifuge.

centrifugal force the amount of force directing parts (like cells) outward from the center of rotation when spinning in a centrifuge.

centriole a cellular structure that plays a role in cellular division.

cephalic vein vein of the forearm that is acceptable for venipuncture.

cerebrospinal fluid (CSF) fluid that surrounds the brain and meninges within the spinal column.

chain of custody process for maintaining control and accountability of a specimen from the point of collection to its final disposition. The process documents the identity of each individual that handles the specimen and each time a specimen is transferred.

chain of infection the process by which infections are transmitted; components include the source of the infection (nonsterile items, contaminated equipment or supplies, etc.), the mode of transmission (direct contact, airborne, medical instruments, etc.), and the susceptible host (patient).

circulatory system body system referring to the heart, blood vessels, and blood; responsible for transporting oxygen and nutrients to cells and transports carbon dioxide and wastes until they are eliminated; transports hormones, regulates body temperature, and helps defend against diseases.

citrate-phosphate-dextrose (CPD) anticoagulant typically used for blood donations.

citrates type of anticoagulant additive for blood collection tubes; prevents the blood clotting sequence by removing calcium and forming calcium salts.

civil law different from criminal law; in civil law, the plaintiff sues for monetary damages.

clean-catch midstream a urine specimen that is used for detecting bacteria and/or for microscopic analysis. Normally, the specimen should be free of contamination because the patient should be instructed to clean and decontaminate themselves prior to urination. The urine specimen should be collected into a sterile container. Urine should be voided and the specimen should be collected midurination.

clinical laboratory a workplace where analytic procedures are performed on blood and body fluids for the detection, monitoring, and treatment of disease.

Clinical Laboratory Improvement Amendments (CLIA) federal guidelines that regulate all clinical laboratories across the United States. Regulations apply to any site that tests human specimens, including small POLs, or screening tests done at the patient's bedside.

clinical pathology major area of laboratory services where blood and other types of body fluids and tissues are analyzed.

coagulation a phase in the blood-clotting sequence in which many factors are released and interact to form a fibrin meshwork, or blood clot.

cocaine an addictive, illegal "street drug" made from leaves of the coca plant.

competency statement performance expectations that include entry-level skills, tasks, and roles performed by the designated health care worker.

confidentiality the protected right and duty of health care workers not to disclose any information acquired about a patient to those who are not directly involved with the care of the patient.

contaminated sharps objects that can penetrate the skin, including needles, scalpels, broken glass, broken capillary tubes, and exposed wires.

contamination presence of blood or potentially infectious substances on an item or surface.

continuous quality improvement (CQI) a theoretical framework and management strategy to improve health care structures, processes, outcomes, and customer satisfaction. It is ongoing and involves all levels of the administrative structure of an organization.

creatinine clearance test analytic procedure to determine whether or not the kidneys are able to remove creatinine from the blood.

criminal actions legal recourse for acts against the public welfare; these actions can lead to imprisonment of the offender.

critical test result a term that should be defined by each health care organization and typically includes test results that are panic values, stat test results, or other results that require an immediate response.

critical value a laboratory result that indicates a pathophysiologic state at such variance with normal as to be life threatening; these values should be defined and reported to the patient's physician as soon as possible; also refered to as a "panic value."

cross-match testing laboratory analysis that involves exposure of a donor's blood to a patient's blood to see if they are compatible or incompatible.

culture a system of values (individualism, importance of education and financial security), beliefs (spiritual, family bonding), and practices (food, music, traditions) that stem from one's concept of reality. Culture influences decisions and behaviors in many aspects of life.

culture and sensitivity (C&S) microbiologic test to determine the growth of infectious microorganisms in bodily specimens (e.g., urine), and to determine which antibiotics are most effective on the microorganism.

Custody and Control Form (CCF) part of the "chain-of-custody" process that requires specific documentation related to donor identification procedures, specimen collection steps, security for the collector, the donor, and the specimen, and tampering with the specimen.

cyanotic bluish in color due to oxygen deficiency.

cytoplasm contained within a cellular membrane, it contains mostly water with dissolved nutrients and contains other structures or organelles of the cell.

decontamination use of physical or chemical means to remove or destroy bloodborne pathogens on a surface (including skin) or item so that pathogens are no longer able to transmit disease. Prior to venipuncture, decontamination involves cleaning with a sterile swab or sponge to prevent microbiological contamination of either the patient or the specimen. This is usually accomplished with a sterile swab containing 70 percent isopropyl alcohol (or isopropanol).

defendant individual (e.g., a health care worker), against whom a legal action (civil or criminal) or lawsuit is filed.

deoxyribonucleic acid (DNA) molecule containing thousands of genes that make up an individual's genetic code. Often referred to as a double helix, DNA is inherited from parents and carries the code for an individual's characteristics such as eye or hair color, height, etc.

Department of Health and Human Services (HHS) federal agency involved in many aspects of health delivery, regulation, and monitoring. One responsibility is the establishment of scientific and technical guidelines for federal drug-testing programs and standards for certification of laboratories engaged in urine drug-testing for federal agencies.

Department of Transportation (DOT) federal agency responsible for the transportation industry in the United States. They develop drug-testing guidelines for specified types of transportation personnel and standards for testing specified categories of drugs.

deposition a legal term referring to the testimony of a witness that is recorded in a written legal format.

diabetes mellitus metabolic disease in which carbohydrate utilization is reduced due to a deficiency in insulin and characterized by hyperglycemia, glycosuria, water and electrolyte loss, ketoacidosis, and in serious conditions, coma. In milder forms of noninsulin-dependent diabetes mellitus, dietary regulation may keep the disorder under control.

diastolic pressure the second measure reported in a blood pressure measurement.

differentials a laboratory test that categorizes blood cells and any abnormalities present.

digestive system body system referring to organs in the gastrointestinal (GI) tract that break down food chemically and physically into nutrients that can be absorbed by the body's cells and allow the elimination of waste products of digestion.

discovery a legal term referring to the right to examine the witness(es) before a trial; it consists of oral testimony under oath and includes cross-examination by lawyers.

disinfectants chemical compounds used to remove or kill pathogenic microorganisms; typically used on medical instruments or countertops.

disposable sterile lancet sterile sharp device, preferably retractable, used in skin puncture collections to penetrate the skin at specified depths (e.g., no more than 2.0 mm for infant heelsticks).

diurnal rhythms opposite of nocturnal (nighttime) rhythms, "diurnal" rhythms are variations in the body's functions or fluids that occur during daylight hours or every 24 hours (e.g., some hormone levels decrease in the afternoon). Also referred to as circadian rhythms.

dizziness lightheadedness, unsteadiness, loss of balance.

dorsal surface region of the body characterized by the back (or posterior) area and including the cranial and spinal cavities.

double bagging practice of using two trash bags for disposing of waste from patient's rooms, particularly those in isolation.

efficacy ability to obtain the desired clinical outcome.

edematous condition in which tissues contain excessive fluid and it often results in localized swelling.

e-mail electronic mail often used in health care facilities. Guidelines for using e-mail, including a patient's consent to use e-mail, are now required of health care facilities.

endocrine glands ductless glands that release their secretions (hormones) directly into the bloodstream.

endoplasmic reticulum cell structure that acts as a transport channel between the cell membrane and the nuclear membrane.

engineering controls refer to devices that isolate or remove bloodborne pathogen hazards from the workplace (e.g., needleless devices, shielded needle devices, plastic capillary tubes, etc.). "Work practice" controls are activities that reduce the risk of exposure (e.g., "no-hands" procedures for discarding sharps, etc.)

Environmental Protection Agency (EPA) federal agency that, among its other responsibilities, regulates the disposal of hazardous substances and monitors and regulates disinfectant products.

erythropoiesis production of erythrocytes, or red blood cells.

erythropoietin (EPO) hormone produced in the kidney that initiates the production of red blood cells.

ethics a branch of philosophy that deals with distinguishing right from wrong and with moral consequences of human actions.

ethylenediamine tetra-acetic acid (EDTA) anticoagulant additive used to prevent the blood-clotting sequence by removing calcium and forming calcium salts. EDTA prevents platelet aggregation and is useful for platelet counts and platelet function tests. Fresh EDTA samples are also useful for making blood films or microscopic slides, because there is minimal distortion of platelets and WBCs.

eutectic mixture of local anesthetics (EMLA) a topical anesthetic (pain reliever) that is an emulsion of lidocaine and prilocaine and can be applied to intact skin.

evacuated tube system method of blood collection using double-sided needles whereby the needle is attached to a holder/adapter and allows for multiple specimen tube fills and changes without blood leakage.

evidence a legal term referring to materials (e.g., tubes, needles, safety devices, waste containers, log books, lab reports, etc.) submitted during a legal case to prove or disprove a lawsuit.

exocrine glands glands that secrete fluids through channels or ducts (e.g., sweat, saliva, mucus, digestive juices).

expert witness a legal term referring to a witness who is specially qualified or has expertise in certain areas pertaining to the case.

exposure control plan a document required in health facilities that details the process for medical treatment, prophylaxis, and/or follow-up after an employee has been exposed to potentially harmful or infectious substances (e.g., in the case of a needle stick injury).

extrinsic factors substances involved in the clotting process that are stimulated when tissue damage occurs.

fainting see *syncope*

false imprisonment a legal term referring to the unjustifiable detention of an individual without a legal warrant for his or her arrest.

Farenheit temperature scale where the freezing point of water is 32° and the boiling point is 112°; normal body temperature is 98°.

fasting blood tests tests performed on blood taken from a patient who has abstained from eating and drinking (except water) for a particular period of time.

fax machines facsimiles are often used to transmit health care information. Guidelines for their use and confidentiality of patient information are required.

feathered edge a term used to describe blood smears on microscopic slides; it is a visible curved edge that thins out smoothly and resembles the tip of a bird's feather.

felony a legal term referring to a public offense that may require a jail sentence.

femoral artery located in the groin area of the leg and lateral to the femur bone, it is the largest artery used as an alternative site for ABG collections. Phlebotomists must be specially trained to perform collections from this site.

fevers of unknown origin (FUO) indicates the patient has an undiagnosed infection, which usually results in ordering blood cultures.

fibrin substance that forms a blood clot.

fibrinolysis the final phase of the hemostatic process whereby repair and regeneration of the injured blood vessel occurs and the clot slowly begins to dissolve or break up (lyse).

fistula an artificial shunt or passage, commonly used in the arm of a patient undergoing kidney dialysis; the vein and artery are fused through a surgical procedure. Only specially trained personnel can collect blood from a fistula.

fomites inanimate objects that can harbor infectious agents and transmit infections (e.g., toilets, sinks, linens, door knobs, glasses, phlebotomy supplies, etc.).

Food and Drug Administration (FDA) federal agency responsible for safety, clinical efficacy, and medical efficacy of the country's food and drug supply. This includes equipment and supplies used in blood collection.

forensic specimens specimens that are involved in civil or criminal legal cases, including specimens for analysis of drugs of abuse.

frontal plane imaginary line running lengthwise on the body from side to side, dividing the body into anterior and posterior sections.

gastric analysis gastric fluid analysis to determine gastric function. Involves passing a tube through the patient's nose and into the stomach. It requires specialized training.

gateway drugs drugs such as tobacco and alcohol, the use of which may lead to the use and abuse of "harder" drugs.

gauge number refers to the size (diameter) of the internal bore of a needle. The larger the number, the smaller the bore size, and vice versa.

gauze loosely woven material used for bandages that are sterile or chemically clean.

genes located on a chromosome, it is a unit of heredity capable of reproducing itself exactly during cell division; it is made of segments of DNA.

gestational diabetes diabetes that begins during pregnancy (often the second or third trimester). It occurs in 1–4% of pregnancies and usually subsides after delivery.

glucose tolerance test (GTT) diagnostic test for detecting diabetes. The test is performed by obtaining blood and urine specimens at timed intervals after fasting, then after ingesting glucose. Each specimen is analyzed for its glucose content to determine if the glucose level returns to normal within 2 hours after ingestion. Diabetic patients' glucose is metabolized differently and may need to be analyzed up to 5 hours after ingestion. Special instructions are needed for the patient, and special training for the phlebotomist should occur if they will be collecting such specimens.

Golgi apparatus cell structure that stores proteins.

granulocytes (basophils, neutrophils, eosinophils) mature leukocytes (WBCs) in the circulating blood; when stained and viewed microscopically, granules are present.

hand hygiene term that applies to hand washing (with non-antimicrobial soap and water), antiseptic hand washing, antiseptic hand rub (with waterless antiseptic), or surgical hand antisepsis.

healthcare-acquired (nosocomial) infections infections acquired after admission into a health facility.

Health Care Financing Administration, renamed the Centers for Medicare and Medicaid Services (CMS) federal agency responsible for oversight of health care financing and regulation in the health care industry. CMS is responsible for Medicare, Medicaid, HIPAA, and CLIA.

Health Insurance Portability and Accountability Act (HIPAA) federal law (1996) expanded in 2000 to protect security, privacy, and confidentiality of personal health information.

heart a key component of the cardiovascular system, it is the pump that forces blood throughout the body.

heelstick pediatric phlebotomy procedure that requires puncturing one of specified areas of an infant's heel.

hematocrit a commonly ordered laboratory test to assess the circulatory system; it describes the concentration of RBCs and therefore provides an indirect measure of the oxygen-carrying capacity of the blood.

hematoma a localized leakage of blood into the tissues or into an organ. In phlebotomy, it can occur as a result of blood leakage during the vein puncture, thereby causing a bruise.

hematopoiesis the process of blood cell formation that occurs in the bone marrow.

hemoconcentration increased localized blood concentration of large molecules such as proteins, cells, and coagulation factors. This can be caused by excessive application of a tourniquet.

hemoglobin the molecules that carry oxygen and carbon dioxide in the RBCs.

hemolysis rupture or lysis of the blood cells.

hemostasis maintenance of circulating blood in the liquid state and retention of blood in the vascular system by prevention of blood loss.

heparin an anticoagulant that prevents blood clotting by inactivating thrombin and thromboplastin, the blood-clotting chemicals in the body.

heparin or saline lock part of a vascular access device, a heparin or saline lock is put in place to be used for medication administration or blood collection. It must be "flushed" routinely to prevent clot formation in the line. Generally speaking, heparin locks are no longer widely used; however, if they are used, blood from this site should not be used for coagulation studies due to possible contamination of the specimen with residual heparin.

histograms bar graphs often used as quality improvement tools.

holder (adapter) plastic apparatus needed in specimen collecting using the evacuated tube method. The adapter/holder secures the double-pointed needle: one end of the needle goes into the patient's vein, and the other end of the needle is placed an evacuated tube.

Hollander test involves gastric fluid to determine gastric function in terms of stomach acid production. It uses insulin to stimulate gastric secretions. Special training is required prior to assisting with this procedure.

home health care services provision of health care services in a patient's home under the direction of a physician.

homeostasis means literally "remaining the same"; also referred to as a steady-state condition, it is a normal state that allows the body to stay in a healthy balance by continually compensating with necessary changes.

hormones body substances secreted from glands that play a role in growth and development, fluid and electrolyte balance, energy balance, and acid–base balance.

human immunodeficiency virus (HIV) a virus spread by sexual contact or exposure to infected blood.

hyperventilation a condition whereby chemoreceptors in the brain cause a faster and deeper rate of respiration in order to blow off excess carbon dioxide.

hypobilirubinemia abnormally low levels of bilirubin in the blood.

hypothyroidism when referring to infantile hypothyroidism, a disorder that may be congenital and results in defective development of an embryo.

hypoxia a condition in which body tissues are not receiving enough oxygen.

illicit drugs illegal drugs including opiates, cocaine, amphetamines, etc.

implanted port type of vascular access device (VAD) surgically implanted beneath the skin; it is a small chamber attached to an indwelling line. Access to these ports must be by specially trained personnel and specially designed noncoring needles.

implied consent a complex legal term that varies from state to state in its interpretation. Basically it entails conditions when immediate action is required to save a patient's life or to prevent impairment of a patient's health (i.e., medical emergency care operates with the notion of implied consent in many cases).

incision a cut into the skin. The term is used to describe the puncture made by an automatic skin puncture device.

infection control programs guidelines designed to address surveillance, reporting, isolation procedures, education, and management of community-acquired and health-care-associated infections.

inferior vena cava one of the two large veins that bring oxygen-poor blood to the heart from the lower trunk of the body (e.g., legs).

informed consent a complex legal term; basically, it refers to voluntary permission by a patient to allow touching, examination, and/or treatment by health care workers after they have been given information about the procedures and potential risks and consequences. It allows patients to decide what may be performed on or to their bodies.

inpatients hospitalized patients.

insulin a chemical produced by the pancreas that is released into the bloodstream to facilitate glucose absorption from the blood into the tissues where it is used for energy. When insulin is not produced (as in diabetes mellitus), blood glucose levels increase because it cannot be absorbed into the tissues.

integumentary system body system referring to skin, hair, sweat and oil glands, teeth, and fingernails; involved in protective and regulatory functions.

interstitial space between tissues and/or organs.

intravenous (IV) catheter vascular access device inserted into a blood vessel for administration of medications, nutrients, and blood collection.

intrinsic system part of the coagulation process that involves the clotting factors contained in the blood.

invasion of privacy a legal term referring to objectionable or personal intrusion upon an individual such that it is offensive (e.g., the publishing of confidential information).

iodine used to make tincture of iodine (2% solution) which is used as a skin disinfectant.

isolation procedures methods used to protect individuals (health care workers) from patients with infectious diseases. Formally divided into two types (category-specific and disease-specific), newer guidelines combine isolation practices for moist and potentially infectious body substances, to be used for all patients. The new categories of isolation are based on the mode of transmission and include airborne, droplet, and contact precautions.

Joint Commission on Accreditation of Healthcare Organizations (JCAHO) independent, non-profit organization that sets quality standards for healthcare.

judicial law legal processes designed to resolve disputes.

lactose tolerance test a test to determine lactose intolerance. Some individuals have difficulty digesting lactose, a milk sugar. This test is similar to the glucose tolerance test (which is usually performed one day before) and requires timed testing for lactose after fasting, then after ingestion of lactose at 1-, 2-, and 3-hour intervals.

lancet/lancing device a sharp apparatus (similar to a needle) used to puncture skin to acquire a capillary blood specimen.

lateral directional term meaning towards the sides of the body.

latex allergy reaction to certain proteins in latex rubber, a natural ingredient in some varieties of gloves. Allergic reactions range from skin redness, rash, hives, or itching to respiratory symptoms and, in rare instances, shock.

law societal rules or regulations designed to protect society and resolve conflicts; laws are rules that must be observed.

liable a legal term that refers to a legal obligation when damages are concerned.

light sensitive refers to laboratory specimens; some chemical constituents (bilirubin, vitamin B_{12}, carotene, and folate, urine porphyrins) decompose if exposed to light and therefore should be protected/covered during transportation and handling.

lipemic when referring to serum, it is a cloudy or milky appearance, usually due to a temporarily elevated lipid level after the ingestion of fatty foods.

lithium iodoacetate antiglycolytic agent and anticoagulant; not to be used for hematology testing or enzymatic determinations.

litigation process a legal action to determine a decision in court. Many malpractice cases are negotiated and settled out of court.

long-term care health care services that are provided for more than 30 days. Usually it is related to chronic conditions (e.g., rehabilitation or services for the elderly in nursing homes).

lymphatic system body system responsible for maintaining fluid balance, providing a defense against disease, and absorption of fats and other substances from the blood stream.

lymphocytes type of white blood cell that is nongranular in appearance; plays a role in immunity and in the production of antibodies.

lymphostasis obstruction and/or lack of flow of the lymph fluid.

lysosomes cell structures that release digestive enzymes into vacuoles, or small pouches, for digestion of food particles.

malice a legal term referring to a reckless disregard for the truth (e.g., knowing that a statement is false).

malpractice a legal term referring to improper or unskillful care of a patient by a member of the health care team, or any professional misconduct, unreasonable lack of skill, or infidelity in professional or judiciary duties; often described as "professional negligence."

marijuana drug derived from the hemp plant, cannabis, that when smoked or eaten causes mood alterations and changes in sensory perceptions and cognitive coordination.

mastectomy removal of a breast.

material safety data sheets (MSDSs) required information about any chemical used in the workplace; MSDSs generally list information about a chemical, precautionary measures, and emergency information about accidental exposures to the chemical.

meconium the first intestinal discharges of the newborn infant, greenish in color; consists of epithelial cells, mucus, and bile.

medial directional term meaning toward the midline of the body.

median cubital vein forearm vein that is most commonly used for venipuncture.

Medicaid a shared federal- and state-funded program designed to provide health insurance for individuals with low income.

medical records definitive documents (paper or electronic) that contain a chronological log of a patient's care. It must include any information that is clinically significant or relevant to the patient's care.

Medicare federal program designed to provide health insurance for the elderly and members of special groups.

megakaryocytes large cells located in the bone from which platelets are formed.

melanin pigment in the skin that provides color and protects underlying tissues from absorbing ultraviolet rays.

meninges protective membranes that cover the brain and spinal cord.

metabolic acidosis a pathologic condition that occurs when the kidneys cannot eliminate acidic substances (e.g., in diabetes mellitus). It can result in kidney (renal) failure and death.

metabolic alkalosis a pathologic condition that results from excessive vomiting or an abnormal secretion of certain hormones that cause's excess elimination of hydrogen ions (from CO_2).

metabolism an important bodily function that allows the formation or breakdown of substances (e.g., proteins) for the purpose of using energy.

microcollection process by which small amounts of blood are collected in small containers or tubes using specially designed devices.

microcontainers specialized collection devices designed for small quantities of blood; some containing anticoagulants. These devices are typically used for pediatric or geriatric patients with fragile or inaccessible veins, and/or for finger sticks.

microorganisms living organisms that are too small to see with the naked eye such as bacteria, viruses, fungi, etc.

misdemeanor a legal term referring to many types of criminal offenses that are not serious enough to be classified as felonies.

mitochondria cell structure that produces energy for the cell.

mode of transmission refers to the method by which pathogenic agents are transmitted (e.g., direct contact, air, medical instruments, other objects, and other vectors).

monocytes type of white blood cell that is nongranular and also plays a role in defense.

multiple-sample needles used with the evacuated tube method of blood collection, these needles are attached to a holder/adapter and allow for multiple specimen tube fills and changes without blood leakage.

muscular system body system referring to all muscles of the body.

National Committee for Clinical Laboratory Standards (NCCLS) nonprofit organization that recommends quality standards and guidelines for clinical laboratory procedures.

National Phlebotomy Association (NPA) professional organization for phlebotomists that offers continuing educational activities and a certification examination for phlebotomists.

needleless system a device that does not use needles for procedures that are normally associated with needle use. This includes collection of bodily fluids or withdrawal of body fluids after initial venous or arterial access is performed. It includes any procedure that has the potential for occupational exposure to bloodborne pathogens from contaminated sharp objects.

needlestick skin puncture using a needle

negligence a legal term referring to the failure to act or perform duties according to the standards of the profession.

neonatal screening typically refers to mandatory (required by law) laboratory testing of infants for specified disorders such as PKU and hypothroidism. There is wide variability in what tests are required by each state.

neonate a newborn infant; term used during the first 28 days after birth.

nervous system body system that includes organs that provide communication in the body, sensations, thoughts, emotions, and memories.

neurons specialized nerve cells that transmit nerve impulses.

nucleolus cell structure located inside the nucleus, aids in cellular metabolism and cellular reproduction.

nucleus cell structure that is the cell's control center; it governs the functions of each individual cell (e.g., growth, repair, reproduction, and metabolism).

obesity an unhealthy abundance of body fat.

occluded veins closed or constricted veins.

occult blood analysis that detects hidden (occult) blood in the stool.

occupational exposure contact via skin, eye, mucous membranes, or parenteral with potentially infectious materials as a result of an individual's work duities.

Occupational Safety and Health Administration (OSHA) an agency of the U.S. Department of Labor requiring employers to provide a safe work environment including measures to protect workers exposed to biological and occupational hazards. OSHA is also responsible for responding to complaints, monitoring employer practices, and imposing sanctions (fines or closure) on employers who are noncompliant.

opiates drugs derived from opium.

osteochondritis inflammation of the bone and its cartilage.

osteomyelitis inflammation of the bone due to bacterial infection.

outcomes used as a quality improvement term to refer to what is accomplished for the patient (e.g., healing, return to wellness, or return to normal functions). Poor patient outcomes have been described as the "5 Ds": death, disease, disability, discomfort, and dissatisfaction.

ova and parasites (O&P) laboratory analysis performed on stool specimens that determines the presence of parasitic microorganisms or eggs of parasitic organisms.

oxalates anticoagulants that prevent blood-clotting sequence by removing calcium and forming calcium salts.

panic value see *critical value*

parental involvement during pediatric phlebotomy procedures, a parent's support and presence during the procedure is often helpful in reducing stress/anxiety for the patient. On the other hand, some parents are reluctant to be involved, so the phlebotomist must assess each situation to determine the level of parental involvement that would optimize the phlebotomy encounter.

parenteral usually refers to delivering medications by piercing mucous membranes or skin through needle stick injections, IVs, etc.

Parkinson's disease a neurological disease characterized by muscular tremors and rigidity of movement.

pathogenic agents disease-causing bacteria, fungi, viruses, or parasites that are transmitted by direct contact, air, medical instruments, other objects, or vectors.

pathology the study of all aspects of disease and abnormal conditions of the body.

patient confidentiality see *confidentiality*

Patient's Bill of Rights a statement originally developed in 1973 by the AHA to affirm the rights of patients. Key elements involve the right to respectful and considerate care; accurate information about diagnoses, treatment, and prognoses; informed consent; refusal of treatment; privacy; confidentiality; advance directives; reviewing records about own treatment; knowing identity and role of personnel involved in care; information about research procedures; billing information; and knowing business relationships of those providing care.

peak a term used for therapeutic drug monitoring to describe the blood sample that is taken when the drug is at its highest concentration in the patient's serum (e.g., "the *peak* level").

pediatric phlebotomies procedures performed on infants and children that require specialized training and management. Often done by skin puncture, pediatric phlebotomies also entail matching the procedure with the specimen requirements for testing, the patient's age and emotional condition, and possible parental involvement.

pericardial fluid fluid from the heart cavity.

peripherally inserted central catheter (PICC) type of vascular access device (VAD) inserted into the peripheral venous system with a lead into the central venous system. A PICC is usually placed in the arm in the basilic or cephalic vein. A PICC should not be used for blood collections because it may collapse during aspiration of the blood.

peristalsis part of the digestive process whereby food is moved in wavelike contractions through the intestines.

peritoneal fluid fluid from the abdominal cavity.

personal protective equipment (PPE) equipment designed to protect the health care worker from hazards in the workplace (e.g., goggles, gloves, gowns, etc.).

petechiae minute, pinpoint hemorrhagic spots in the skin that may be indicative of a coagulation abnormality. For phlebotomists, it should be a warning sign that the patient may bleed excessively.

phenylketonuria (PKU) a congenital disorder, usually diagnosed at birth, that can cause brain damage resulting in severe retardation, often with seizures and other neurologic abnormalities.

phlebotomist individual who practices phlebotomy (i.e., a blood collector); *phlebo* is related to "vein," and *tomy* relates to "cutting."

physician-patient relationship the association between the patient and the physician providing clinical and consultative services; the communication between them is private and confidential.

physician's office laboratories (POLs) non-hospital laboratories usually based in a physician's office/clinic at the private practice.

physiology study of the functional components of the body.

pituitary gland also referred to as the master gland, stimulates other glands to produce hormones as needed. It controls and regulates hormone production through chemical feedback.

plaintiff a legal term referring to the person who initiates a lawsuit or legal action.

plasma liquid portion of the blood in which blood cells are suspended.

platelets (thrombocytes) blood cells that aid in blood clot formation.

pleural fluid fluid from the lung cavity.

pneumatic tube systems transportation system used in many health care facilities for specimens and paper-based documentation. Considerations for use of these systems involves evaluation of speed, distance, control mechanisms, shock absorbency, sizes of carriers, and breakage/spillage rates.

point-of-care refers to tests and procedures that are actually performed at the patient's bedside or at the "point of care." The tests are not sent to a laboratory in a remote location; rather, they are rapid methods designed to produce quick results.

post centrifugation phase period of time after a specimen has been centrifuged but before serum or plasma has been removed for testing

posterior surface region of the body characterized by the back (or dorsal) area and including the cranial and spinal cavities.

postprandial glucose test a glucose test performed after ingestion of a meal; useful for screening patients for diabetes, because glucose levels in serum specimens drawn 2 hours after a meal are rarely elevated in normal patients. In contrast, diabetic patients have elevated glucose values 2 hours after a meal.

preanalytical phase refers to the laboratory testing phases in which tests are ordered and specimens are collected and prepared for testing. Preanalytical variables include patient variables (fasting versus nonfasting, stress, availability, etc.), transportation variables (specimen leakage, tube breakage, excessive shaking, etc.), specimen processing variables (centrifugation, delays, contamination of the specimen, exposure to heat or light), and specimen variables (hemolysis, inadequate volume, inadequate mixing of the tube, etc.).

precentrifugation phase period of time after a specimen has been collected but before centrifugation.

premature infant an infant born before 37 weeks of gestation (normal gestation is 40 weeks).

preventive law a legal term referring to the use of education and planning to avoid legal conflicts.

primary care health care services that are provided to maintain and monitor normal health and provide preventive services.

primary tube tube containing the patient's blood sample.

privacy the patient's right to respectful consideration of the confidential nature of his or her health information.

process used as a quality improvement term to refer to what is actually done to the patient in a health care encounter. Process assessments are common throughout the specimen collection process to see if proper procedures and standards were followed.

proficiency testing (PT) testing that is part of the quality management of laboratory services and involves subscribing to an outside source to provide "unknown" or "blind" specimens to see how one laboratory's results compare with other laboratories' results. Performance reviews on proficiency tests are part of the accrediting process for most laboratories.

protective (reverse) isolation precautionary measures and procedures designed to protect patients who are particularly susceptible or at increased risk of acquiring infections (e.g., patients with low WBC counts (neutropenic or leukopenic), patients with burns, and/or immunosuppressed patients).

pulmonary circuit when blood leaves the heart and enters the right and left pulmonary arteries, they carry deoxygenated blood.

pulse rate rate used to assess normal functioning of the cardiovascular system; it is measured off the pulse located in an artery. Normal pulse rate is about 75 beats per minute.

puncture proof a surface that can withstand punctures from sharp objects such as needles.

quality control material daily controls that are used in analytic testing to determine acceptable ranges of test results (i.e., tolerance limits).

qualitative test pertains to the presence or absence (positive or negative) of a substance in the specimen.

quantitative test pertains to the exact measurement or quantity of substance in the specimen

radial artery located on the thumb side of the wrist, this artery is most commonly used to collect blood specimens for arterial blood gases. Phlebotomists must be specially trained to perform collections from this site.

random urine sample urine sample taken at random time(s).

red blood cells (RBCs or erythrocytes) blood cells that function to transport oxygen and carbon dioxide in the body.

reference ranges when referring to laboratory values, these are laboratory test values that are considered within "normal" limits.

reproductive system body system referring to organs involved in sperm production, secretion of hormones (e.g., testosterone, estrogens, and progesterone), ovulation, fertilization, menstruation, pregnancy, labor, and lactation.

requisition form paper-based method for requesting laboratory tests.

respiratory acidosis a pathologic condition that results when the respiratory system is unable to eliminate adequate amounts of CO_2 (e.g., a collapsed lung or blocked respiratory passages).

respiratory alkalosis a pathologic condition that results from hyperventilation or the loss of too much CO_2 from the lungs.

respiratory system body system referring to parts that assist in respiration or breathing (e.g., nose, pharynx, larynx, trachea, bronchi, and lungs).

respondeat superior a legal term referring to the concept by which the actions of an individual are attributed to the supervisors or employers in control. In these cases, the supervisor may be liable for the negligent actions of their employee. It is also referred to as "vicarious liability."

Rh factor a method to categorize blood according to the presence or absence of the Rh antigen.

ribosomes cell structure that assembles amino acids into proteins.

risk management management programs to reduce risks associated with health care delivery. Risk management programs reduce preventable injuries and accidents, and minimize financial loss to the organization.

sagittal plane imaginary line running lengthwise on the body from front to back, dividing the body into right and left halves.

sclerosed veins veins that have become hardened.

secondary care specialized health care services usually provided by a physician who is an expert on a particular group of diseases, organ systems, or an organ (e.g., an ophthalmologist diagnoses and treats disorders of the eyes).

secondary tube tube containing removed plasma/serum (an aliquot) *after* specimen centrifugation of a primary tube containing the patient's blood sample.

separated plasma/serum serum or plasma that has been removed or separated from contact with blood cells. It is refered to as an "aliquot." It can be removed from the primary tube after centrifugation using a pipette, or separated from cellular contact with a chemical or physical barrier.

septicemia formally called "blood poisoning," the term now means the presence of toxins or multiplying bacteria in the blood.

serum when blood is allowed to clot, sera separates from the blood cells, which are meshed in a fibrin clot. Serum contains the same constituents as plasma except that the clotting factors are contained within the clot.

sexually transmitted diseases (STDs) pathogenic diseases that are transmitted via sexual contact (e.g., gonorrhea, genital herpes, syphilis, and human immunodeficiency virus).

sharps any devices or tools that can potentially cut, puncture, or cause injury.

single-sample needle used for collecting a blood sample from a syringe.

single-specimen collection term commonly used for urine drug testing to refer to a single-specimen requirement.

skeletal (striated voluntary) muscles muscles that are attached to bones.

skeletal system body system referring to all bones and joints.

skin puncture a cut into the skin (e.g., of the finger or heel) with a retractable puncture device or a nonretractable lancet.

skin test test that determines whether a patient has had contact with a particular antigen and therefore has produced antibodies to that antigen. A wide range of disease states stimulate antibody responses in individuals. Examples of skin tests

include tuberculosis and fungal, ragweed, and milk allergies.

sodium fluoride an additive (antiglycolytic agent) present in specific blood collection tubes that is used for glycolytic inhibition tests.

sodium polyanethole sulfonate (SPS) an additive typically used in blood culture bottles to prevent clotting.

source the origin of an infection (e.g., human hands, lab coats or other clothing, contaminated medical instruments, etc.).

specimen collection manual electronic or paper-based document required by accrediting agencies that includes instructions for patient preparation, type of collection containers, amounts of specimen required for specified tests, timing requirements, preservatives or anticoagulants needed, special handling instructions, proper labeling requirements, and other test-specific or situation-specific requirements for specimens.

split-specimen collection term commonly used for urine drug testing to refer to the specimen requirement for two specimens. The donor should not be allowed to "split" his or her own specimen; the specimen should be split by the "collector" using one original specimen and depending on the volume and integrity of the original specimen.

sputum fluid from the lungs that often contains pus.

stakeholders individuals, groups, organizations, and/or communities that have an interest in or are influenced by health care services. Stakeholders can be internal to the organization or external (i.e., outside the organization).

standard of care the practices or guidelines that a reasonably prudent person would follow in any particular circumstance. Many agencies, licensing boards, certifying boards, and accrediting organizations write standards of care or standards of practice to guide health care workers in their duties.

Standard Precautions a set of safeguards designed to reduce the risk of transmission of microorganisms; guidelines apply to *all patients and all body fluids, nonintact skin, and mucous mem-*

branes and include the use of barrier protection *(protective equipment such as gloves, gowns, etc.), hand hygiene, and proper use and disposal of needles and other sharps.* Standard precautions are more comprehensive than "Universal Precautions" which apply only to transmission of blood-borne pathogens. Policies must comply with OSHA Standards. Standard Precautions and Universal Precautions are available from the U.S. Centers for Disease Control and Prevention.

STAT an emergency situation that requires immediate action; in the case of blood collection and analysis, tests that are ordered "STAT" should be given the highest priority for collection, delivery to the laboratory, analysis, and reporting.

statute of limitations a legal term referring to the time limit after an injury that a plaintiff must file a lawsuit or be forever barred from doing so. The statute of limitations for professional negligence in most states is 2 years.

statutory laws statutes and ordinances that are legally binding but in certain instances may require the courts (judicial law) to step in.

steady state also referred to as homeostasis, it is a condition that allows the normal body to stay in balance by continually compensating with necessary changes, thereby remaining in a healthy condition.

sterile gauze pads typically used in blood collection procedures either during the decontamination process and/or after blood collection to aid in stopping the bleeding; it is a sterile cotton mesh pad that is packaged in individual units.

sterile technique use of procedures that produce an aseptic condition (i.e., free from all living microorganisms and their spores).

structure used as a quality improvement term to refer to the physical or organizational properties of the setting where health care is provided.

substance abuse over use and/or addiction to drugs and/or alcohol.

sucrose nipple or pacifier a sucking device for infants and toddlers that is used to pacify or comfort the child.

superior vena cava one of the two large veins that brings oxygen-poor blood to the heart from the head, neck, arms, and chest region.

supine reclining position.

surveillance monitoring and data collection on specific populations that are at risk for infections; have previously acquired infections; have been accidentally exposed to a communicable disease, contaminated equipment, or hazardous reagents; and patients in specified areas of the facility.

susceptible host a component in the "chain of infection"; the degree to which an individual is at risk for acquiring an infection. Factors affecting susceptibility are age, drug use, degree and nature of the patient's illness, and status of the patient's immune system.

sweat chloride test used in the diagnosis of cystic fibrosis.

syncope the transient (and frequently sudden) loss of consciousness due to a lack of oxygen to the brain (i.e., fainting) and resulting in an inability to stay in an upright position. Patients usually recover their orientation quickly, but injuries (e.g., abrasions, lacerations) often result from falling to the ground. Syncope may be caused by a variety of things including hypoglycemia, hyperventilation, cardiac, neurologic, or psychiatric conditions, or medications. Many patients become dizzy and faint (i.e., become "weak in the knees") at the thought or sight of blood.

synovial fluid joint fluid.

syringe method method of venipuncture whereby a syringe is used to collect blood that is then transferred to collection tubes.

systemic circuit part of the cardiovascular system that carries blood to the tissues of the body.

systolic pressure the first reading reported for a blood pressure measurement.

tamper resistant container or device that is unalterable.

tertiary care health care that is highly specialized and oriented toward unusual and complex diagnoses and therapies. Sophisticated instrumentation and technology or invasive procedures are used in an acute care facility.

therapeutic drug monitoring (TDM) testing procedures to evaluate drug levels in a patient's blood. This is valuable for drug dosage and to monitor the patient for a variety of other factors (clinical effectiveness, toxicity, etc.).

therapeutic phlebotomy removal of blood for therapeutic reasons (i.e., in conditions where there is an excessive production of blood cells).

thrombi blood clots formed somewhere within the cardiovascular system; they may occlude a vessel or attach to the wall of a vessel.

tissue (interstitial) fluid fluids found in between and around tissues that are not blood.

tort a legal wrong in which the person who commits it is liable for damages in civil, not criminal, court. The tort system is part of the judicial system concerned with resolving two-party disputes over whether some harm has been committed to one party or his/her property.

tourniquet a soft rubber strip typically about 1 inch wide and 15 to 18 inches long used on the arm to help find a site for venipuncture. The ends are stretched around a patient's arm about 3 inches above the venipuncture area. The tightening of the tourniquet causes venous filling in the veins and enables better visualization and feel of the prominent veins in the area.

toxicology scientific study of poisons (including drugs), how they are detected, their actions in the human body and treatment of the conditions they produce.

trace evidence evidence found at the scene of a crime or on a person involved in a crime (e.g., fingerprints, hairs, fibers, glass fragments, drugs, firearms, etc.).

trace metals elements such as aluminum or lead that may be present in the blood. Specially prepared blood collection tubes are required during phlebotomy so they are free of metals that may cause interference with the testing process.

transmission precautions categories of precautionary measures based on the route of transmission of disease. Three types of transmission-based precautions are airborne, droplet, and contact precautions.

transverse plane imaginary line running crosswise, or horizontally, on the body, dividing the body into upper and lower sections.

troponin T a protein released and detected after a myocardial infarction (MI); it is elevated only when heart damage has occurred; thus, it is valuable in the early diagnosis of MI and in monitoring the effectiveness of therapy after an MI.

trough a term used for therapeutic drug monitoring to describe the blood sample that is taken just prior to the next dose, or when the drug is at a low concentration in the patient's serum (i.e., the "trough" level).

turbid cloudy or milky in appearance.

Universal Precautions (also called "Standard precautions" or "Standard Universal Precautions"). Refers to an infection control concept of bloodborne disease control, requiring that all human blood and other potentially infectious materials be treated as if known to be infectious for HIV, HBV, HCV, or other bloodborne pathogens, regardless of the perceived risk. Other concepts in infection control are referred to as "Body Substance Isolation" (BSI) and Standard Precautions, meaning that all body fluids and substances are potentially infectious.

urinary system body system referring to processes enabling the production and elimination of urine. Consists of kidneys, ureters, bladder, and urethra.

vacuum (evacuated) tube color-coded specimen collection tube that contains a vacuum so as to aspirate blood when a needle enters a patient's vein. The tubes are part of a blood collection method that also requires a double-pointed needle and a special plastic holder (adapter). One end of the double-pointed needle enters the vein, the other pierces the top of the tube, and the vacuum aspirates the blood into the tube. Tubes may contain anticoagulants.

vascular access devices (VADs) a variety of specially designed devices to allow entrance into a vein or artery. One of the most commonly used VADs is a central venous catheter (CVC), which is usually inserted into the subclavian vein (in the chest area below the clavical), the jugular vein, or the superior vena cava.

vasoconstriction rapid constriction of the blood vessels to decrease blood flow to the area.

veins blood vessels that carry blood toward the heart after oxygen has been delivered to the tissues.

venae cavae largest veins of the body.

ventral surface region of the body characterized by the front (or anterior) area and including the thoracic, abdominal, and pelvic cavities.

ventricles two of the four chambers of the heart.

venules minute veins that flow into larger veins.

vertigo the sensation of moving around in space or having objects move around a person, caused by a variety of illnesses including middle ear disease, toxemia due to food poisoning, and infectious diseases.

vicarious liability a legal term whereby actions of one individual may be imputed to another person having control (e.g., the actions of an employee may be blamed on the supervisor in charge). The term is synonymous with *respondeat superior.*

visceral (nonstriated, smooth, involuntary) muscles muscles that line the walls of internal structures (e.g., veins and arteries).

volume space occupied by a liquid and usually measured in liters or milliliters.

whistle blowing disclosure of a legal wrongdoing by an employee of the same organization (i.e., an illegal action is reported by an employee to appropriate authorities such as a governmental agency, accreditation agency, etc.). Employees who speak out to reveal illegal actions may fear reprisals that could jeopardize their safety or their job. Thus, numerous laws are in place to protect employees who report legitimate wrongdoings.

white blood cells (WBCs or leukocytes) blood cells that provide for defense against infectious agents.

winged infusion system also called a butterfly set or scalp needle set, the system can be used for difficult venipunctures due to small or fragile veins. The needle is typically smaller, and it has a thin tubing with a Luer adapter at the end so that it can be used on a syringe or an evacuated tube system during venipuncture.

work practice controls practices that diminish the likelihood of exposure to hazards by altering the manner in which the work is performed (e.g., prohibiting the recapping of needles with a two-handed approach.

zone of comfort area of space surrounding a person/patient that is considered "private or personal"; if a stranger (or phlebotomist) gets too close to the individual (i.e., beyond the zone of comfort), the person/patient may begin to feel uncomfortable.

INDEX

lactose tolerance test, 381
lancets, 230–34
Lasette device, 231
latex products safety, 172, 173t, 226, 228, 338
law, governmental, 44
lawsuits
  avoiding, 51, 52
  cases pertaining to clinical labopratory activities, 54–55
  depositions during, 49–50
  evidence for, 50
  improper techniques/negligence, cases resulting from, 55–56
  statement of case, 49
Lazernick v. General Hospital of Monroe Country, 54
legal terminology, 45, 46
leukocytes. See white blood cells
liability, legal issues, 45, 46
listening, active, 27, 28t. See also communication
lithium heparin tubes, 212–13
lubricant powder, 226
lymphatic system
  diagram, 86f
  disorders, 86
  laboratory tests, 86
  structure and function, 85–86
lymphocytes, 85, 96. See also lymphatic system
lysosomes, 67

M

malpractice
  definition, 46
  depositions regarding, 49–50
  insurance, 56–57
  medical director/physician, by, 46–47
  steps following filing, 50
mastectomy patients, blood drawing of, 268
Material Safety Data Sheets, 166–67

medical records, 182. See also documentation
  confidentiality issues, 53
  importance, 51
  purposes of, 53
  uses of, 51
melanin, 69
melanoma, 70
metabolism, 67, 79
microspecimens, 228, 233f, 234–36
mitochondria, 67
monocytes, 96
Monoject Monoletter Safety Lancet, 232f
muscular dystrophy, 72
muscular system, 72, 74f

N

needle disposal, 223
needlestick injury, 222
  butterfly system, stemming from, 271
  prevention strategies, 247, 252
  reporting, 247
negligence, factors when considering, 45
nerve damage, from phlebotomy procedures, 69, 267
nervous system
  diagram of, 76f
  disorders, 75
  laboratory testing related to, 75
  structure and function, 73, 75
nosocomial infections. (See healthcare-acquired infections)

O

occult blood screening, fecal, home, 421
oral sucrose, 337
OSHA
  blood-borne exposure follow-up, 128, 130, 132
  waste disposal regulations, 161
osteomylelitis, 71

SINGLE PC LICENSE AGREEMENT AND LIMITED WARRANTY

READ THIS LICENSE CAREFULLY BEFORE OPENING THIS PACKAGE. BY OPENING THIS PACKAGE, YOU ARE AGREEING TO THE TERMS AND CONDITIONS OF THIS LICENSE. IF YOU DO NOT AGREE, DO NOT OPEN THE PACKAGE. PROMPTLY RETURN THE UNOPENED PACKAGE AND ALL ACCOMPANYING ITEMS TO THE PLACE YOU OBTAINED THEM. *THESE TERMS APPLY TO ALL LICENSED SOFTWARE ON THE DISK EXCEPT THAT THE TERMS FOR USE OF ANY SHAREWARE OR FREEWARE ON THE DISKETTES ARE AS SET FORTH IN THE ELECTRONIC LICENSE LOCATED ON THE DISK:*

1. GRANT OF LICENSE and OWNERSHIP: The enclosed computer programs and data ("Software") are licensed, not sold, to you by Pearson Education, Inc. ("We" or the "Company") and in consideration of your purchase or adoption of the accompanying Company textbooks and/or other materials, and your agreement to these terms. We reserve any rights not granted to you. You own only the disk(s) but we and/or our licensors own the Software itself. This license allows you to use and display your copy of the Software on a single computer (i.e., with a single CPU) at a single location for <u>academic</u> use only, so long as you comply with the terms of this Agreement. You may make one copy for back up, or transfer your copy to another CPU, provided that the Software is usable on only one computer

2. RESTRICTIONS: You may <u>not</u> transfer or distribute the Software or documentation to anyone else. Except for backup, you may <u>not</u> copy the documentation or the Software. You may <u>not</u> network the Software or otherwise use it on more than one computer or computer terminal at the same time. You may <u>not</u> reverse engineer, disassemble, decompile, modify, adapt, translate, or create derivative works based on the Software or the Documentation. You may be held legally responsible for any copying or copyright infringement which is caused by your failure to abide by the terms of these restrictions.

3. TERMINATION: This license is effective until terminated. This license will terminate automatically without notice from the Company if you fail to comply with any provisions or limitations of this license. Upon termination, you shall destroy the Documentation and all copies of the Software. All provisions of this Agreement as to limitation and disclaimer of warranties, limitation of liability, remedies or damages, and our ownership rights shall survive termination.

4. LIMITED WARRANTY AND DISCLAIMER OF WARRANTY: Company warrants that for a period of 60 days from the date you purchase this SOFTWARE (or purchase or adopt the accompanying textbook), the Software, when properly installed and used in accordance with the Documentation, will operate in substantial conformity with the description of the Software set forth in the Documentation, and that for a period of 30 days the disk(s) on which the Software is delivered shall be free from defects in materials and workmanship under normal use. The Company does not warrant that the Software will meet your requirements or that the operation of the Software will be uninterrupted or error-free. Your only remedy and the Company's only obligation under these limited warranties is, at the Company's

option, return of the disk for a refund of any amounts paid for it by you or replacement of the disk. THIS LIMITED WARRANTY IS THE ONLY WARRANTY PROVIDED BY THE COMPANY AND ITS LICENSORS, AND THE COMPANY AND ITS LICENSORS DISCLAIM ALL OTHER WARRANTIES, EXPRESS OR IMPLIED, INCLUDING WITHOUT LIMITATION, THE IMPLIED WARRANTIES OF MERCHANTABILITY AND FITNESS FOR A PARTICULAR PURPOSE. THE COMPANY DOES NOT WARRANT, GUARANTEE OR MAKE ANY REPRESENTATION REGARDING THE ACCURACY, RELIABILITY, CURRENTNESS, USE, OR RESULTS OF USE, OF THE SOFTWARE.

5. LIMITATION OF REMEDIES AND DAMAGES: IN NO EVENT, SHALL THE COMPANY OR ITS EMPLOYEES, AGENTS, LICENSORS, OR CONTRACTORS BE LIABLE FOR ANY INCIDENTAL, INDIRECT, SPECIAL, OR CONSEQUENTIAL DAMAGES ARISING OUT OF OR IN CONNECTION WITH THIS LICENSE OR THE SOFTWARE, INCLUDING FOR LOSS OF USE, LOSS OF DATA, LOSS OF INCOME OR PROFIT, OR OTHER LOSSES, SUSTAINED AS A RESULT OF INJURY TO ANY PERSON, OR LOSS OF OR DAMAGE TO PROPERTY, OR CLAIMS OF THIRD PARTIES, EVEN IF THE COMPANY OR AN AUTHORIZED REPRESENTATIVE OF THE COMPANY HAS BEEN ADVISED OF THE POSSIBILITY OF SUCH DAMAGES. IN NO EVENT SHALL THE LIABILITY OF THE COMPANY FOR DAMAGES WITH RESPECT TO THE SOFTWARE EXCEED THE AMOUNTS ACTUALLY PAID BY YOU, IF ANY, FOR THE SOFTWARE OR THE ACCOMPANYING TEXTBOOK. BECAUSE SOME JURISDICTIONS DO NOT ALLOW THE LIMITATION OF LIABILITY IN CERTAIN CIRCUMSTANCES, THE ABOVE LIMITATIONS MAY NOT ALWAYS APPLY TO YOU.

6. GENERAL: THIS AGREEMENT SHALL BE CONSTRUED IN ACCORDANCE WITH THE LAWS OF THE UNITED STATES OF AMERICA AND THE STATE OF NEW YORK, APPLICABLE TO CONTRACTS MADE IN NEW YORK, AND SHALL BENEFIT THE COMPANY, ITS AFFILIATES AND ASSIGNEES. HIS AGREEMENT IS THE COMPLETE AND EXCLUSIVE STATEMENT OF THE AGREEMENT BETWEEN YOU AND THE COMPANY AND SUPERSEDES ALL PROPOSALS OR PRIOR AGREEMENTS, ORAL, OR WRITTEN, AND ANY OTHER COMMUNICATIONS BETWEEN YOU AND THE COMPANY OR ANY REPRESENTATIVE OF THE COMPANY RELATING TO THE SUBJECT MATTER OF THIS AGREEMENT. If you are a U.S. Government user, this Software is licensed with "restricted rights" as set forth in subparagraphs (a)-(d) of the Commercial Computer-Restricted Rights clause at FAR 52.227-19 or in subparagraphs (c)(1)(ii) of the Rights in Technical Data and Computer Software clause at DFARS 252.227-7013, and similar clauses, as applicable.

Should you have any questions concerning this agreement or if you wish to contact the Company for any reason, please contact in writing: Prentice-Hall, New Media Department, One Lake Street, Upper Saddle River, NJ 07458.